# IMAGING IN ONCOLOGY

Edited by

## Walter L. Curati

MD FRCR

Senior Lecturer and Consultant
Department of Imaging
Hammersmith Hospital, London, UK

## Martin J. Lipton

MD

Professor of Radiology and Medicine
Chairman, Department of Radiology
The University of Chicago, Chicago, Illinois,
USA

## David O. Cosgrove

MA MSc FRCP FRCR

Department of Imaging
Hammersmith Hospital,
London, UK

## David J. Allison

BSc MD FRCR FRCP

Director and Professor
Department of Imaging
Hammersmith Hospital, London, UK

GREENWICH MEDICAL MEDIA LTD
219 The Linen Hall
162-168 Regent Street
London
W1R 5TB

ISBN 1 900 151030

First Published 1998

**British Library Cataloguing in Publication Data**
A catalogue record for this book is available from the British Library.

Distributed worldwide by
Oxford University Press

Typeset by Saxon Graphics Ltd, Derby

Printed in Great Britain by
Ashford Colour Press

# CONTENTS

Contributors ......................................................................................... vii

Forewords ............................................................................................ ix

**CHAPTER 1**

**Introduction** ...................................................................................... 1

*Walter L. Curati, David O. Cosgrove, Martin J. Lipton and David J. Allison*

**CHAPTER 2**

**The central nervous system** ............................................................. 7

*Lloyd E. Savy and Ivan F. Moseley*

**CHAPTER 3**

**The head and neck** .......................................................................... 33

*Antonio Chiesa, Roberto Maroldi, Giuseppe Battaglia, Patrizia Maculotti and Davide Farina*

**CHAPTER 4**

**The lung and mediastinum** ............................................................. 47

*Geraldine Walsh and Christopher D. R. Flower*

**CHAPTER 5**

**The breast** ....................................................................................... 63

*William E. Svensson*

**CHAPTER 6**

**The oesophagus, stomach, duodenum and small intestine** .............. 79

*Daniel J. Nolan*

**CHAPTER 7**

**The colon and rectum** ..................................................................... 99

*Clive I. Bartram*

**CHAPTER 8**

### The liver, biliary system and pancreas ............................................. 111

*Michel Lafortune and Luigi Lepanto*

**CHAPTER 9**

### The kidney, bladder, prostate and testes ......................................... 125

*Walter L. Curati and Gordon Williams*

**CHAPTER 10**

### The endocrine system .................................................................... 139

*Daniel A. Darko and Karim Meeran*

**CHAPTER 11**

### The ovaries, endometrium and cervix ............................................. 153

*Nandita M. deSouza and W. P. Soutter*

**CHAPTER 12**

### The lymphatic system ................................................................... 167

*Walter L. Curati*

**CHAPTER 13**

### The bone and soft tissue .............................................................. 175

*Asif Saifuddin*

**CHAPTER 14**

### The cardiovascular system ............................................................ 189

*Craig A. Hackworth and Martin J. Lipton*

### Index ............................................................................................ 203

# CONTRIBUTORS

**David J. Allison**
*Director and Professor*
*Department of Imaging*
*Hammersmith Hospital*
*London*
*UK*

**Clive I. Bartram**
*Consultant Radiologist*
*St Mark's Hospital*
*Northwick Park*
*Harrow*
*UK*

**Giuseppe Battaglia**
*Assistant*
*Department of Radiology*
*University of Brescia*
*Brescia*
*Italy*

**Antonio Chiesa**
*Professor and Chairman*
*Department of Radiology*
*University of Brescia*
*Brescia*
*Italy*

**David O. Cosgrove**
*Department of Imaging*
*Hammersmith Hospital*
*London*
*UK*

**Walter L. Curati**
*Senior Lecturer and Consultant*
*Department of Imaging*
*Hammersmith Hospital*
*London*
*UK*

**Daniel A. Darko**
*Honorary Clinical Research Fellow*
*Endocrine Unit*
*Hammersmith Hospital*
*London*
*UK*

**Nandita M. deSouza**
*Senior Lecturer and Consultant*
*The Robert Steiner MRI Unit*
*Hammersmith Hospital*
*London*
*UK*

**Davide Farina**
*Resident*
*Department of Radiology*
*University of Brescia*
*Brescia*
*Italy*

**Christopher D. R. Flower**
*Consultant Radiologist*
*Addenbrooke's Hospital*
*Cambridge*
*UK*

**Craig A. Hackworth**
*Assistant Professor of Radiology*
*The University of Chicago*
*Chicago*
*Illinois*
*USA*

**Michel Lafortune**
*Professor of Radiology*
*Centre Hospitalier de l'Université de*
*Montréal*
*Quebec*
*Canada*

**Luigi Lepanto**
*Assistant Professor of Radiology*
*Centre Hospitalier de l'Université de*
*Montréal*
*Quebec*
*Canada*

**Martin J. Lipton**
*Professor of Radiology and Medicine*
*Chairman, Department of Radiology*
*The University of Chicago*
*Chicago*
*Illinois*
*USA*

**Patrizia Maculotti**
*Assistant*
*Department of Radiology*
*University of Brescia*
*Brescia*
*Italy*

**Roberto Maroldi**
*Assistant*
*Department of Radiology*
*University of Brescia*
*Brescia*
*Italy*

**Karim Meeran**
*Consultant Physician and Endocrinologist*
*Endocrine Unit*
*Hammersmith Hospital*
*London*
*UK*

**Ivan R. Moseley**
*Consultant Neuroradiologist*
*National Hospital, Queen Square &*
*Moorfield Eye Hospital*
*London*
*UK*

**Daniel J. Nolan**
*Consultant Radiologist*
*Department of Radiology*
*Radcliffe Hospital*
*Oxford*
*UK*

**Lloyd E. Savy**
*Consultant Neuroradiologist*
*Royal Free Hospital & Royal National*
*Throat Nose and Ear Hospital*
*London*
*UK*

**Asif Siaffudin**
*Consultant Radiologist*
*Royal National Orthopaedic Hospital*
*Stanmore, Middlesex*
*UK*

**William E. Svensson**
*Director of Radiology*
*Ealing Hospital*
*Honorary Senior Lecturer*
*Hammersmith Hospital*
*London*
*UK*

**W. P. Soutter**
*Reader and Consultant*
*Gynaecological Oncology*
*Hammersmith Hospital*
*London*
*UK*

**Geraldine Walsh**
*Senior Registrar*
*Addenbrooke's Hospital*
*Cambridge*
*UK*

**Gordon Williams**
*Consultant and Honorary Senior Lecturer*
*Urology and Renal Transplant Unit*
*Hammersmith Hospital*
*London*
*UK*

# FOREWORD
## *by Professor Karol Sikora*

The key to the successful treatment of most patients with cancer is a detailed understanding of the location of the primary tumour and its likely routes of spread. Surgery and radical radiotherapy are still the main curative modalities for cancer although chemotherapy is increasing its potential both in the adjuvant setting and as primary therapy. For the surgeon and radiotherapist accurate, detailed and comprehensible anatomical information is essential. New technologies such as minimally invasive organ conservation, tele-surgery, robotics and conformal radiotherapy make such information even more important.

This book provides a succinct summary of tumour imaging, considering each organ system in turn. It is well illustrated by good quality clinical images which in themselves provide a useful educational tool. The discussion by well known experts, helps to guide the clinician to the most appropriate test under different circumstances. As healthcare systems globally become increasingly cost conscious it is vital that carefully selected, high yield investigations are used rather than the blunderbuss approach with the clinician requesting everything possible. Too often patients with well documented, essentially untreatable, metastatic disease still linger inappropriately on medical wards being further investigated rather than being offered appropriate palliative care. And yet accurate tumour staging is essential if the correct treatment is to be chosen and data from different centres reliably compared. Here you will find excellent guidance for the most appropriate investigation for many different oncological problems. Useful algorithms for diagnostic work-up and subsequent management are included for several common clinical scenarios.

Most importantly this book demonstrates the vital need for continual dialogue between those involved in clinical decision making and the imaging team. In cancer medicine, diagnosis is only useful as a guide to treatment. Constant interaction and teamwork is an essential component of good patient care in this increasingly important area of medicine.

*Karol Sikora*
*Chief, WHO Cancer Programme and Professor of Clinical Oncology,*
*Imperial College School of Medicine, Hammersmith Hospital, London*
*1998*

# FOREWORD

*by Professor Stephen Bloom*

For a long time imaging has been the province of specialists. This is clearly wrong. Of all branches of medicine surely imaging is the one where it is easiest to appreciate both the normal and the abnormal. Recent advances have been dramatic. It is now well within the ken of the average doctor both to appreciate the beauty of normal structure and to identify a particular abnormality in his patient. This exciting new book is the celebration of those advances and an opportunity for all clinicians to participate in the action. It sets out in an easy to understand and clear way how to detect the *major human diseases*. It has been predicted that once infections are covered by a range of effective antibiotics, a state that we are close to achieving, and the degenerative arterial diseases, currently the cause of much early mortality and morbidity, are abolished by new cholesterol lowering agents, our biggest enemy will be *cancer*. It is thus in the field of cancer diagnosis that we should focus our attention. This book offers a superb opportunity to get involved personally and at the cutting edge. The chapters are written by world experts, not only as experts in their field, but as experts in communication. They have been specifically chosen as good communicators, able to bring to every physician an understanding of the latest diagnostic techniques and how the reader can personally be able to contribute on behalf of his patient. Read and enjoy.

*Stephen Bloom*
*Chairman, Division of Investigative Science*
*Imperial College School of Medicine*
*1998*

# 1

# IMAGING IN ONCOLOGY

Introduction

*'Education is at the foundation of many initiatives to improve the health.'[1]*

*One of many quotations linking health and education, this was selected for its publication date on the centenary of the discovery of X-rays by W. C. Roentgen in 1895 and with this work we now celebrate 100 years of clinical-radiological correlation as Antoine Béclère (1856 – 1939) was the first physician to use fluoroscopy to diagnose pulmonary tuberculosis in 1897, only 2 years after Roentgen's discovery. [2]*

# Introduction

## Imaging Strategies

*'A well designed imaging strategy is an implicit component of the approach to a patient with cancer'. [3]*

This quotation summarises the origin of the motivation to write and edit this book which is aimed at medical students and colleagues in clinical practice. It seeks to improve the management of patients with cancer by providing the essentials of modern imaging techniques as applied to organ-based investigations.

The book adopts an integrative approach to the use of the most recent imaging modalities in both the initial assessment of a patient presenting with the symptoms and/or signs of cancer, and in further diagnostic and staging procedures.

In modern imaging we possess both the requisite technology and the clinical expertise to do a great deal for our patients. There is, however, a third factor to be considered, the so-called 'cost-benefit' equation for patient and society. The cost element of this concept is not based only on the financial impact of imaging techniques, but also on the risks of ionizing radiation for both the patient and the population as a whole. This problem was first addressed in detail in 'Critical Diagnostic Pathways in Radiology', [4] a publication which has had a strong influence on the way we conduct and teach modern imaging investigations. These issues are, if anything, even more important now than when they were first raised.

Medical decision analysis, discussed in more detail below, also depends on evidence-based medicine for sources of information and can, with appropriate techniques, individualise the treatment of data, follow up the consequences of decisions over long periods of time and generate cost effectiveness ratios. [5]

## Algorithms

Algorithms or critical diagnostic pathways became a

necessity for the day to day running of an Imaging Department in the late '70s when CT scanning installations in the industrialised world provided a novel means of investigating the human body. While CT of the brain provided an entirely new technique for the imaging of the skull contents and replaced previous invasive techniques (often requiring general anaesthesia), the study of the rest of the body by CT – Body CT – had to compete in a more serious fashion with traditional techniques. The use of the word traditional has a negative connotation in a domain in which progress is generally taken to be synonymous with the alleviation of suffering. The essence, the 'raison d'être' of research in medicine, is the broadening of knowledge from molecular biology to surgical technique or medical therapy including a spectrum of imaging procedures ranging from the simple X-ray beam to complex Positron-Emission Tomography (PET scanning) and Magnetic Resonance Spectroscopy (MRS imaging).

The French phrase 'arsenal diagnostique' embraces the dual concept of both a range of techniques and a choice of techniques. What may in an ideal set of circumstances be the best investigation may not, in the real world, be available owing to scarcity of resources, different political priorities, etc., and the appropriate selection of tests from those which are available will be determined by considerations of cost/efficacy, where efficacy is generally measured in terms of life duration, and cost/utility, where the duration of life is weighted according to its quality. [5] In addition to these considerations the cost-benefit ratio of imaging in financial terms is a constant reminder that we do not live in Utopia and in the non-industrialised world major epidemiological factors usually tend to direct resource allocation away from high technology medicine.

The defence of established techniques for the imaging of the chest and abdomen is undermined by two factors: *time* and, paradoxically (because existent 'conventional' studies are usually less expensive to implement), *cost*. The *time* factor is the essence of algorithm philosophy: a more sophisticated one-step modality which can image a tumour and furnish the means of obtaining a tissue diagnosis is preferable to a chain of simple techniques which would ultimately still require a further (perhaps endoscopic) step to achieve access to a specimen of tissue. The other factor, *cost,* plays a part in all diagnostic investigations whether undertaken during the course of a hospital admission or in a series of outpatient attendances. In comparing the 'fast lane' with the 'slow lane' the benefit of the time-factor is superficially obvious but we must not lose sight of its true implications: earlier treatment and a genuine reduction in pain, emotional distress and morbidity. The prolonged occupation of a hospital bed is financially and socially 'expensive'. The social implications (quality of life for the patient and for his/her family, and for subsequent patients on the waiting list) merge with political implications with their own widespread consequences ranging from popularity issues with the electorate to the potentially difficult reallocation of budget resources.

The last argument in favour of algorithms, but definitely not the least in our priority list, is the maxim 'primum nil nocere'. This applies to diagnostic techniques using ionizing or high energy radiations and to all interventional procedures. A non-stochastic effect (not related to chance, but measurable with thresholds of reversible and irreversible damage) is bad enough and requires discipline in radiation protection, but the stochastic effect (related to chance, the 'lottery of life'), implies the avoidance of any potentially harmful technique and alone imposes the concept of the proper justification of any radiological procedure.

Going back 100 years to Roentgen and Béclère, the use of X-rays for the diagnosis and follow-up of pulmonary TB is universally accepted, but we do not use fluoroscopy for this indication any more and should we now need to do so, we would choose equipment with a modern image intensifier.

## LOGIC IN MEDICINE AND ALGORITHMS

What is 'logic in medicine'? Logic, according to Paul Tomassi [6] is, in the most general sense of the term, simply the study of the nature of reasoning, of argument. But the term is more often used in a much narrower sense as the study of *deductive* reasoning and deductive argument. We must also recognise another kind of logic which is not deductive in character but inductive and probabilistic which proceeds from a finite list of particular observations to a concluding generalisation.

Algorithms consist of a series of questions linked by lines labelled with the answers, which lead to the next question or to the diagnosis. (7) The terminology varies according to language; the French term 'analyse decisionelle', for instance, is linked to the 'arbre de capture' which is equivalent to the English 'flow chart' or 'computer sequencing'.

Inverting a algorithm step-by-step leads to a process known today as audit. Audit has become an unavoidable process implemented in order to counteract the questionable argument: 'this is what good radiologists do, therefore it has to be right'. The concept of

Continuing Medical Education (CME) as applied by current (self)-regulatory bodies replaces the more traditional self-disciplined approach of reading the current literature and a few recent books, and attending staff rounds and a few national and international meetings.

Algorithms can be either:

1) A step beyond simple interpretation of images acquired by radiologists 'consultants' in managerial terminology – in the process of helping clinicians (A recent article by Robinson [8] addresses this issue: 'Radiology's Achilles' Heel: error and variation in the interpretation of the Roentgen image')

and/or

2) the integration of imaging modalities (and their 'consultant') into the concept of organ-based medicine. Not so long ago the Oncologist was the close relative of the radiologist as both shared a common basic knowledge in physics and imaging interpretation. In the algorithms for many oncological situations multiple other investigative 'windows' should be opened: e.g. the diagnosis of a lung tumour includes not only the initial abnormal chest X-ray but also CT and bronchoscopy, or bronchoscopy and CT. The symptoms and signs of gastric carcinoma justify endoscopy and/or contrast studies, and further imaging for staging, etc.

We – the editors of this book – have been very fortunate in gathering together a formidable group of imaging experts, each, within his or her special area, as comfortable in their knowledge of radiology as in clinical medicine. We extend to all of them our most sincere thanks for their outstanding contribution, and to our partners and families our thanks for their support and understanding.

After so many months of gestation, the book is ready. Allow me in a final quote to paraphrase and (for once) disagree with my favourite author, Antoine de Saint-Exupéry in the 'Petit Prince': it is not the time we have *lost* but the time we have *given* this book which makes it so important.

# References

1. Craft, N. Lifespan: Conception to Adolescence. *BMJ* 1997; **315**: 12 027–12 030 (8 November 1997).

2. Curati-Alasonatti, W. Modern Imaging techniques: 100 years of clinical radiological correlations. *Postgrad Doctor* 1997; **13**: 237–240.

3. Bragg, DJ. *Imaging Strategies for Oncologic Diagnosis and Staging in: Oncologic Imaging*. Bragg DJ, Rubin P, Youker JE. Editors – Pergamon Press (New York) 1985.

4.  Eisenberg RL & Amberg JR. *Critical Diagnostic Pathways in Radiology*. JB Lippincott Co. (Philadelphia) 1981.

5.  Junod AF. Decision analysis and/or evidence based medicine. *Med et Hyg* 1997; **55:** 2027–9.

6.  Tomassi P. *Logic in Medicine, in logic in medicine* (second edition) Phillips CI Editor. BMJ Publishing Group (London) 1995.

7.  Williams BT. *Computer aids to clinical decisions*. Vol I and II. Florida: CRC Press, 1982.

8.  Robinson PJA. Radiology's Achilles' Heel: error and variation in the interpretation of the Roentgen image. *BJR* 1997, **70:** 1085–98

# 2

# THE CENTRAL NERVOUS SYSTEM

Lloyd Savy and Ivan Moseley

Intra-axial brain tumours
Extra-axial brain tumours
The pituitary region and visual pathway
The pineal region
The skull base
The spine
Postoperative imaging and radiation effects
New imaging techniques

Cross-sectional imaging has revolutionized the investigation and diagnosis of tumours affecting the central nervous system. Computed tomography (CT) and subsequently magnetic resonance imaging (MRI) have entirely supplanted conventional methods of visualizing intracranial neoplasia and dramatic improvements in resolution and scanning speed have increased diagnostic sensitivity and lowered the clinical threshold for investigation. Radiographs still play a small part in the diagnosis of spinal tumours, especially vertebral metastases, but MRI has almost completely replaced myelography and CT as the definitive initial investigation for suspected neoplastic disease of the spine. MR spectroscopy and functional MRI can now provide important information about the composition of tumours and effects on adjacent brain respectively and image-guided interactive systems have greatly facilitated the surgical treatment of brain tumours.

# Intra-axial brain tumours

The first and most important diagnostic step in the analysis of intracranial tumours on CT or MRI is the differentiation between intra- and extra-axial location, i.e. whether the tumour lies within or outside brain parenchyma. This distinction has important prognostic implications as many of the former are malignant with poor long-term prospects, whereas the latter tend to be benign for which a surgical cure is frequently realistic. MRI is somewhat more sensitive than CT in the detection and characterization of intra-axial tumours.[1] It allows multiplanar imaging and does not subject the patient to ionizing radiation. However, cost and availability may favour CT, which can also demonstrate some diagnostic features such as tumour calcification better than MRI. It may also be the investigation of choice in critically ill or confused patients and is usually more practical for guiding biopsy.

## *Astrocytoma*

An important criterion in the analysis of intra-axial tumours radiologically is the differentiation between diffuse, infiltrative astrocytic tumours and localized, non-infiltrative tumours. The former have a worse prognosis; they include fibrillary astrocytoma, anaplastic astrocytoma, glioblastoma multiforme and gliomatosis cerebri, in order of severity.[2]

*Fibrillary astrocytomas* have poorly defined margins. On CT they are usually of lower density than brain; about 20% calcify and up to 50% may show irregular enhance-

ment. On MRI they show non-specific high signal on T2-weighted (T2W) and proton density (PD) sequences and mild low signal on T1W sequences. They may contain areas of subtle high signal on T1W images, due possibly to calcification or microhaemorrhage. Apparent tumour cysts cannot be differentiated from microcystic change by signal characteristics, but the presence of internal septa, partition levels between fluids or fluid and debris, and fluid motion effects, may signify a drainable cyst.[3] Peritumoural vasogenic oedema is rare, but tumour cells may exist outside the region of abnormal density or signal.[4] A minority dedifferentiate to become more malignant tumours after an indolent period of many years.

*Anaplastic astrocytoma* is more likely to show enhancement and vasogenic oedema (Fig. 2.1).

*Glioblastoma multiforme* usually occurs in patients over 50 years old. It almost always enhances on CT and MRI, usually with a thick ring of enhancement, which can be irregular or partly nodular, around a central area of non-enhancing necrosis. This central area shows low density on CT and T2/PD high, T1 low intensity on MRI.[5] These aggressive tumours usually have extensive surrounding vasogenic oedema, which tracks through white matter and may cross the midline at the corpus callosum. Intratumoural haemorrhage may occur and spread via the subarachnoid space as well as direct invasion of bone may be seen. There is frequently midline shift and contralateral hydrocephalus due to compression of the foramen of Monro. Other pathology which can mimic glioblastoma includes solitary metastasis, anaplastic oligodendroglioma, lymphoma, radiation necrosis, abscess and cavernoma with recent haemorrhage.

*Gliomatosis cerebri* is a very diffuse gliomatous process involving both white and grey matter, causing little or no reduction in attenuation on CT, but much more conspicuous confluent or multifocal T2/PD high signal change on MRI.[6] Little or no mass effect may be evident and only rarely enhancement. Neurological deficits may initially be relatively mild, but there is remorseless progression and invariably a poor prognosis. The differential diagnosis radiologically may include encephalitis and demyelination.

*Localized, non-infiltrative astrocytic tumours* have a more favourable prognosis.[7] Histologically they are frequently pilocytic. Radiologically they are sharply demarcated and lobular, often with a cystic component, and almost always some enhancement; they rarely exhibit oedema, calcification or haemorrhage. Other tumours in this

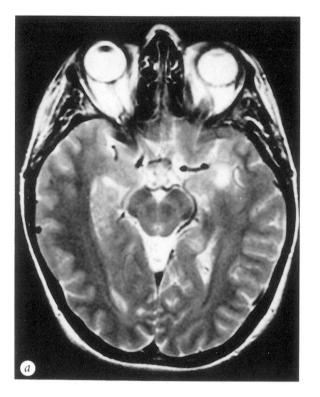

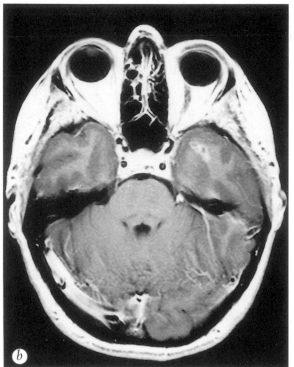

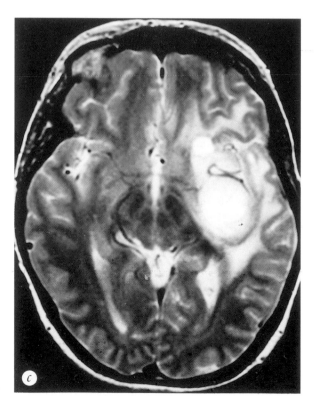

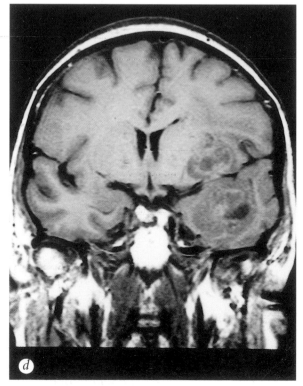

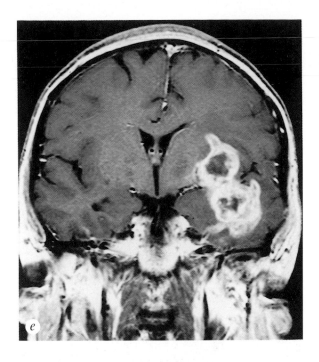

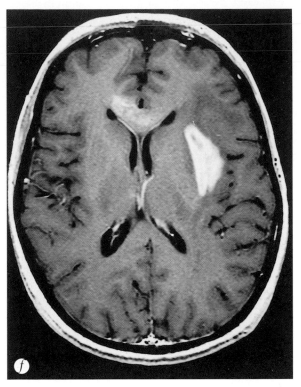

*Figure 2.1* — Anaplastic astrocytoma in a 55-year-old woman, who presented with a single seizure. Initial MRI – axial T2W (a), enhanced axial T1W (b) - revealed a small enhancing intrinsic lesion within the left anterior temporal lobe white matter. Four months later there had been dramatic progression: axial T2W (c), unenhanced coronal T1W (d), enhanced coronal (e) and axial (f) T1W images. A large tumour now involves left frontal and tem- poral lobes and insula. There is irregular rim enhancement, cen- tral non-enhancing T1 low signal due to necrosis and extensive vasogenic oedema, although only mild mass effect. The genu of corpus callosum is thickened despite normal signal on both T1W and T2W images and there is a further area of tumour enhance- ment to the right of the midline.

category include pleomorphic xanthoastrocytoma (a relatively benign, superficially-located glioma of young adults, often presenting with seizures), and subependy- mal giant cell astrocytoma, seen characteristically adja- cent to the foramen of Monro in up to 10% of patients with tuberous sclerosis.

## Oligodendroglioma

Calcification is the hallmark of oligodendroglioma, seen best on CT (50–90%) and optimally on MRI as low signal on T2W gradient echo images. This tumour is usually located in frontal or temporal lobes, often superficially.[8] It is often slow-growing and has a better prognosis than infiltrative astrocytoma, with an overall 5-year survival rate of approximately 50%, although the degree of malignancy is variable. On CT, oligoden- droglioma is usually a mixed hypo/isodense mass con- taining calcification, which may show enhancement, focal cysts or haemorrhage. There are no specific signal characteristics on MRI, although the observation of cal- cification is useful. Differential diagnosis includes astrocytoma, glioblastoma and dysembryoplastic neu- roepithelial tumour.

## Neuronal tumours

Ganglion cell tumours such as ganglioglioma and gan- gliocytoma or mixed neural/glial cell tumours may be indistinguishable from gliomas radiologically, with similar density and signal characteristics to astrocy- tomas. They typically present in children and young adults as supratentorial intrinsic masses, frequently in the temporal lobes.[9] About half contain cysts and 30% calcification. The solid component usually enhances but surrounding oedema is not typical. Occasionally they are of grey matter density and signal and may mimic grey matter heterotopia.

A relatively rare tumour of neural origin with characteristic imaging appearances is central neurocytoma. This benign tumour usually presents in young adults. CT and MR demonstrate a well-circumscribed, inhomogeneous, partly calcified mass, typically within the third or lateral ventricles, close to the foramen of Monro or septum pellucidum (Fig. 2.2).[10] There is characteristically a broad-based attachment to the superolateral ventricular wall.[11] The tumour may return high signal or signal close to that of grey matter on T2W MRI. Hydrocephalus is almost always present. Differential diagnosis includes other intraventricular tumours, such as ependymoma; oligodendroglioma and astrocytoma may also lie predominantly or completely within the ventricles.

Dysembryoplastic neuroepithelial tumour (DNT) is another relatively recently characterized tumour of glioneuronal origin.[12,13] This totally benign tumour which occurs most frequently in temporal lobe grey matter can be the cause of complex partial seizures, which may be cured by its excision. Usually small at presentation, it may be overlooked on CT, although

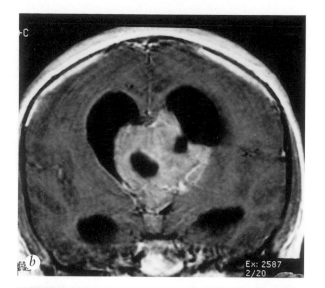

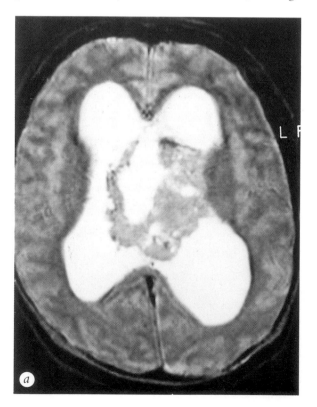

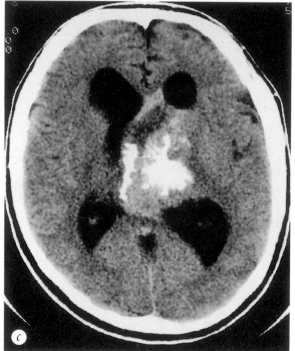

*Figure 2.2* — Central neurocytoma in a 29-year-old man. Axial T2W MRI (a) shows a large inhomogeneous mass within the third and lateral ventricles, much of which is of the same intensity as cortex. It causes obstructive hydrocephalus. The majority of the tumour enhances on post-gadolinium T1W image (b). Areas of T1 low, T2 high signal suggest cystic or microcystic components. Dense calcification is seen within parts of the tumour on CT (c).

larger lesions may be evident as a low density area with little if any mass effect; 50% calcify. On MRI the cortical location is characteristic; high signal on T2W and PD and equal to or slightly lower than grey matter on T1W images is seen. A DNT often cannot be distinguished from low grade glioma.

## Ependymoma

Ependymomas are usually slow-growing, lobulated tumours, which arise from the ependymal lining of the ventricles or central canal of the spinal cord. They are more common in children than adults, and in children most frequently lie within the fourth ventricle. The tumour characteristically has a 'plastic' appearance on imaging: it may extend through the outlet foramina of the ventricle and surround the brainstem and upper cord with only minor distortion of the neuraxis (Fig. 2.3). In adults the majority of ependymomas are supratentorial and these are usually extraventricular, although they may be partly or completely intraventricular. On CT ependymomas are usually isodense; 50% calcify; most show moderate inhomogeneous enhancement; haemorrhage is uncommon. On MRI they yield T1 low, T2 high signal, and the location and shape provide more specific clues to the diagnosis than signal and enhancement characteristics.[14] There is a spectrum of anaplasia; the observation of central necrosis on CT or MRI suggests a more aggressive tumour. Cerebral spinal fluid (CSF) seeding is not uncommon and is detected most accurately by MRI with gadolinium enhancement.

## Haemangioblastoma

This uncommon tumour may occur in isolation, but 10–20% occur as part of von Hippel Lindau syndrome. The characteristic appearance on CT or MRI is of an intrinsic cerebellar mass consisting of a relatively small, intensely enhancing nodule, often with a larger cyst adjacent to it:[15] a solid enhancing mass may be seen. Location in the brainstem or supratentorial compartment is rare. The tumour nodules are multiple in a minority of cases and MRI is more sensitive than CT in demonstrating these small lesions in the posterior fossa, as well as vascular signal voids which may be closely related to them. Only symptomatic lesions are treated surgically.

## Lymphoma

The incidence of primary CNS lymphoma is increasing, both in patients who are immunodeficient, such

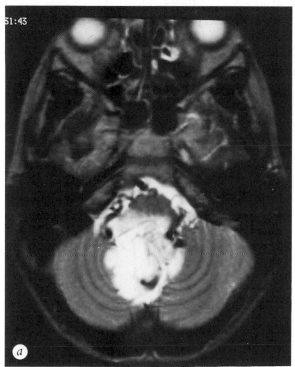

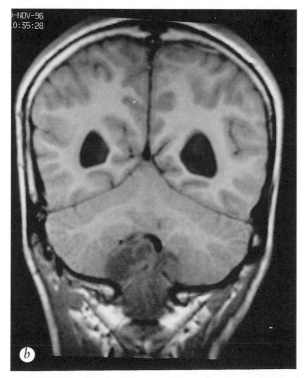

*Figure 2.3* — caption overleaf

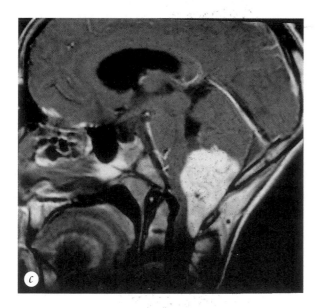

*Figure 2.3* — Posterior fossa ependymoma in a 16-year-old boy. Axial T2W MRI (a) shows a mixed signal intensity mass within the inferior part of the fourth ventricle, which extended through the outlet foramina. Coronal T1W image (b) shows tumour of mixed signal, slightly lower than that of grey matter, extending below the foramen magnum. The post-gadolinium sagittal image (c) shows intense, inhomogeneous enhancement of the tumour, the shape of which conforms to the subarachnoid space around the neuraxis. Serpiginous areas of signal void are due to distended posterior fossa veins.

as those with AIDS, organ transplant or congenital immunodeficiency, and in immunocompetent patients. In the latter the peak incidence is in the sixth decade. The tumour is nearly always non-Hodgkin's lymphoma and has a dismal prognosis, although radiotherapy can prolong life, particularly in patients with AIDS.

Lymphoma is typically located close to the ventricles, either in deep white matter or basal ganglia. Calcification is absent and haemorrhage very uncommon.[16] On CT the mass is usually isodense or slightly denser than grey matter, often spherical, and shows dense homogeneous or thick ring enhancement. Oedema occurs, but is usually less in degree than with metastases or aggressive gliomas. In 20–40% of cases multiple sites are affected. On MRI tumour signal characteristics are similar to grey matter, although either high or low signal on T2W sequences may be seen (the latter due to dense cellularity).

In AIDS lymphoma, central necrosis and peritumoural oedema are more common,[17] and the main differential diagnosis is toxoplasmosis. Subependymal spread and enhancement along perivascular (Virchow-Robin) spaces are features which favour lymphoma,[18] whereas haemorrhage favours toxoplasmosis, despite occurring more frequently in AIDS than non-AIDS lymphoma.

Primary CNS lymphoma can also show a more diffuse, infiltrative pattern, which may be indistinguishable from gliomatosis cerebri.

## Metastases

Intra-axial metastases comprise 20% of clinically detected brain tumours and occur most frequently in the fourth to seventh decades; 80% are supratentorial. The lung, breast, skin (melanoma), gastrointestinal tract and genitourinary tract are the commonest primary sites. The optimal imaging method for detection of small metastases is gadolinium-enhanced MRI,[19] which can also differentiate small metastases from ischaemic areas. CT still has an important role in investigating the acutely ill patient. The grey/white matter interface is a site of predilection, as there is significant narrowing of cerebral arterioles at this level.[20] Metastases exhibit florid vasogenic oedema, although this tends not to cross the corpus callosum or involve cortex, in contradistinction to that associated with primary tumours. Cortical metastases may show little or no surrounding oedema. Most metastases are of low density, T2/PD high and T1 low signal, but haemorrhage is present in 20% (particularly melanoma, choriocarcinoma and renal cancer). Melanin itself has a characteristic MRI signal (T1 high, T2 low intermediate signal), although primary brain tumours as well as metastases may be melanotic (Fig. 2.4); mucinous adenocarcinoma often yields T2 low signal. Metastases may calcify or even ossify (especially osteosarcoma). Enhancement occurs on both CT and MRI: it may be nodular or consist of a thick irregular ring, with a central non-enhancing area due to necrosis. This contrasts with the characteristically thin enhancing rim of cerebral abscess, although the radiological appearance may be similar.

Recently, the advent of stereotactic radiosurgery for solitary metastases and the use of adjuvant radiotherapy after surgery have increased the importance of detecting small metastases.

## Posterior fossa neoplasms of childhood

In children infratentorial neoplasms are more prevalent than supratentorial neoplasms and present with symptoms of hydrocephalus, cranial nerve palsies or cerebellar syndromes. The commonest tumours are juvenile pilocytic astrocytoma, primitive neuroectodermal tumour (PNET) — previously termed medulloblastoma, ependymoma and brainstem glioma. MR is the most useful imaging modality, due to its clear depiction of posterior fossa anatomy[21] and facility to perform enhanced scans of the brain and whole spine at the time of initial diagnosis, to demonstrate small leptomeningeal metastases which have spread via CSF.

Pilocytic astrocytoma frequently arises in the cerebellar vermis or hemisphere in children and young adults and is typically partly cystic, partly solid. About 10% are calcified; enhancement is variable. PNET (medulloblas-

toma) occurs in a similar location, also mainly in children, and may be indistinguishable, although it tends to be more homogeneous; it is usually relatively dense on CT and may be of low signal on T2W MRI, due to dense cellularity. Enhancement is usually intense; haemorrhage and calcification are rare. PNET shows early CSF dissemination, and preoperative gadolinium enhanced scans of the whole neuraxis are useful as postoperatively small foci of leptomeningeal haemorrhage may be present. Like metastases these can also appear as tiny high signal areas on enhanced images, but unlike metastases they are usually also of high signal on unenhanced T1W images.

Brainstem gliomas may be pilocytic or fibrillary astrocytomas. They are usually solid, low grade tumours, which expand the brainstem, and are much more easily detected on MRI than CT.

# Extra-axial brain tumours

Neoplasms arising from structures around the brain are usually benign, but may cause neurological deficit

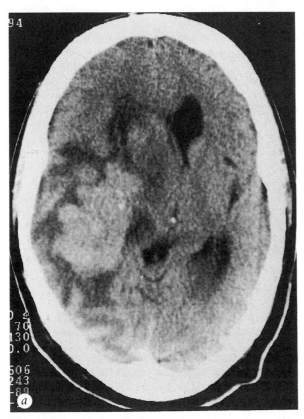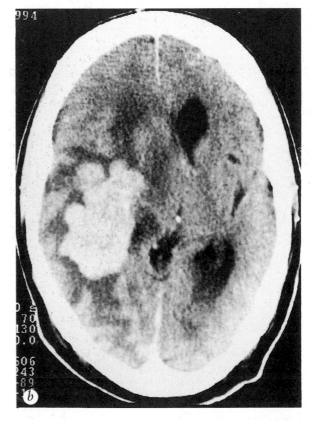

*Figure 2.4* — caption overleaf

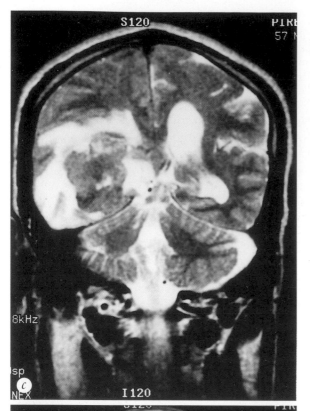

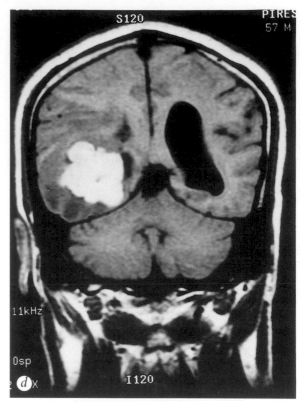

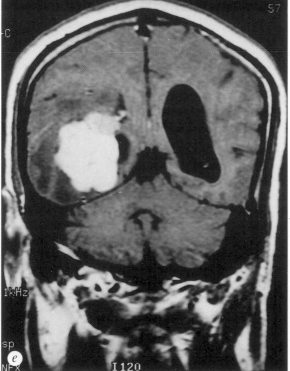

*Figure 2.4* — Intraventricular tumour with unusual signal characteristics which was shown histologically to be a melanotic ependymoma. Unenhanced CT (a) demonstrates a very large multilobular hyperdense mass containing a little calcification, which enhances homogeneously (b). There is severe vasogenic oedema in the right cerebral hemisphere (note the sparing of caudate and lentiform nuclei), subfalcine herniation to the left, compression of the ipsilateral lateral ventricle and contralateral hydrocephalus. MRI strongly suggests the intraventricular location of the mass. Its low signal on the T2W image (c) and high signal on the T1W image (d) are highly unusual for ependymoma, and are due to the presence of melanin in this case. Gadolinium enhancement of the mass (e) is masked by its high signal, except for a small tumour component which is isointense to brain on the unenhanced scan.

or even death by compressing the neuraxis. The mode of therapy and the prognosis depend on the location of the tumour. It is therefore important for imaging studies to distinguish between extra- and intra-axial tumours, although this can be difficult. MRI is superior to CT in this respect as it can demonstrate displaced cortex lying deep to extra-axial tumours, compression of adjacent gyri, and also small intervening structures such as pial blood vessels, dura and pockets of CSF, lying between tumour and brain (Fig. 2.5). It is particularly useful for suspected posterior fossa tumours as its multiplanar capability helps to demonstrate the relationship of an extra-axial mass to the brainstem and cerebellum. Furthermore, the beam hardening artefacts which degrade CT in the posterior fossa are avoided. MRI is also better than CT at defining the margins of extension of extra-axial tumours, arterial encasement and dural sinus compression or invasion. Gadolinium aids tissue characterization (meningioma and metastasis enhance whereas dermoid and epidermoid do not), and also increases sensitivity for detection of small extrinsic tumours such as metastases and lymphoma.

## Meningioma

Meningioma is by far the commonest primary extra-axial intracranial tumour. It is twice as prevalent in women as men, and presents most frequently in the fourth to seventh decades. It is very rare in children, in whom it is more likely to be a manifestation of neurofibromatosis. Areas where arachnoid granulations are abundant are sites of predilection for meningioma, including the parasagittal region and the meninges close to the pterion. The tumour can also arise from pial meningeal cells and therefore can occur within the ventricles or Sylvian fissures.

CT shows an isodense or dense mass with a broad base to the overlying dura mater. Internal calcification is present in 20% and may be punctate or dense. There is almost always dense homogeneous enhancement. Oedema in adjacent brain is common and variable in extent. An important sign on CT is thickening of adjacent bone (hyperostosis), which if present is a strong pointer to the diagnosis. This may involve paranasal sinuses, particularly the posterior ethmoid air cells adjacent to a meningioma of the planum sphenoidale, known as pneumosinus dilatans. The hyperostosis is usually a reactive rather than neoplastic phenomenon, although infiltration and expansion of the skull vault or base by tumour itself may also be seen; indeed meningioma can be solely intradiploic, arising from arachnoid cell rests in the diploic space.

On MRI meningiomas usually yield signal close to that of grey matter on all sequences and if small may be inconspicuous and easily overlooked. As on CT there is intense homogeneous enhancement of the mass and an enhancing 'dural tail' extending away from its base is characteristic, but not specific. The dural tail frequently does not contain tumour cells.[22] Peripheral cysts may be seen on MRI and CT and can be intratumoural or subarachnoid.

To some extent meningioma subtypes can be identified by MRI signal.[23] Angioblastic or syncytial tumours tend to exhibit higher signal than cortex on T2W images; transitional tumours are isointense; fibroblastic tumours may show lower T2W signal than cortex, due to calcification within psammoma bodies. The rare lipomatous form of meningioma yields high signal on T1W images and is of low density on CT due to its fat content. Malignant meningioma is difficult to predict radiologically. Invasion of the brain suggests it, but transcalvarial spread does not.[24] Haemangiopericytoma is usually indistinguishable from meningioma radiologically, but may be suggested by the absence of hyperostosis or tumoural calcification.[25]

Angiography still occasionally plays a part in the preoperative assessment of meningiomas, both to indicate the degree of tumour vascularity and to determine the patency or otherwise of adjacent dural sinuses, although MRI and MR angiography (MRA) can also provide similar information. Angiography is also necessary in planning preoperative embolization using particulates, to reduce the vascularity of the tumour and facilitate haemostasis at surgery.

Differential diagnosis depends on location: 8th nerve Schwannoma in the cerebellopontine angle; pituitary adenoma in the suprasellar region; choroid plexus papilloma within the ventricles; metastasis, lymphoma or granuloma at any extra-axial site are examples.

## Nerve sheath tumours

The commonest intracranial nerve sheath tumour is 8th nerve Schwannoma. It usually arises from the superior vestibular nerve rather than the acoustic nerve and presents with sensorineural deafness and/or tinnitus. It is typically bilateral in neurofibromatosis II. MRI has replaced CT in screening for this tumour as it is more sensitive and does not subject a potentially large screened population to ionizing radiation. On 1.5 Tesla MRI, fast T2 sequences with high spatial resolution may be sufficient to exclude small 8th nerve tumours, if the whole length of the nerve can be visualized.[26] If not, or on lower field strength systems, gadolinium-enhanced T1W sequences may be required. Small lesions are of similar

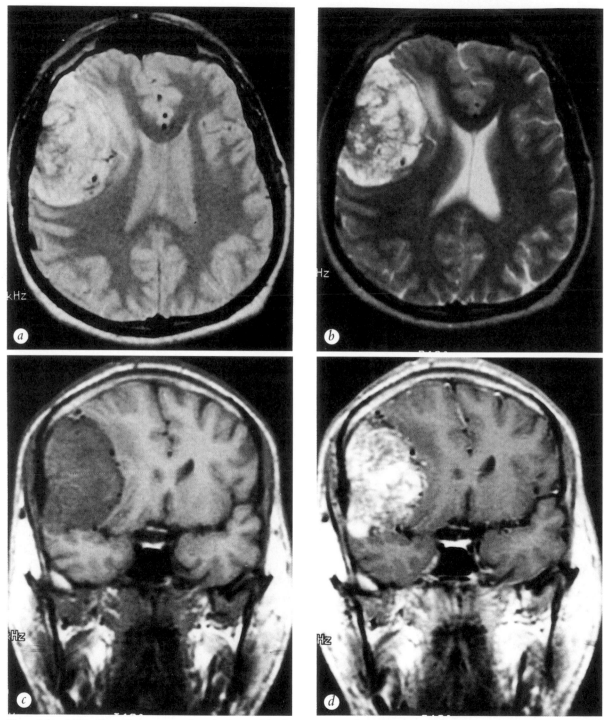

***Figure 2.5*** — MRI of large frontotemporal meningioma arising in the region of the pterion in a 31-year-old man. Axial proton density (a) and T2W (b) images. Coronal T1W images (c) before and (d) after gadolinium. Both the signal of the tumour on PD and T2W images and the enhancement pattern are less homogeneous than usual. The extra-axial location is signified by the displace-ment and compression of adjacent gyri and the presence of pial vessels between tumour and brain, seen as small signal voids. Hyperostosis of the adjacent skull vault is evident, in comparison with the opposite side. Vasogenic oedema within the underlying white matter is clearly seen on the T2W image.

intensity to brain on all sequences and therefore stand out against the high intensity of surrounding CSF on T2W images. CSF motion effects may simulate a mass in the cerebellopontine angle, but lack of contrast enhancement will exclude tumour. 8th nerve Schwannoma (Fig. 2.6) is characteristically cone-shaped, lying partly within the expanded internal auditory meatus and partly within the cerebellopontine angle cistern. Larger tumours can compress the brain stem and cause hydrocephalus. They may undergo central necrosis and form cysts and therefore show T2 high, T1 low signal and central non-enhancement. Calcification is extremely rare, in contrast with meningioma, but haemorrhage is more common. The shape of the tumour and absence of hyperostosis are also useful discriminators. Other tumours which occur in the cerebellopontine angle include metastasis, epidermoid, exophytic glioma and ependymoma.

5th nerve (trigeminal) Schwannoma is the second commonest intracranial nerve sheath tumour and may be recognized on MRI by its orientation along the line of the nerve.

## Maldevelopmental tumours and cysts

Arachnoid cyst, lipoma, epidermoid and dermoid are all extra-axial masses which may compress the brain. However, arachnoid cysts are common incidental findings on imaging, usually without clinical significance. Midline lipomas occur in conjunction with developmental abnormalities, typically dysgenesis of the corpus callo-

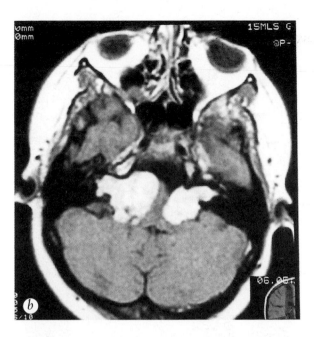

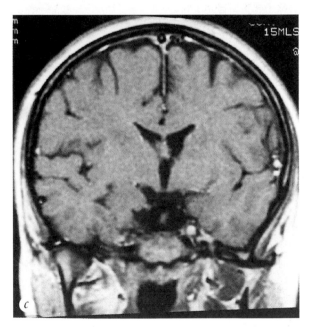

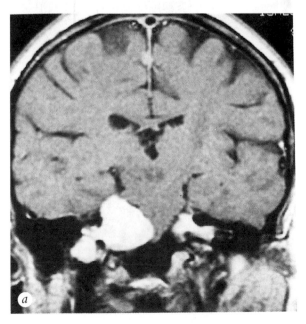

*Figure 2.6* — Bilateral 8th nerve Schwannomata in a patient with neurofibromatosis type II. Coronal T1W MRI (a) and axial T1W image after gadolinium injection (b). Note the characteristic 'ice-cream cone' shape of the tumours, which occupy the expanded internal auditory meatus and cerebellopontine angles and compress the brain stem. Smaller Schwannomas are shown in the right jugular foramen and (c) involving the left trigeminal nerve.

sum. Epidermoids may grow and cause symptoms and require surgery or radiotherapy. They are characterized on imaging by density and signal close to CSF, lack of calcification or enhancement, and — unlike arachnoid cysts — lobulated margins.[27] Dermoids are inhomogeneous masses which tend to occur in the midline and may be identified on MRI or CT by the presence of fat, or differentiated structures such as teeth within the mass.

## Choroid plexus papilloma

This highly vascular benign intraventricular tumour accounts for 0.5% of intracranial neoplasms, but is one of the commonest brain tumours in infants. It occurs most frequently in the lateral ventricle in children and the 4th ventricle in adults, but also occurs in the 3rd ventricle. It may extend through the 4th ventricular outlet foramina and can also be located solely within the cerebellopontine angle. Apart from intense homogeneous enhancement, the most characteristic feature on imaging is a lobular, fronded appearance to its surface, more readily appreciated on MRI than CT. Calcification is common and cyst formation and haemorrhage also occur. Hydrocephalus is also usually present and may be secondary to repeated intraventricular haemorrhage or CSF oversecretion.[28] Carcinoma of the choroid plexus is much less common. It has similar appearances on imaging and features such as invasion of the brain and dissemination via CSF do not distinguish it from papilloma.

## Metastases

Intracranial metastases may be solely extra-axial, particularly breast and prostate carcinoma and neuroblastoma, and cannot be reliably demonstrated without intravenous contrast enhancement.[29] Enhanced MRI is much more sensitive than CT. Lymphomatous involvement of the leptomeninges or dura mater (Fig. 2.7) may be primary or secondary, solitary or multiple and occurs in a third of patients with systemic lymphoma.

Extra-axial metastases can have many deleterious effects on the CNS, including brain compression, cranial nerve involvement, venous thrombosis, haemorrhagic meningitis and hydrocephalus, and all of these can be demonstrated by MRI.

# The pituitary region and visual pathway

MRI has almost completely replaced CT for the assessment of chiasmal compression by tumours in the pitu-

itary region. Pituitary macroadenoma is by far the commonest cause, but meningioma, craniopharyngioma, teratodermoid and metastasis may also involve the chiasmatic cistern, as well as intrinsic tumours of the optic pathway such as glioma (usually pilocytic astrocytoma). The pituitary infundibulum may be the site of lymphoma or germinoma, as well as adenoma and very rarely other primary tumours such as glioma and choristoma (granular cell tumour).[30] The latter is usually evident as an enhancing infundibular mass of similar density and signal to brain.

The multiplanar capability of MRI allows excellent demonstration of the relationship of a large pituitary tumour to the cavernous sinuses and internal carotid arteries, and has obviated the need for angiography. On postoperative scans artefact from surgical clips may obscure the region of interest less than on CT.

In the orbit CT still plays an important part in the diagnosis of tumours affecting the optic nerve/sheath complex. The demonstration of calcification of the nerve sheath is virtually pathognomonic of meningioma; erosion or hyperostosis of the optic canals or bony walls at the orbital apex are more readily identified than on MRI; fat within the rectus muscle cone provides good inherent contrast with the nerves; narrow sections of 1–2 mm provide good spatial resolution for small tumours. However, MRI usually separately identifies the nerve and its dural sheath, will show pathology within the nerve more sensitively than CT, and avoids radiation to the lens. Gadolinium-enhanced, fat-suppression techniques are sensitive to tumours of the nerve sheath such as meningioma. The patient's age at presentation is a good discriminator of glioma and meningioma of the optic nerve/sheath complex: the former usually present in the first two decades and the latter after this time. Orbital lymphoma is most prevalent in elderly women and typically has the appearance of a diffuse, usually extraconal mass in the anterior part of the orbit, which is difficult to distinguish from orbital granuloma.

## Pituitary adenoma

Microadenomas are defined as tumours less than 10 mm in diameter and typically present with endocrine symptoms, although many are asymptomatic, and they are a common incidental finding at autopsy. About 50% are prolactinomas and for these, in the absence of visual signs, both the initial diagnosis and monitoring following medical therapy can be achieved biochemically, without any need for imaging. Patients with acromegaly or Cushing's syndrome, or rarely syndromes related to thyrotrophic or gonadotrophic hormone hypersecretion, may require imaging to locate the tumour within the pituitary gland prior to surgery. This requires MRI using thin slices, small field of view and a fine matrix. Microadenomas are usually of high signal compared with the pituitary on T2 fast spin echo images and of low signal on T1W images. They enhance less than the remainder of the gland in the early phase following gadolinium injection and more than the gland in the late phase.[31] Alteration in shape of the pituitary, signified by a bulge in its superior surface, depression of part of the floor of the fossa, or displacement of the infundibulum, may help to locate a microadenoma but are less sensitive signs than signal change and can be misleading. Rarely petrous vein sampling by catheterization via the femoral vein may be required to distinguish Cushing's syndrome from syndromes of extraneous corticosteroid overproduction and to assist in lateralization of tumour.

Pituitary macroadenoma may present with symptoms of optic pathway compression, but alternatively with

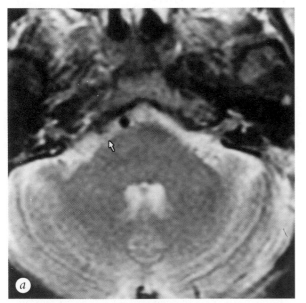

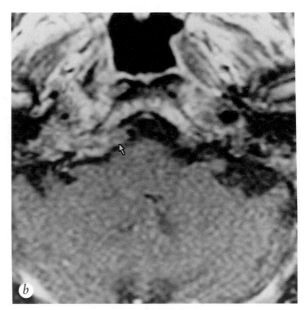

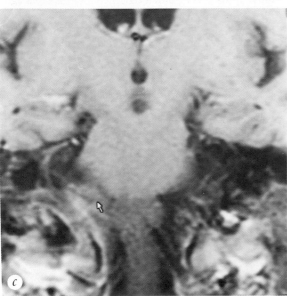

*Figure 2.7* — A man of 70 years with systemic non-Hodgkin's lymphoma, who presented with right 6th and 7th nerve palsies. Axial T2W MR (a) shows no definite abnormality in the cerebellopontine angle. The basilar artery can cause slightly reduced signal in adjacent CSF due to the effects of pulsation (arrow). However, a gadolinium-enhanced T1W image (b) clearly demonstrates enhancing tumour involving the meninges at this site (arrow), and in contact with the basilar artery. Enhanced coronal scan (c) also shows the extent of tumour within the cistern.

symptoms or signs of 3rd or 5th nerve compression, hypopituitarism, diabetes insipidus or pituitary apoplexy; in the latter case, haemorrhage or infarct within the tumour may be seen on MRI (Fig. 2.8). These tumours enhance with gadolinium, but unenhanced T1W images suffice for monitoring tumour size. On CT macroadenomas are isodense and show intense enhancement, but rarely calcify.

## Craniopharyngioma

Craniopharyngioma arises from squamous epithelial rests along Rathke's cleft and is usually predominantly suprasellar, with an intrasellar component. It is more common in children than adults. On CT 90% show calcification, cyst formation and nodular or rim enhancement. MRI may show multiple cysts of different signal intensity.[32,33] The presence of calcification and a solid component helps to differentiate this entity from Rathke's cleft cyst.

# The pineal region

Pineal tumours constitute less than 1% of intracranial tumours. They may present with symptoms of hydro-

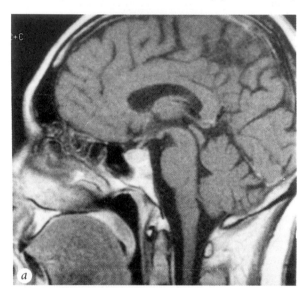

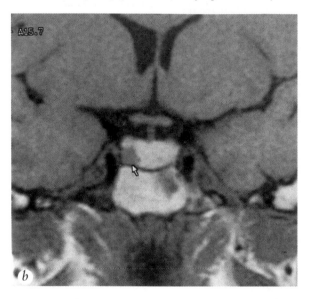

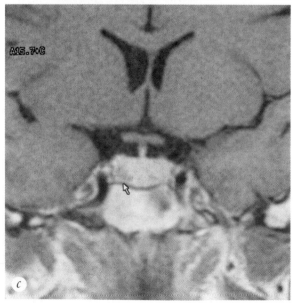

*Figure 2.8* — Unenhanced T1W MR images showing a haemorrhagic pituitary adenoma. Sagittal scan (a) demonstrates an enlarged pituitary gland of abnormally high signal causing expansion of the pituitary fossa. The haemorrhagic tumour is of similar signal to adjacent fatty marrow within the basisphenoid. Coronal scans (b) before and (c) after gadolinium show an area of normal signal within the right side of the gland (arrow); however, this enhances to a lesser degree than the cavernous sinus, suggesting that it represents non-haemorrhagic tumour rather than normal pituitary tissue.

cephalus due to compression of the aqueduct, Parinaud's syndrome due to tectal plate compression, or endocrine symptoms such as precocious puberty. They include pineal cell tumours (pinealoblastoma and pinealocytoma) and germ cell tumours (germinoma and teratoma). These may be difficult to distinguish radiologically, but some features aid in differential diagnosis.[34,35]

Teratoma typically presents in the first decade, predominantly in boys. It may be calcified, cystic or haemorrhagic, and the presence of fat or differentiated structures such as teeth signifies the diagnosis. Germinoma usually has a more homogeneous appearance on CT and MRI, is dense on CT and can be of the same intensity as grey matter on T2W images. Its diagnosis is important as it responds to low-dose radiotherapy. It occurs most frequently in the first three decades and 90% of patients are male. The primary tumour may arise in the suprasellar region or within the third ventricle as well as from the pineal gland. Seeding through the CSF space is common, but such metastases may also respond well to radiotherapy.

Pineal cell tumours are less common: pinealocytoma is a benign tumour of adults. Pinealoblastoma is a less well differentiated malignant neoplasm found in young children. It is a subtype of primitive neuroepithelial tumour (PNET) and has a strong tendency to metastasize within the subarachnoid space. It may appear less well encapsulated than other pineal tumours, enhances less homogeneously and may invade adjacent brain, but there are no pathognomonic radiological features.

Pineal cysts are a common incidental finding, seen in at least 5% of the population on MRI, and found much more frequently at autopsy. They should have a signal close to or slightly higher than CSF with all MR sequences and have a thin, well-defined, round capsule. They may show peripheral contrast enhancement. Any cyst greater than 1.5 cm in diameter, however, should be regarded with suspicion.

# The skull base

Neoplastic skull base lesions cause a wide variety of CNS symptoms depending on their location. They may compress the base of the brain and brainstem and may involve cranial nerves, cavernous, lateral and sigmoid sinuses, or carotid arteries. Meningioma and metastases can occur anywhere at the base of the skull. Nasal and sinus malignancy such as carcinoma, rhabdomyosarcoma[36] and olfactory neuroblastoma (esthesioneuroblastoma)[37] can invade the anterior cranial fossa. Each of these tumours exhibits bone destruction, but there are no specific density or signal characteristics on CT or MRI, with non-specific T2 high, T1 low signal and enhancement following contrast medium; biopsy is almost always required. MRI is more reliable for demonstrating the extent of the lesion.

Central skull base tumours involve the sphenoid and basioccipital regions. Pituitary tumours have been described above. Chordoma is a relatively benign but locally invasive neoplasm, often with a poor outcome. It arises from the remnants of the notochord and tends to involve the clivus in the midline. Apart from the location it does have other characteristic imaging features: on CT a high percentage are calcified and severe bone destruction is usually evident; on T2W MRI[38] it returns a very high signal, which may be higher than that of CSF and often has a strikingly inhomogeneous appearance (Fig. 2.9); it enhances avidly. Chondrosarcoma is a very similar tumour histologically as well as radiologically and orthographically, but typically arises lateral to the clivus. Either of these tumours can invade the middle or posterior cranial fossae, as can nasopharyngeal carcinoma. The upper cervical spine may also be involved. Other tumours which can involve the central skull base include trigeminal Schwannoma and juvenile angiofibroma.

Posterolateral skull base tumours involve the temporal bone. Glomus jugulare tumours may compress the neuraxis and cause cranial nerve palsies. The irregular erosion of the jugular foramen and extent of petrous bone destruction are best assessed by high resolution CT using narrow sections, but the relationship of the tumour to brain is seen more clearly on MR. Angiography is used to define which branches of the external carotid artery supply the tumour and preoperative embolization can reduce the size of the mass and aid haemostasis at surgery. Glomus tympanicum, like glomus jugulare, is a highly vascular paraganglioma, but arises in the middle ear cleft. Either of these can reach the cerebellopontine angle. Other tumours arising in the temporal bone region include squamous carcinoma of the external auditory meatus and nerve sheath tumours arising from the 7th to 12th cranial nerves. Meningioma may occur at the surface of the clivus or at the foramen magnum and can compress the brain stem or upper cord, often with relatively mild neurological signs due to its slow growth.

# The spine

MRI is now the primary imaging modality in the diagnosis of spinal tumours. It is more sensitive and specific than scintigraphy in the detection of vertebral

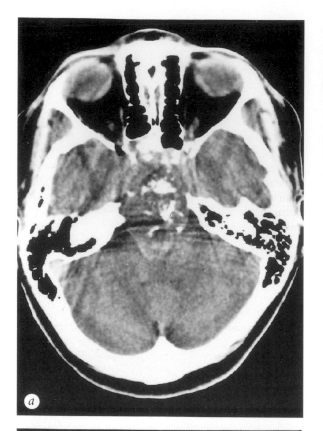

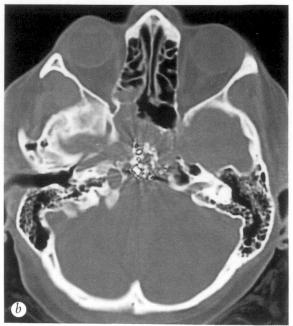

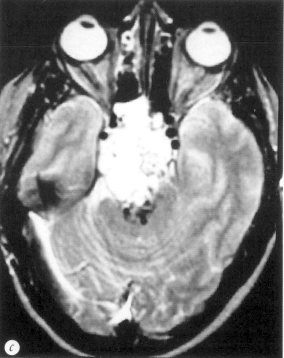

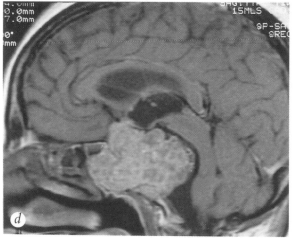

*Figure 2.9* — Skull base chordoma. (a,b) Unenhanced CT shows a large mass containing punctate calcification, causing destruction of the basisphenoid and compression of the brainstem. Axial T2W MRI (c) shows the typical mottled signal of chordoma, higher than that of CSF, and displacement of carotid and basilar arteries. Sagittal T1W image following gadolinium (d) shows inhomogeneous tumour enhancement and clearly displays the extent of skull base destruction and compression of the pons.

metastases[39] and superior to CT myelography in the assessment of intraspinal tumours. CT still has a role in the assessment of bone architecture prior to surgery for metastases and in the differential diagnosis of primary tumours of the vertebrae.

## Intramedullary tumours

MRI is by far the best method of demonstrating features of intramedullary tumours such as subtle cord enlargement, parenchymal oedema, haemorrhage and haemosiderin. Gadolinium enhancement may help to discriminate tumour from surrounding oedema, particularly for metastases and haemangioblastoma.

The commonest intramedullary tumours are gliomas, of which astrocytoma and ependymoma are difficult to differentiate on MRI. Each usually demonstrates focal expansion of the cord and non-specific T2W high signal, and normal or low T1W signal, with variable, ill-defined enhancement.[40] Signs favouring ependymoma over astrocytoma are; location in the lower cord or conus, central rather than eccentric position within the cord, a well-defined plane of cleavage between tumour and normal cord and intratumoural haemorrhage: astrocytomas tend to be longer but less bulky. Despite these differences, distinction between the two is frequently impossible.

Intramedullary cysts above or below the tumour may be lined by neoplastic cells, in which case the cyst wall may be enhanced, or they may be due to a syringomyelic cavity filled with CSF.

Astrocytoma of the cord varies considerably in its degree of anaplasia. Most adult tumours are benign, but for malignant tumours survival is usually less than 2 years. The overall survival rate following surgery and radiotherapy is approximately 60% at 5 years and 23% at 10 years. The outcome for ependymoma is better and only 15% recur following complete excision.

Haemangioblastoma constitutes 3% of intramedullary tumours and 30% of these patients have von Hippel Lindau syndrome. The MRI appearance is more characteristic,[41] with a small intensely enhancing nodule within or on the surface of the cord (more often posteriorly), the majority with a large adjacent non-enhancing cyst, which is usually non-neoplastic. Haemangioblastomas may be multiple. Meningeal varicosities on the dorsal surface of the cord are a further pointer to the diagnosis. Treatment is usually surgical.

Intramedullary metastases (Fig. 2.10) are rare; the lung is the commonest source. Patients present with rapid clinical progression of a cord syndrome. MRI typically demonstrates a small T2 high signal, enhancing lesion with adjacent oedema which may be invisible on CT myelography. Unfortunately, despite radiotherapy, the majority of these patients die within 6 months.

## Intradural, extramedullary tumours

As with extra-axial brain tumours, the recognition of an extramedullary location for spinal tumours is important, as the majority are benign, and surgical cure and alleviation of symptoms of cord compression are often realistic. The commonest tumours located within the subarachnoid space are meningiomas and neurofibromas.[42]

Spinal meningioma is most prevalent in the 5th and 6th decades; 60–80% occur in women, in whom the thoracic spine is usually affected. Symptoms are usually myelopathic rather than radiculopathic. The tumour is occasionally solely extradural, in which case malignant histology is more likely. Plain radiography or CT may demonstrate erosion of pedicles or enlargement of neural foramina. Like intracranial meningiomas, on CT the mass is usually iso- or hyperdense, with homogeneous enhancement and sometimes dense calcification, although it may be impossible to detect without intrathecal contrast medium (CT myelography). On MRI it is usually of similar signal to the cord or may yield slightly higher signal on T2W and lower signal on T1W sequences. Gadolinium enhancement is usually intense and can help to define the tumour margins. Signal may be very low if there is dense tumour calcification.

Characteristic features that differentiate meningioma from neurofibroma are a broad base on the dura mater, a single tumour and location posterolateral to the cord. Neurofibromas are characteristically dumb-bell shaped as they transgress the neural foramen along the line of the nerve; they therefore may be both intradural and extradural. They may be multiple and tend to lie slightly anterior to the cord. There is considerable overlap in these characteristics however.

Neurofibroma is the commonest intraspinal tumour and usually occurs as part of neurofibromatosis, whereas spinal Schwannoma (neurinoma) is usually solitary and in patients without neurofibromatosis. Neurofibroma usually presents in the fourth decade, most commonly in the cervical region, with pain and radiculopathy. On imaging it can sometimes be differentiated from meningioma by the characteristic shape, a higher signal on T2W images, and absence of calcification (Fig. 2.11).

*a*
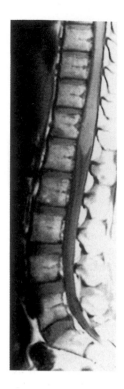

*b*
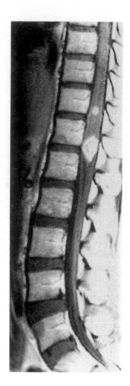

*c*
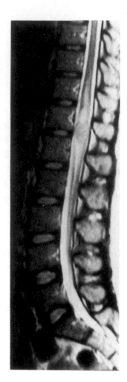

*d*
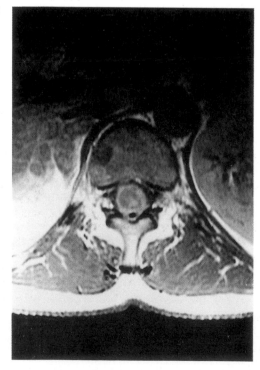

*Figure 2.10* — Intramedullary and extradural metastases from breast carcinoma. Sagittal T1W images (a) before and (b) after gadolinium injection. The lumbar expansion of the cord is larger than normal and two enhancing intramedullary masses are shown. In addition small low signal deposits are present in the D12 and L5 vertebral bodies; these enhance with gadolinium and therefore become less conspicuous relative to the surrounding marrow. On sagittal T2W image (c) the intramedullary lesions are of similar signal to cord, but the larger one is identified because of the high signal oedema above and below it. The vertebral body deposits are very inconspicuous, which is often the case on T2W images. Axial post-gadolinium T1W image (d) shows the larger enhancing intramedullary mass. The D12 vertebral body deposit, despite some enhancement, is still of lower signal than marrow.

Spinal intradural extramedullary metastases occur with many CNS tumours by seeding through the subarachnoid space (Fig. 2.12). These are frequently tiny lesions which require gadolinium-enhanced MR for their detection, and this demonstrates tumour nodules in only about a fifth of cases with tumour cells within the CSF. The commonest primary tumour is medulloblastoma in children, but glioblastoma, ependymoma, oligodendroglioma, astrocytoma and retinal, pineal and choroid plexus tumours can all spread in this way. Malignant tumours from outside the CNS can metastasize to the spinal meninges by direct invasion, lymphatic or haematogenous routes.

## Extradural tumours

Metastases are the commonest extradural tumours to cause cord compression and thecal impingement by such metastases occurs in 5% of all systemic cancer. Frequent sites of primary tumour are prostate, lung and breast, and vertebral lymphoma and myeloma also cause cord compression.

Plain radiography may demonstrate a lytic or sclerotic metastasis, sometimes with collapse of the vertebral body, and in the thoracic spine paravertebral soft tissue swelling may be evident. CT shows paravertebral masses in more detail and provides accurate information on the bone architecture of collapsed vertebrae, and in particular the integrity or otherwise of posterior elements, as well as those of adjacent vertebrae, which may be infiltrated to a lesser degree. This information may be important if surgical decompression and stabilization is contemplated. However, CT without intrathecal contrast does not show the intraspinal extent of tumour or site and degree of cord compression, for which CT myelography or MRI is required.

MRI is the optimal investigation in suspected metastatic cord compression. It is more sensitive than scintigraphy in detection of vertebral metastases. It is much easier to perform than CT myelography in patients who are often immobile and in severe pain, and will demonstrate intramedullary as well as extramedullary pathology. Most metastases yield low signal on T1W images, and high, normal or low signal on T2W images, depending partly on whether they are lytic or sclerotic.[43] Some fast T2W sequences are poor at differentiating metastases from marrow. Most metastases enhance following gadolinium, but this can mask the lesion as it may then return the same signal as surrounding marrow, therefore fat saturation techniques should be used for enhanced images. Gadolinium is also useful for characterizing the exact site of epidural tumour spread within the spinal canal, differentiating epidural tumour from other pathology such as prolapsed disc, and differentiating other causes of T1 low signal in vertebral bodies.

Spinal lymphoma is usually extradural, characteristically with vertebral body involvement, a paraspinal mass and diffuse infiltration of the extradural space via neural foramina.

Vertebral haemangiomas are common incidental findings on spinal MR and usually return high signal on both T1W and T2W images. They rarely affect the spinal cord, but if so surgery, radiotherapy or embolization may be necessary.

Other primary bone tumours very rarely cause cord compression. Most occur more frequently in the posterior elements than in vertebral bodies, including osteoid osteoma, osteochondroma, osteoblastoma, aneurysmal bone cyst and giant cell tumour. Malignant tumours such as chondrosarcoma, osteosarcoma and Ewing's tumour may be seen, but the latter two are usually metastatic in the spine. In children, paravertebral tumours of neural origin such as neuroblastoma, ganglioneuroblastoma and ganglioneuroma, may extend through neural foramina into the epidural space and cause cord compression. Vertebral body chordoma is usually more malignant than clival or sacral chordoma, but shows similar radiological characteristics.

# Postoperative imaging and radiation effects

Expected postoperative changes following resection or biopsy of intracranial tumours include haemorrhage at the tumour bed and oedema and swelling around it. Signal change on MRI and enhancement in the line of resection may persist for several weeks. Thus early postoperative imaging for assessment of residual tumour can be misleading, although it has been suggested that imaging earlier than 48 hours postoperatively may avoid this.

Radiotherapy to the central nervous system can cause transient white matter oedema or permanent diffuse leucomalacia, as well as focal brain necrosis; the latter can be particularly difficult to distinguish from residual or recurrent tumour. Calcifying microangiopathy and eventually focal or diffuse brain atrophy may occur. Necrosis is usually apparent at the tumour bed on imaging between 6 months and 2 years after radiation treatment, depending on the dosage and rate of delivery. It is

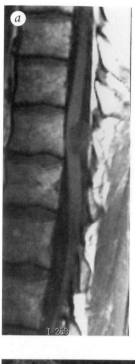
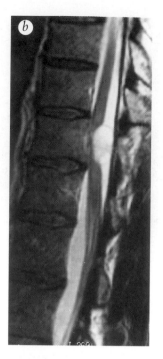
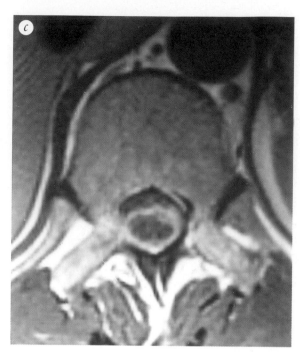
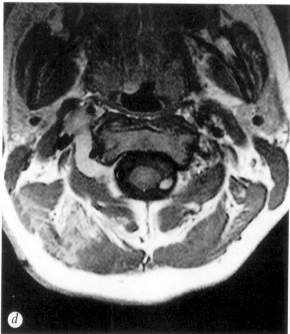

**Figure 2.11** — A 50-year-old man previously treated for Hodgkin's lymphoma presented with a 6-week history of progressive leg weakness and back pain. MR showed a very well-defined extramedullary, intradural mass causing severe cord displacement and compression. The tumour returns low/intermediate signal on T1W (a) and high signal on T2W (b) images. Axial post-gadolinium T1W image (c) shows rim enhancement of the mass. The intradural location and shape are untypical of lymphoma, but characteristic of neurofibroma; this was confirmed histologically following surgery. (d) A different patient with neurofibromatosis II. Axial post-gadolinium T1W image shows a small extramedullary Schwannoma to the left of the cord. A larger tumour is seen passing through the right neural foramen and into the carotid sheath and a further small tumour is present in the oropharynx.

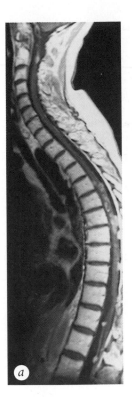
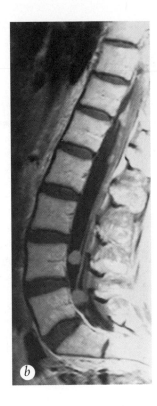
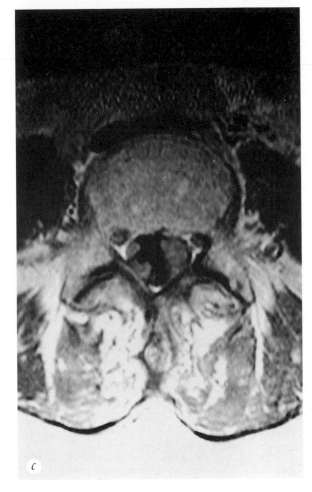

*Figure 2.12* — Intradural, extramedullary spinal metastases from pineal germinoma. a,b) Sagittal and c) axial T1W post-gadolinium images. Numerous enhancing nodules are seen on the surface of the cord, and involving the cauda equina.

common after radiation seed placement. It may coexist with recurrent tumour and both may cause mass effect and ring enhancement on CT and MR. More specific signs to signify recurrent tumour are progressive enlargement of a focal mass lesion on serial scans, an anatomic pattern such as a butterfly distribution, and new enhancement at the tumour site. In general MRI is poor at differentiating tumour from radiation effects, but techniques such as MR spectroscopy, positron emission tomography (PET), single photon emission computed tomography (SPECT)[44] and functional MRI all offer the potential to discriminate between them in some cases. Newer techniques which measure local cerebral blood volume may be useful, such as echoplanar MRI with bolus gadolinium injection,[45] and these seem to correlate with indices of local cerebral metabolism provided by fluorodeoxyglucose-PET. However, these functional methods may still be confounded by coexistent radiation necrosis and recurrent tumour.

Abnormal meningeal enhancement may be non-neoplastic, as a result of either surgery, shunt insertion or a previous extracerebral collection. This is usually linear and diffuse and tends to persist unchanged, often for many years, whereas nodular or increasing meningeal enhancement is more suggestive of residual or recurrent meningeal tumour.

Radiation to the brain can also induce neoplasia and it is important to be aware of the potential development of both meningiomas and gliomas many years after intracranial radiotherapy for other tumours.

# New imaging techniques

MR angiography (MRA) can contribute to the preoperative assessment of intracranial tumours by demonstrating displacement, compression, encasement or occlusion of major arteries, veins and dural sinuses, especially if used in conjunction with MRI. Specific examples of its use are in the parasellar region, to show the relationship of the internal carotid arteries to pituitary tumours; in the posterior fossa, the relation between a large 8th nerve Schwannoma and surrounding veins and sinuses; and in the superior sagittal sinus, to show whether adjacent tumours such as meningioma partially or completely occlude the sinus. MRA has largely replaced conventional cerebral angiography in these instances.

Stereotactic CT is used to guide biopsy of brain tumours by calculating the precise three-dimensional position of an intracranial probe tip using a frame fixed to the skull vault. Frameless MR stereotaxy utilizes skin markers on the scalp and face to calculate the position of the probe tip during surgery. This allows real-time multiplanar display of the extent of tumour resection to be depicted on preoperative gadolinium-enhanced scans.

Much research is being performed into the imaging and analysis of biochemical and physiological characteristics of brain tumours, with the goal of tissue characterization to detect and grade malignant neoplasms, differentiate recurrence from iatrogenic change, and differentiate neoplasm from other pathology, such as lymphoma and inflammatory disease in AIDS.[46] Fluorodeoxyglucose-PET is sensitive but relatively non-specific in the diagnosis of high grade neoplasms, as the radiopharmaceutical is also taken up by inflammatory processes and areas of cellular necrosis. Thallium is concentrated in tumour but not in necrosis, and thallium-SPECT has been shown to be more accurate than CT but less accurate than gadolinium-enhanced MR in detection and follow-up of gliomas.[47]

MR spectroscopy measures metabolite levels within a unit volume of brain tissue and can be targetted at specific areas of abnormality on MRI. Gliomas are characterized by a reduction in N-acetyl aspartate, which is a neuronal marker, and by raised choline levels, due to increased membrane turnover. However, these and other single metabolite resonances do not classify tumours in terms of grade, whereas multiparametric statistical analysis may do so in future.[48,49]

Functional MRI (fMRI) has potential clinical application in several aspects of the management of brain neoplasms. Maps of regional cerebral blood flow are provided by functional MR perfusion studies, and tumour grade seems to correlate with blood flow;[45] this technique can therefore signify a higher tumour grade than suggested by MRI and prompt biopsy or surgery. It can also direct biopsy to the more malignant part of a neoplasm and avoid the common problem of undergrading. Another fMRI technique is diffusion imaging, which can help to distinguish the cystic and solid components of a tumour. Surgical debulking of gliomas may be aided by task activation studies, which can demonstrate the precise location of eloquent areas of motor or sensory cortex. These may be displaced or may have relocated secondary to tumour.[50] Functional MRI can be performed at the same time as conventional MRI and may thus become a cost-effective alternative to PET and SPECT.

# Acknowledgement

The authors gratefully acknowledge the assistance of radiographers at the Queens Square Imaging Centre and the Addenbrooke's Hospital MRI Unit, Cambridge.

# References

1. Lee BCP, Kneeland JB, Cahill PT, Deck MDF. MRI recognition of supratentorial tumors. *AJNR* 1985; **6**: 871–878.

2. World Health Organization. *Classification of Brain Tumours*. Zurich: WHO, 1990.

3. Kjos BO, Brant-Zawadzki M, Kucharczyk W, Kelly WM, Norman D, Newton TH. Cystic intracranial lesions: magnetic resonance imaging. *Radiology* 1985; **155**: 363–369.

4. Earnest FIV, Kelly PJ, Scheithauer BW et al. Cerebral astrocytomas: histopathological correlation of MRI and CT contrast enhancement with stereotactic biopsy. *Radiology* 1988; **166**: 823–827.

5. Kieffer SA, Salibi NA, Kim RC et al. Multifocal glioblastoma: diagnostic implications. *Radiology* 1982; **143**: 709–710.

6. Spagnoli MV, Grossman RI, Packer RJ et al. Magnetic resonance imaging determination of gliomatosis cerebri. *Neuroradiology* 1987: **29**: 15–18.

7. Forsyth P, Shaw E, Scheithauer B, O'Fallon J, Layton D, Katzmann J. 51 cases of supratentorial pilocytic astrocytoma: a clinicopathologic, prognostic and flow cytometric study. *Cancer* 1993; **72**: 1335–1342.

8. Lee Y, Tassel PV. Intracranial oligodendrogliomas: imaging findings in 35 untreated cases. *AJNR* 1989; **10**: 119–127.

9. Castillo M, Davis PC, Takei Y, Hoffman JC Jr. Intracranial gan-glioglioma: MRI, CT and clinical findings in 18 patients. *AJNR* 1990; **11**: 109–114.

10. Goergen SK, Gonzales MF, McLean CA. Intraventricular neuro-cytoma: radiologic features and review of the literature. *Radiology* 1992; **182**: 787–792.

11. Wichmann W, Schubiger O, von Demling A *et al*. Neuroradiology of central neurocytoma. *Neuroradiology* 1991; **33**: 143–148.

12. Koeller KK, Dillon WP. Dysembryoplastic neuroepithelial tumors: MR appearance. *AJNR* 1992; **13**: 1319–1325.

13. Ostertun B, Wolf HK, Campos MG *et al*. Dysembryoplastic neu-roepithelial tumors: MR and CT evaluation. *AJNR* 1996; **17**: 419–430.

14. Spoto GP, Press GA, Hesselink JR, Solomon M. Intracranial ependymoma and subependymoma: MR manifestations. *AJNR* 1990; **11**: 83–91.

15. Neumann HPH, Eggert HR, Schumacker M *et al*. Central nervous system lesions in von Hippel Lindau syndrome. *J Neurol Neurosurg Psychiatry* 1992; **55**: 898–901.

16. Jack CR Jr, O'Neill BP, Banks PM, Reese DF. Central nervous system lymphoma: histologic types and CT appearance. *Radiology* 1988; **167**: 211–215.

17. Johnson BA, Fram EK, Johnson PC, Jacobowitz R. The variable MR appearance of primary lymphoma of the central nervous sys-tem: comparison with histopathologic features. *AJNR* 1997; **18**: 563–572.

18. Dina T. Primary central nervous system lymphoma versus toxo-plasmosis in AIDS. *Radiology* 1991; **179**: 823–828.

19. Healy ME, Hesselink JR, Press GA, Middleton MS. Increased detection of intracranial metastases with intravenous Gd-DTPA. *Radiology* 1987; **165**: 619–624.

20. Russel DS, Rubinstein LJ. *Pathology of Tumors of the Nervous System*, 5th edn. Baltimore: Williams and Wilkins; 1989.

21. Lee BCP, Kneeland JB, Deck MDF, Cahill PT. Posterior fossa lesions: magnetic resonance imaging. *Radiology* 1984; **153**: 137–143.

22. Tien RD, Yang PJ, Chu PK. 'Dural tail sign': a specific MR sign for meningioma? *J Comput Assist Tomogr* 1991; **15**: 64–66.

23. Elster AD, Challa VR, Gilbert TH, Richardson DN, Contento JC. Meningiomas: MR and histopathological features. *Radiology* 1989; **170**: 857–862.

24. Burger PC, Scheithauer BW. Tumours of meningothelial cells. In: *Tumors of the Central Nervous System*. Washington DC: Armed Forces Institute of Pathology; 1994, pp.259–286.

25. Chiechi MV, Smirniotopoulos JG, Mena H. Intracranial haeman-giopericytomas: MR and CT features. *AJNR* 1996; **17**: 1365–1371.

26. Press GA, Hesselink JR. MR imaging of cerebellopontine angle and internal auditory canal lesions at 1.5T. *AJNR* 1988; **9**: 241–251.

27. Tampieri D, Melanson D, Ethier R. MR imaging of epidermoid cysts. *AJNR* 1989; **10**: 351–356.

28. Jelenik J, Smirniotopoulos JG, Parisi JE, Kanzer M. Lateral ven-tricular neoplasms of the brain: differential diagnosis based on clinical, CT and MR findings. *AJNR* 1990; **11**: 567–574.

29. Sze G, Soletsky S, Bronen R, Krol G. MR imaging of the cranial meninges with emphasis on contrast enhancement and meningeal carcinomatosis. *AJNR* 1989; **10**: 965–975.

30. Cone L, Srinivasan M, Romanul FCA. Granular cell tumor (cho-ristoma) of the neurohypophysis: two cases and a review of the lit-erature. *AJNR* 1990; **11**: 403–406.

31. Yuh WTC, Tali ET, Nguyen H *et al*. Sequential MR enhancement pattern in normal pituitary gland and pituitary adenoma. SMRM Annual Meeting 1993, New York.

32. Pusey E, Kortman KE, Flannigan BD *et al*. MR of craniopharyn-giomas: tumor delineation and characterisation. *AJNR* 1987; **8**: 439–444.

33. Eldevik OP, Blaivas M, Gabrielsen TO, Hald JK, Chandler WF. Craniopharyngioma: radiologic and histologic findings and recur-rence. *AJNR* 1996; **17**: 1427–1439.

34. Chang T, Teng MMH, Guo W-Y, Sheng W-C. CT of pineal tumors and intracranial germ-cell tumors. *AJNR* 1989; **10**: 1039–1044.

35. Tien RD, Barkovich AJ, Edwards MSB. MR imaging of pineal tumous. *AJNR* 1990; **11**: 557–565.

36. Latack JT, Hutchinson RJ, Heyn RM. Imaging of rhabdomyosar-comas of the head and neck. *AJNR* 1987; **8**: 353–359.

37. Regenbogen VS, Zinreich J, Kim KS *et al*. Hyperostotic esthe-sioneuroblastoma: CT and MR findings. *J Comput Assist Tomogr* 1988; **12**: 52–56.

38. Meyers SP, Hirsch WL Jr, Curtin HD *et al*. Chordomas of the skull base: MR features. *AJNR* 1992; **13**: 1627–1636.

39. Avrahami E, Tadmor R, Dally O *et al*. Early MR demonstration of spinal metastases in patients with normal radiographs and CT and radionuclide bone scans. *J Comput Assist Tomogr* 1989; **13**: 598–602.

40. Sze G, Stimac GK, Bartlett C *et al*. Multicenter study of gadopen-tetate dimeglumine as an MR contrast agent: evaluation in patients with spinal cord tumors. *AJNR* 1990; **11**: 967–974.

41. Kaffenberger DA, Sah CP, Mortagh FR, Wilson C, Silbiger ML. MR imaging of spinal cord haemangioblastoma associated with syringomyelia. *J Comput Assist Tomogr* 1988; **12**: 495–498.

42. Matsumoto S, Hasu K, Uchino A *et al*. MRI of intradural extramedullary spinal neurinomas and meningiomas. *Clin Imag* 1993; **17**: 46–52.

43. Kamholtz R, Sze G. Current imaging in spinal metastatic disease. *Sem Oncol* 1991; **18**: 158–169.

44. Carvalho P, Schwartz R, Alexander E *et al*. Detection of recurrent gliomas with quantitative thalium-201/technetiom 99m HMPAO single photon emission computerized tomography. *J Neurosurg* 1992; **77**: 565–570.

45. Aronen H, Gazit IE, Louis DN *et al*. Cerebral blood volume maps of gliomas: comparison with tumour grade and histologic findings. *Radiology* 1994; **191**: 41–51.

46. Slosman DO, Lazeyras F. Metabolic imaging in the diagnosis of brain tumors. *Curr Opin Neurol* 1996; **9**: 429–435.

47. Rollins NK, Lowry PA, Shapiro KN. Comparison of gadolinium-enhanced MR and thallium-201 single photon emission comput-ed tomography in pediatric brain tumors. *Pediatr Neurosurg* 1995; **22**: 8–14.

48. Preul MC, Caramanos Z, Collins DL *et al*. Accurate non-invasive diagnosis of human brain tumors by using proton magnetic resonance spectroscopy. *Nature Med* 1996; **2**: 323–325.

49. Shimizu H, Kumabe T, Tominaga T *et al*. Noninvasive evaluation of malignancy of brain tumors with proton MR spectroscopy. *AJNR* 1996; **17**: 737–747.

50. Atlas SW, Howard RS, Maldjian J *et al*. Functional MRI of regional brain activity in patients with intracerebral gliomas: findings and implications for clinical management. *Neurosurgery* 1996; **38**: 329–338.

# 3

# THE HEAD AND NECK

Antonio Chiesa, Roberto Maroldi, Giuseppe Battaglia,
Patrizia Maculotti and Davide Farina

**Neoplasms arising from the upper aerodigestive mucosa**
**Neoplasms arising from nasosinusal mucosa**
**Non-mucosal and salivary gland lesions**

Some common features allow most head and neck neoplasms to be grouped into one of three homogeneous classes: lesions arising from upper airway mucosa; lesions arising from the mucosa of paranasal sinuses; and extra-mucosal and salivary gland lesions.

A number of significant clinical advantages have resulted from the application of CT, MR and ultrasound in the management of these neoplasms. As most head and neck malignancies arise from the mucosal epithelium, mainly the upper aerodigestive tract, diagnosis can usually be made from direct or endoscopically-guided biopsy. Clinical examination is essential for evaluating either superficial spread of neoplasms or functional data, e.g. impaired motility of vocal cords. The goals of imaging are the precise assessment of deep tissues invasion and the detection of nodal metastases.

In addition, it should be noted that the prognosis of head and neck malignancies depends on several factors. None of the biological properties of the neoplasm (grading, mitotic index) can be studied with imaging techniques, although positron emission tomography (PET) and MR spectroscopy are promising modalities. The other significant prognostic factors are related to the local extent of the neoplasm (T), and to nodal (N) or distant (M) metastases[1] and the assessment of TNM staging represents the central goal of imaging in most head and neck malignancies.

# Neoplasms arising from the upper aerodigestive mucosa

Neoplasms arising from the upper aerodigestive mucosa share four common features:

- squamous cell carcinoma is the most common histotype;

- the superficial spread of a neoplasm can be adequately assessed by direct examination or endoscopy;

- a typical pattern of deep, extramucosal extent of neoplasms can be observed;

- nodal metastases are frequent.

As a general rule, the deep spread of squamous cell carcinoma follows two different patterns:

- progressive invasion through the submucosa, the muscular layer (e.g. the constrictor muscle at the

level of the pharynx) and, further, into fat tissue, vessels, nerves and bones of adjacent structures;

- spread along pre-existing pathways, such as nerves and vessels.

As a consequence, an imaging technique is very dependent on the contrast it can achieve between tumour and fat tissue layers, muscles, bones, vessels and nerves.

## Detection of the degree of wall invasion in upper aerodigestive tract neoplasms

This problem applies to malignant neoplasms arising from the nasopharynx, orohypopharynx, larynx and oesophagus. Its solution requires discrimination between the abnormal signal of neoplasm and the normal wall. The thickness of the wall (which determines its main signal) depends on its muscular content, e.g. the complex of constrictor muscles in the pharynx.

Generally, the contrast resolution of CT is inadequate for distinguishing the muscle from the abnormal density of the adjacent tumour.[1] MR can, however, demonstrate the different signal intensities between the muscular layer (hypointense) and the neoplasm (moderately hyperintense) (Fig. 3.1), particularly when spin echo (SE) turbo T2-weighted sequences are used[2] and MRI should be chosen for the precise evaluation of muscular wall invasion.[3]

## Detection of neoplastic spread beyond the walls (equivalent to class T4 of TNM staging)

Demonstration of the replacement of fat tissue surrounding the wall by the tumour is the key indicator of neoplastic spread beyond the upper aerodigestive tract walls. Usually, this information is adequately provided either by CT or MR.

## Detection of neoplastic invasion of muscles and other 'key areas'

This problem applies, for example, to the floor of the mouth muscles in cases of tongue neoplasms and to the vocal cords and paraglottic spaces in cases of laryngeal neoplasms. Again, the replacement of muscle or fat tissue signal by the tumour indicates neoplastic invasion. It should be noted that fat tissue actually behaves as a natural contrast agent both for CT and MR.

This finding is critical if intrinsic muscles invasion by *tongue neoplasms* is to be accurately quantified. Since the fat content of these muscles is noticeable, solid neo-

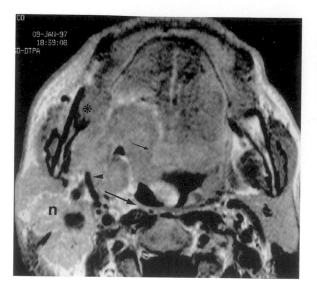

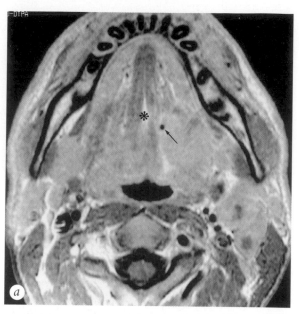

***Figure 3.1*** — Glosso-tonsillar squamous cell carcinoma. On MR the tumour spreads circumferentially along the walls of the glosso-tonsillar sulcus extending deep into the adjacent structures. After Gd-DTPA injection the tumour enhances. Base of the tongue has been invaded (short arrow). The neoplasm spreads into the parapharyngeal space and invades the medial pterygoid muscle. The external carotid artery appears to be surrounded by neoplastic tissue (arrowhead). The abnormal signal intensity of the posterior oropharyngeal wall on the right side indicates inflammation and oedema (long arrow). Level II partly necrotic lymphatic metastasis (n). Abnormal hypointensity of the medullary space of right mandibular ramus was associated with neoplastic invasion (✳).

plastic tissue replacing fat can be detected. Spin echo T1-weighted sequences show the hypointense neoplasms obliterating the regular texture of the muscular fibres, normally separated by thin fat layers.[2,4]

In addition, an accurate assessment of tumour margins can be achieved by enhancement of neoplastic tissue with intravenous administration of contrast agents (iodine for CT studies and gadolinium (Gd)-based for MR).[1] Both CT and MR clearly show the precise relationship between the tumour and lingual septum, because of the latter's fat content. Finally, MR is definitely superior to CT in defining the degree of neoplastic invasion of the muscles of the floor of the mouth muscles (Fig. 3.2).[5]

The vocal cord should be considered a crucial structure in the management of *laryngeal neoplasms*, since its extensive invasion often requires aggressive surgical management (vertical hemilaryngectomies, supracricoid laryngectomies, total laryngectomy) (Fig. 3.3).[6] Furthermore,

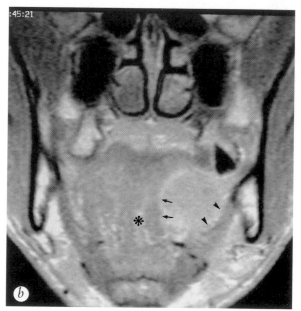

***Figure 3.2*** — Base-of-tongue squamous cell carcinoma. a) On enhanced axial T1 MR sequence, the neoplasm extends from the left tongue base into the floor of the mouth muscles. The tumour surrounds the left lingual artery (arrow) and invades the styloglossus muscle (a boundary between base of the tongue and floor of the mouth) and a landmark for the XII nerve. Two non-homogeneous adenopathies are at level II. b) Displacement of both the genioglossus muscle (arrows) and mylohyoid muscle (arrowheads) by the neoplasm is better demonstrated on the coronal plane. On both axial and coronal images the lingual septum (✳) appears not to have been invaded by the tumour.

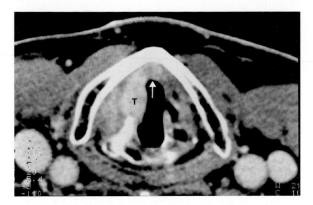

*Figure 3.3* — Right glottic squamous cell carcinoma. On enhanced CT the hyperdense neoplasm (T) extends along the entire surface of the right vocal cord. The vocal muscle is partly invaded. The enhancing neoplastic tissue spreads into the anterior commissur, which is abnormally thickened (arrow). The asymmetrical thinning of the right paralaryngeal space results from oedema of the thyroarytenoid muscle. The tumour approaches the vocal process of the right arytenoid cartilage (sclerotic). No abnormality of the thyroid cartilage is detectable.

surgical treatment is influenced by the demonstration of neoplastic spread into submucosal fat spaces of the larynx deep to the lateral walls (paralaryngeal spaces). Conversely, deep invasion through the epiglottis into the pre-epiglottic space does not change the surgical management, since the entire space is usually removed by conservative surgical techniques. In contrast, this information is useful for planning radiation therapy. CT is reliable in calculating the volume of a tumour invading the pre-epiglottic space, which is a valuable predictor of successful control of the disease (Fig. 3.4).

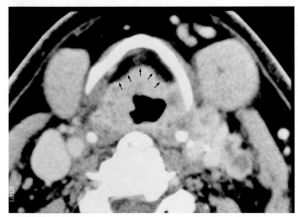

*Figure 3.4* — Supraglottic squamous cell carcinoma. The neoplasm arises from the infrahyoid epiglottis and spreads circumferentially into both aryepiglottic folds. Partial invasion of the pre-epiglottic space is shown (arrows).

## Detection of perineural or perivascular spread

This information is crucial in the management of *nasopharyngeal neoplasms* (because of the possible invasion of trigeminal nerve, internal carotid artery and cavernous sinus), *oral cavity* and *base-of-tongue neoplasms* (hypoglossus and laryngeal nerves, carotid artery). Direct signs of spread include changes in diameter or density/signal of nerves and vessel walls.[7] Indirect signs are changes in bone structures (diameter or shape of skull base foramina and fissures), obliteration of fat tissue within foramina or fissures and muscular atrophy indicating denervation.

CT usually only shows indirect signs, such as remodelling/erosion of skull base foramina or pterygo-palatine fissure walls. MRI can demonstrate some cranial nerves (particularly the trigeminal nerve and its branches), both within or outside the cranial cavity, and abnormalities of the walls of the internal carotid artery and jugular vein or cavernous sinus.[8] These advantages of MR allow earlier detection of perineural and perivascular spread (Fig. 3.5). Intravenous contrast injection highlights the abnormal signal/density of the nerves or vessel walls involved. However, both CT and MR are sometimes unable to distinguish neuritis from perineural neoplastic spread.

## Detection of bone or cartilage invasion

This information is critical for the management of neoplasms arising from the *nasopharynx* (because of the possible involvement of the skull base and Eustachian tube), *oral cavity* (mandible, infrastructure, pterygoid plates) and *larynx* (cartilage and hyoid bone). Detection requires the demonstration of the destruction of bones, ossified (provided by cortical rims lining a medullary space) and non-ossified cartilage.

It should be noted that neoplastic invasion by squamous cell carcinoma seldom results in sclerosis of bone or cartilage. Sclerosis usually indicates inflammatory changes caused by tumour, rather than invasion. This finding can be observed either in the skull base and facial bones or in the ossified laryngeal cartilages.

CT is particularly useful in assessing bone destruction. Neoplasms seldom spread into the medullary space of bone and cartilage (especially thyroid cartilage) without extensive destruction of the cortical rim. In these cases CT shows a thinning of the cortical bone/ossified cartilage and an abnormal tissue density replacing the fat with-

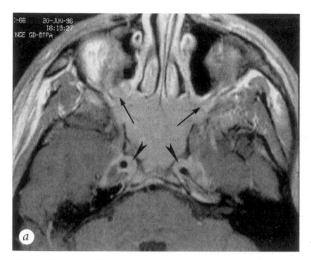

**Figure 3.5** — Undifferentiated carcinoma of the nasopharynx. a) On axial T1-weighted MRI sequence, the homogeneous tumour fills the sphenoid sinus and extends into the fat tissue of both inferior orbital fissures (arrows). Bilateral intracranial spread through the foramen lacerum and perivascular invasion of the carotid arteries are demonstrated on axial (arrowheads) and b) coronal MR views (arrowheads). Level V adenopathy on the left side (n) and bilateral retropharyngeal metastatic lymph nodes (n) are shown.

in the medullary space (Fig. 3.6). The reliability of MR in detecting intramedullary (and intracartilaginous) tumour spread is definitely superior to CT (Fig. 3.7).[9–12]

MRI is more sensitive but less specific than CT in detecting neoplastic cartilage invasion in laryngeal neoplasms. MR tends to overestimate neoplastic cartilage invasion and may result in overtreatment, whereas CT tends to underestimate invasion and may lead to inadequate therapy. Proton density SE MR sequences are particularly useful in the evaluation of the more resistant non-ossified cartilage of the larynx.[9,6,13]

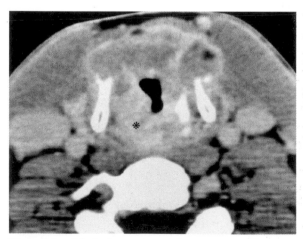

**Figure 3.6** — T4 glottic squamous cell carcinoma. Diffuse invasion of thyroid cartilage by tumour is shown by the destruction of the ossified rims and replacement of the medullary space by soft tissue. The barrier provided by the outer perichondrium has prevented neoplastic spread into the soft tissues of the neck (pathologic observation). Destruction of the right side of cricoid cartilage is demonstrated (✱).

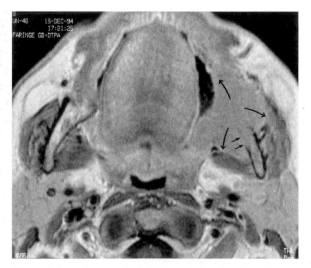

**Figure 3.7** — Retromolar trigon squamous cell carcinoma. Tumour erases the 'black' signal of the cortical rim of the mandible (short arrows) and extends into the medullary space, replacing its fat content. Infiltration of the medial pterygoid, the masseter and the buccinator (curved arrows) muscle is also present.

## Detection of occult adenopathies in clinically negative (N0) necks

Patients treated for cancer arising from the upper aerodigestive tract often die of a disease related to the presence of cervical nodal metastases, despite successful control of the primary tumour. The overall prognosis for these patients is directly related to the presence or absence of metastatic adenopathies.[14,15] Moreover, the most relevant prognostic factor for predicting recurrent cervical lymph node metastases is the presence of nodal disease at the initial diagnosis.

In about 20% of clinically negative necks, histological examination reported positive lymph nodes, multiple metastatic nodes were detected in 13% and a single positive node in 16%. These data are in keeping with the clinical observation that about 15% of N0 necks will eventually develop nodal recurrence (all primary sites of the neck considered).[16] Different strategies have been developed by clinicians to manage N0 neck patients who have this 15% risk of occult metastases. Surgery or radiotherapy would constitute unnecessary therapy for 85% of these patients but delaying treatment until nodal disease is detected would entail a slightly worse prognosis for 15% of them. However, regardless of the particular treatment strategy adopted for clinical N0 necks, the accurate detection and staging of cervical metastases is crucial to patient survival.

Diagnosis relies on the detection of even microscopic neoplastic deposits within normal sized lymph nodes. However, as approximately 25% of electively operated on sides of the neck contain exclusively metastases smaller than 3 mm, the sensitivity of all imaging modalities in these necks is limited to 75%. Currently, the reliable imaging criteria used in assessing abnormal lymph nodes are a minimal axial diameter of the node not exceeding 11 mm in the jugulo-digastric group and 10 mm elsewhere (Table 3.1). It has been proposed that retropharyngeal nodes should not exceed 8 mm in diameter. However, MRI can easily detect nodes of 4–5 mm and if they show the same signal intensity as the primary nasopharyngeal tumour on T1- and T2-weighted images they are probably invaded.[17] It has also been suggested that the ratio of the maximal longitudinal length to nodal width should be >2 for normal hyperplastic nodes and <2 for metastases (which are more often spherical in shape). Moreover, groups of three or more lymph nodes with maximal diameters of 8–15 mm or minimal axial diameter of 9–10 mm in the jugulo-digastric area and of 8–9 mm elsewhere are suggestive of lymph node metastases. Regardless of the lymph node size, the most reliable imaging feature of metastatic disease is 'nodal necrosis', detected on both enhanced CT and T1-weighted MR images as a low density (CT) or low intensity (MR) area > 3 mm (Fig. 3.8).[18] The overall error rate of these size criteria for both false-positive and false-negative CT and MR diagnoses is in the range is 10–20%.

Ultrasound has an accuracy of no more than 80%; however, when used to guide cytological sampling, its diagnostic accuracy rises to 95%. In the follow-up of treated patients, ultrasound is useful in the assessment of those patients in whom post-treatment fibrotic changes do not allow correct clinical assessment. Retropharyngeal nodes cannot be evaluated by ultrasound.

New imaging modalities, such as immunoimaging with SPECT, thallium SPECT, PET and fused images, are developing rapidly. Although these techniques are likely to become very accurate for the staging of the neck, it is doubtful whether they will be used routinely because

**Table 3.1** Modified American Joint Committee on Cancer radiological nodal staging guidelines.

| Stage | Definition |
| --- | --- |
| N0 | All nodes <15 mm in diameter with no central low density (on CT) or central low intensity (on MR) |
| N1 | Single ipsilateral node 15–29 mm in diameter; or single ipsilateral node <15 mm with central low density (on CT) or central inhomogeneous intensity (on MR) |
| N2 | Single ipsilateral node 3–6 cm in diameter or multiple ipsilateral nodes all <6 cm; |
| N2a | Single ipsilateral node 3–6 cm in diameter |
| N2b | Multiple ipsilateral nodes all <6 cm |
| N2c | Bilateral or contralateral nodes, none of which is >6 cm in diameter |
| N3 | Node or nodes >6 cm in diameter |

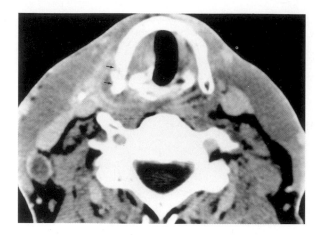

*Figure 3.8* — Right piriform sinus squamous cell carcinoma. On enhanced CT the neoplasm extends into the apex of the piriform sinus and spreads along the inferior constrictor muscle, which inserts on the outer surface of the thyroid cartilage ala. Therefore the neoplasm destroys the cartilage from the outside (arrows). An abnormal node presenting a central hypodense area with rim enhancement is detectable on the ipsilateral side at level III. The adenopathy has a normal diameter.

of cost and availability. Their role will probably be more important in the detection of unknown primaries, distant metastases and follow-up after radiotherapy in case where there is clinical doubt. (Table 3.1).

Extranodal spread is present in more than 50% of nodes that are 20–30 mm in their greatest dimension and in more than 70% of lymph nodes that are >30 mm. Extranodal spread is more reliably detected on contrast-enhanced CT than on MR: they consist of irregular nodal rim-enhancement with infiltration of adjacent fat planes. Once the neoplasm has spread beyond the lymph node capsule, the most reliable criterion of vascular invasion is the degree of arterial/vein circumferential involvement by neoplastic tissue: if the vessel is completely surrounded by tumour it is probably invaded. When the fat planes are also totally effaced by the signal intensity of neoplastic tissue, the vessel is almost certainly invaded.

## Neoplasms arising from nasosinusal mucosa

Nasosinusal neoplasms account for only 3% of all cancers of the head and neck area. They arise from the mucosal surface of the nasal cavity and paranasal sinuses. The tumour may extend beyond the bony 'boxes' of the facial framework, either by destroying the walls or spreading along nerves and vessels that run through fissures and foramina within the craniofacial bones.

Key to treatment planning is the determination of the following features:

- nature (benign vs. malignant);

- histotype: squamous cell carcinoma is the most fre-

quent malignant lesion and it usually arises from the maxillary sinus, whereas adenocarcinoma arises from the ethmoid sinus;

- superficial and deep (extramucosal) extent of the lesion.

In most cases, endoscopy allows tissue diagnosis through percutaneous biopsy and accurate staging of the superficial spread. Therefore, differentiation between different neoplasms is not a main goal of CT or MR. Both techniques are useful in the investigation of anatomical structures that cannot be reached by endoscopy, either because they are submucosal (bones, vessels, orbital and intracranial contents) or because they are located deep in the paranasal sinuses.

The *en bloc* removal of neoplasm within normal adjacent tissues successfully controls the lesion. The development of combined surgical approaches through the nasal cavity and the anterior cranial fossa was made possible by the precise radiological mapping of submucosal spread towards the anterior cranial fossa, the orbit, the pterygo-palatine and the superior orbital fissures. The degree of spatial/anatomical detail required in treatment planning, however, differs significantly between surgery and radiotherapy.[19] A number of elementary questions can be used as a guide.

### How important is the determination of the most probable site of origin of a nasosinusal neoplasm?

Patterns of spread of nasosinusal neoplasms depend on their site of origin. For this reason, it is useful to discriminate between low (maxillonasal) and high (nasoethmoidal) lesions. A key point is to assess the most probable centre of growth of lesions. While this is easy for small neoplasms, it can be very difficult in advanced neoplasms.

Critical sites in 'low' lesions include the posterior wall of the maxillary sinus, a pathway to the infratemporal fossa and pterygo-palatine fissure and the orbital floor. In 'high' neoplasms, these include the posterior aspect of the lamina papyracea, the orbital roof, the anterior skull base floor and the sphenoid sinus, particularly its roof.

Generally, the probable site of origin of the lesion can be inferred from CT and MR findings, combined with history and clinical data. MR is better than CT at discriminating between the tumour and intrasinusal retained secretions or mucoperiosteal inflammatory changes.

## Is it crucial to differentiate lesions limited to the sinusal walls from those extending beyond these boundaries?

It should be noted that the periosteum is the most effective barrier to the spread of aggressive lesions, neoplastic or inflammatory, beyond sinusal walls. It is particularly resistant in two of the most critical sinonasal areas: the skull base (where it links to the dura) and the orbit (where the periosteum of seven bones becomes a continuous layer, the periorbita). Therefore, an assessment of neoplastic spread beyond the periosteum of sinusal walls is critical for therapeutic planning because it is related to dural or orbital infiltration.

Although MR cannot directly show the mineral content of bones, in some areas it can detect the connectival/periosteal layer which limits the sinusal walls.[20] The sinusal walls in contact with the neoplasm may present various signal changes. On MR, a thick hypointense sinusal wall (on T1 and T2 SE sequences), with focal areas of erosion, usually indicates chronic inflammation. Again, periosteal thickening appears as an hypointense line parallel to the outer surface of the sinusal wall. Inflammatory changes of the sinusal mucosa are always associated: they usually appear as a diffuse mucoperiosteal thickening which is homogeneously hyperintense on T2-weighted sequences, and as a double layer of signal intensities, enhanced mucosa, non-enhancing submucosa on CT or SE T1-weighted sequences after Gd-DTPA.

Bowing and displacement of a normal and continuous hypointense sinusal wall by the tumour excludes neoplastic spread beyond the bony periosteal barrier. When

the displacement is not caused by the tumour, a mucocele represents the most likely explanation. Mucoceles generally arise from neoplastic obstruction of the sinusal ostium. Signal intensity of mucoceles may vary widely vary on T2- and T1-weighted images, depending on the protein content of the fluid, which is usually higher in older lesions.

Replacement of the hypointense signal of the sinusal walls by neoplastic tissue is a reliable sign of invasion.

## Can imaging reliably predict orbital exenteration?

A key point is that the orbit is usually preserved at surgery, provided the periorbita is not (or only minimally) invaded, even though the bone has been completely eroded. In fact, a more aggressive approach does not improve survival. The assessment of the thin bony lamina papyracea should not be underestimated; however, it is not crucial, since the lamina itself is in most cases partly or completely resected at surgery for pathologic examination.

MR is of particular value in demonstrating the thin hypointensity of the non-invaded periorbita, which can still be detected after erosion of the mineral content of the orbital walls (Fig. 3.9). An accurate MRI evaluation of the orbit requires comparison between different sequences and planes since the walls have an oblique orientation.

Despite attempts to assess the integrity of orbital walls, the information provided by CT or MR has only limited

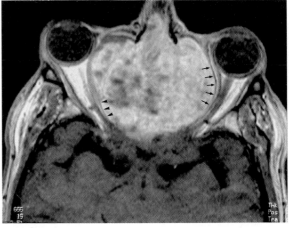

***Figure 3.9*** — Ethmoid sinus adenocarcinoma. The huge tumour displaces both medial orbital walls causing bilateral exophthalmos. On the left side, the hypointense line separating the tumour from the intraorbital fat is still detectable (arrows). On the right side, the same finding can be identified only at the posterior third of the lamina papyracea (arrowheads).

impact on the surgeon's decision to resect the orbit or to save it, as this decision depends not only on imaging data but also on other factors (e.g. intraoperative staging, vision of the contralateral eye, presence of metastases). Nevertheless, if imaging suggests orbital infiltration, the patient should be informed that an *exenteratio orbitae* may be required. Indeed, the final decision depends on the intraoperative staging. If the probability of exenteration were based only on ophthalmic symptoms, the lesion would be overestimated in over 50% of cases. Conversely, the negative predictive value of MRI — residual hypointense line between tumour and orbital fat — is effective. Focal areas of abnormal signal intensity of the hypointense periorbita can be overestimated.

## Are there any indications for anterior craniofacial resection?

This problem applies to neoplasms in contact with the structures that separate the paranasal sinuses from the anterior and middle cranial fossae. Generally, craniofacial resection (CFR) is recommended if the tumour extends to the mucosal surface of these sinusal walls. If intracranial spread occurs, the precise grading of the lesion — tumour confined to the dura mater or invading the brain tissue — affects not only surgical planning but also the patient's prognosis. In fact, while CFR is more likely to control neoplasms, it carries the substantial risks of an aggressive surgical procedure. Whether the precise extent of brain infiltration – amount of brain resection, contralateral spread to the olfactory/frontal lobes, middle cranial fossa invasion – should contraindicate surgery remains controversial.

CT and MRI findings are good indicators of the feasibility of CFR.[19] MR is of remarkable value in grading the neoplastic spread to the anterior cranial fossa, particularly when focal areas of skull base invasion are detected.[21] A key diagnostic observation concerns the signal intensity of the three tissue layers at the interface between the ethmoid roof and the brain at the anterior cranial fossa: cribriform plate and its periosteum, dura mater, and subarachnoid space. On enhanced sagittal and coronal spin echo T1-weighted MR sequences, the three layers give rise to a 'sandwich' of different signals (bone—periosteum complex, dura and cerebrospinal fluid), where dural hyperintensity is due to a hypervascular inflammatory reaction.[22]

Generally, three different patterns of neoplastic involvement of the skull base are observed: the neoplasm is in close contact with an uninterrupted, hypointense cribriform plate; the neoplasm erases the hypointensity of the cribriform plate, extending into the anterior cranial fossa (ACF) and displacing an uninterrupted, hyperintense and thickened dura; the neoplasm encroaches on the dural hyperintensity, the hypointense CSF invades brain tissue. The latter finding is easier to detect if the signal intensity of the neoplasm is lower than the enhanced dura surrounding the invaded segment.

Oedema surrounding the involved area and replacement of cerebral parenchyma by the signal intensity of neoplastic tissue indicate brain invasion on MRI and CT (Fig. 3.10).[22]

Finally, it is essential to assess perineural or perivascular spread toward the middle cranial fossa, usually through pterygo-palatine and orbital fissures (Fig. 3.11).

## Discrimination of an inflammatory reaction and retained secretions from neoplastic tissue

MR can discriminate a neoplastic mass from surrounding retained secretions better than CT. On SE T2-weighted sequences there is usually a significant difference in signal intensity between the neoplasm (exhibiting intermediate signal because it is highly cel-

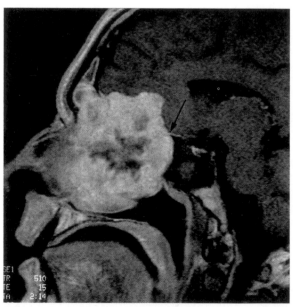

***Figure 3.10*** — Ethmoid sinus adenocarcinoma. On a sagittal enhanced T1 MR sequence the neoplasm destroys the floor of anterior skull base. A residual 'sandwich' of bone and hyperintense dura is still detectable at the planum sphenoidalis (arrow). The enhancing tumour extends into a blocked (hypointense fluid content with mucosal rim enhancement) frontal sinus. Retained secretions fill the blocked sphenoid sinus.

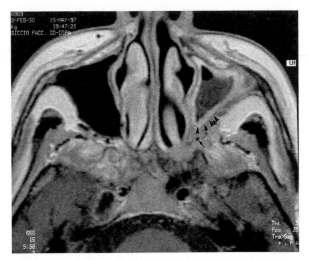

***Figure 3.11*** — Left maxillary sinus squamous cell carcinoma. Follow-up CT after chemotherapy. Patient complains of pain in the area of the second branch of the trigeminal nerve. Perineural spread into the inferior orbital and pterygopalatine fissures appears as soft tissue surrounding the signal void of the pterygopalatine artery (arrow). Retained secretions and inflammatory changes of the maxillary sinus mucosa are present. The hypointensity of the posterior maxillary wall is not detectable (arrowheads).

lular), adjacent structures (bone, muscles and fat tissue) and retained secretions (generally markedly hyperintense). However, retained secretions may vary widely in signal intensity depending on their protein content.[21] Moreover, variable enhancement of neoplastic tissue is obtained by Gd-DTPA infusion, usually resulting in a better discrimination of tumour from adjacent tissues on SE T1-weighted images (Fig. 3.10).

# Non-mucosal and salivary gland lesions

This heterogeneous group includes neoplasms that generally present as soft-tissue masses in the neck. They must be differentiated from a number of benign lesions that arise from the different anatomical structures of the neck.

Understanding the anatomical organization of the neck is helped by thinking of it first as an axle, along which vessels, nerves, airways and the upper digestive tract run from the cranium to the trunk, anchored to a robust musculoskeletal support. Secondly, focus on the deep cervical fascia, which splits into three different layers that define several spaces. These layers behave as barriers, preventing lesions from crossing their boundaries. Although the individual layers cannot be detected on normal CT or MR scans, they are of great importance, since knowledge of the precise boundaries and of the contents of the spaces allows a differential diagnosis unique to each particular space. Within these spaces there are two important groups of glands: the exocrine glands, distributed around the oral cavity (parotid, submandibular, sublingual) and the endocrine glands, located at the thoracic inlet (thyroid and parathyroids). Furthermore, it should be noted that the neck is the body region with the greatest number and complexity of lymph nodes: of the 800 in the entire body, 300 are located in this region.

A simple physical examination permits the diagnosis of several soft-tissue masses of the neck because of the superficial site of the lesion. Ultrasound is useful in assessing the content of lesion — solid vs. liquid — and it accurately evaluates lymph nodes and guides cytological sampling. CT and MR are usually indicated to stage nodal spread of squamous cell carcinoma of the upper aerodigestive tract. They are seldom required for the differential diagnosis of the soft-tissue masses of the neck.

## Neck masses in children

In most cases, the correct diagnosis can be obtained by simple clinical examination. Moreover, when clinical data suggest acute lymphadenitis, imaging is not usually indicated and the case generally resolves after antibiotic treatment. Non-mucosal and salivary gland neoplasms are rare among children, rhabdomyosarcoma and lymphoma being the two most frequent head and neck malignancies. The differential diagnosis includes not only inflammatory diseases but also congenital lesions (thyroglossal duct cysts, lymphangiomas, branchial cleft cysts).[23]

## Thyroid masses

Discovery of a single nodule or nodules in the thyroid on palpation in a non-hyperthyroid patient requires, as a first step, a simple needle aspiration which, besides distinguishing solid or liquid content, permits cytological sampling, essential for diagnosis. Ultrasound-guided sampling is indicated when fine needle aspiration cytology yields non-diagnostic material.[24]

Neither radioactive scanning nor ultrasound can distinguish a malignant neoplasm, even if a 'cold' lesion is suspected (in 16% of cases the nodule is malignant). Radionuclide scanning is the procedure of choice for the work-up of a diffusely enlarged thyroid and for hyperthyroid patients presenting single or multiple nodules.

Malignant thyroid neoplasms are rare: their prognosis mainly depends on the histotype, sex, age and local extent of disease. The assessment of local spread is usually accomplished by ultrasound (lesion limited to the capsule, detection of nodal metastases). Aggressive neoplasms extending beyond the capsule may require CT or MRI to assess invasion of the trachea, vessels and adjacent muscles, before surgical treatment (Fig. 3.12).[25]

## Extent of salivary gland masses

Again, clinical examination and fine needle aspiration cytology can achieve all the information required for this work-up. Ultrasound can accurately evaluate the gland parenchyma. If a deep lobe neoplasm is suspected or a large malignant lesion is detected, CT or MR are appropriate.[4] In fact, the tumour extent into the parapharyngeal space or the invasion of the adjacent skull base are not detectable by clinical examination or ultrasound: they require scanning techniques. Nevertheless, malignant salivary gland neoplasms are rare. Adenoidcystic carcinoma tends to spread slowly along neural pathways and an MRI survey is therefore indicated.

## Approach to rarer soft-tissue masses

Most are nerve sheath neoplasms: schwannomas or neurofibromas. Common sites include the vagus nerve, the cervical roots and the sympathetic chain. A schwannoma usually presents as a painless, slow-growing mass in the anterolateral neck. On MR, a schwannoma demonstrates a fusiform shape, absence of flow void within its tissue (differential diagnosis with paragangliomas), well-circumscribed margins, uniform enhancement on T1-weighted sequences and variable hyperintensity on T2 (Fig. 3.13). The features of neurofibroma are indistinguishable from those of schwannoma, except for the diffuse plexiform type that demonstrates an infiltrative pattern of growth.

Few lesions exhibit a specific density/signal. Among these, lipoma is the most frequent. Typical findings include a well-circumscribed lesion showing the same density/signal as adjacent fat. In most soft-tissue masses, however, biopsy confirmation is necessary to obtain a definitive diagnosis.

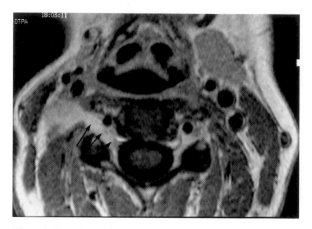

*Figure 3.13* — Cervical root neuroma. The lesion appears hyperintense after Gd-DTPA injection on a T1 MRI sequence. The typical fusiform shape of the lesion along the course of a cervical root is detectable (arrows). The vertebral artery is displaced anteriorly.

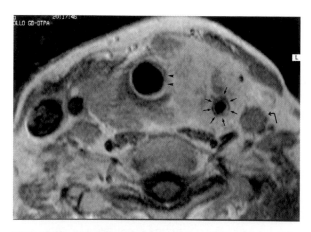

*Figure 3.12* — Undifferentiated carcinoma of the left lobe of the thyroid gland. On an axial T1 MR sequence the neoplasm enhances and extends beyond the capsule invading the common carotid artery (encased)(short arrows). The left tracheal wall is infiltrated (arrowheads). Thrombosis of the left internal jugular vein is detected (curved arrow).

# References

1. Aspestrand F, Boysen M, Engh V. Prognostic significance of contrast enhancement and tumor demarcation at CT of squamous cell carcinomas of the oral cavity and oropharynx. *Acta Radiol* 1994; **35**: 217–221.

2. Held P, Breit A. MRI and CT of tumors of the pharynx: comparison of the two imaging procedures including fast and ultrafast MR sequences. *Eur J Radiol* 1994; **18**: 81–91.

3. Madison MT, Remley KB, Latchaw RE, Mitchell SL. Radiologic diagnosis and staging of the head and neck squamous cell carcinoma. *Radiol Clin North Am* 1994; **32**: 163–181.

4. Campbell RS, Baker E, Chippindale AJ *et al*. MRI T staging of squamous cell carcinoma of the oral cavity: radiological-pathological correlation. *Clin Radiol* 1995; **50**: 533–540.

5. Bootz F. Lenz M, Skalej M, Bongers H. Computed tomography (CT) and magnetic resonance imaging (MRI) in T-stage evaluation of oral and oropharyngeal carcinomas. *Clin Otolaryngol* 1992; **17**: 421–429.

6. Castelijns JA, Becker M, Hermans R. Impact of cartilage invasion on treatment and prognosis of laryngeal cancer. *Eur Radiol* 1996; **6**: 156–169.

7. Mukherji SK, Weeks SM, Castillo M, Yankaskas BC, Krishnan LA, Schiro S. Squamous cell carcinomas that arise in the oral cavity and tongue base: can CT help predict perineural or vascular invasion? *Radiology* 1996; **198**: 157–162.

8. Laccourreye O, BÄly N, Halimi P, Guimaraes R, Brasnu D. Cavernous sinus involvement from recurrent adenoid cystic carcinoma. *Ann Otol Rhinol Laryngol* 1994; **103**: 822–825.

9. Becker M, Zbaren P, Laeng H, Stoupis C, Porcellini B, Vock P. Neoplastic invasion of the laryngeal cartilage: comparison of MR imaging and CT with histopathologic correlation. *Radiology* 1995; **194**: 661–669.

10. Castelijns JA, Brekel MW. Magnetic resonance imaging evaluation of extracranial head and neck tumors. *Magn Reson Q* 1993; **9**: 113–128.

11. Hermans R, Lenz M. Imaging of the oropharynx and oral cavity. Part I: Normal anatomy. *Eur Radiol* 1996; **6**: 362–368.

12. Lenz M, Hermans R. Imaging of the oropharynx and oral cavity. Part II: Pathology. *Eur Radiol* 1996; **6**: 536–549.

13. Zbaren P, Becker M, Laeng H. Pretherapeutic staging of laryngeal carcinoma. Clinical findings, computed tomography and magnetic resonance imaging compared with histopathology. *Cancer* 1996; **77**: 1263–1273.

14. Foote RL, Olsen KD, Davis DL *et al*. Base of tongue carcinoma: patterns of failure and predictors of recurrence after surgery alone. *Head Neck* 1993; **15**: 300–307.

15. McLaughlin MP, Mendenhall WM, Mancuso AA *et al*. Retropharyngeal adenopathy as a predictor of outcome in squamous cell carcinoma of the head and neck. *Head Neck* 1995; **17**: 190–198.

16. Jaulerry C, Rodriguez J, Brunin F *et al*. Results of radiation therapy in carcinoma of the base of the tongue. The Curie Institute experience with about 166 cases. *Cancer* 1991; **67**: 1532–1538.

17. Ross MR, Schomer DF, Chappell P, Enzmann DR. MR imaging of head and neck tumors: comparison of T1-weighted contrast-enhanced fat-suppressed images with conventional T2-weighted and fast spin-echo T2-weighted images. *AJR* 1994; **163**: 173–178.

18. Som PM. Detection of metastasis in cervical lymph nodes: CT and MR criteria and differential diagnosis. *AJR* 1992; **158**: 961–966.

19. Reisner K, Uhlig U. The influence of computer tomography on treatment strategies and follow-up in tumors of the nasopharynx and the paranasal sinuses. A retrospective study on 104 patients. *Strahlentherapie Onkologie* 1996; **172**: 1–8

20. Chong LY, Fan YF. Skull base erosion in nasopharyngeal carcinoma: Detection by CT and MRI. *Clin Radiol* 1996; **51**: 625–631.

21. Allbery SM, Chaljub G, Cho NL, Rassekh CH, John SD, Guinto FC. MR imaging of nasal masses. *Radiographics* 1995; **15**: 1311–1327.

22. Ahmadi J, Hinton DR, Segall HD, Couldwell WT. Surgical implications of magnetic resonance-enhanced dura. *Neurosurgery* 1994; **35**: 370–377.

23. Vazquez E, Enriquez G, Castellote A *et al*. US, CT, and MR imaging of neck lesions in children. *Radiographics* 1995; **15**: 105–122.

24. Vassilopoulou Sellin R. Management of papillary thyroid cancer. *Oncology Huntingt* 1995; **9**: 145–151.

25. Takashima S, Nomura N, Noguchi Y, Matsuzuka F, Inoue T. Primary thyroid lymphoma: evaluation with US, CT, and MRI. *J Comput Assist Tomogr* 1995; **19**: 282–288.

# 4

# THE LUNG AND MEDIASTINUM

Geraldine Walsh and Christopher Flower

**Bronchial carcinoma**
**The solitary pulmonary nodule**
**Superior sulcus tumour**
**Pulmonary metastases**
**Lymphoma and haematological malignancies**
**Mediastinal tumours**
**Pleural malignancy**

A wide range of neoplasms arise in or secondarily involve the thorax. These include primary lung cancer, mediastinal tumours, pleural malignancy and thoracic spread of extrathoracic malignancies. Frontal and lateral chest radiographs remain the initial imaging investigation in suspected intrathoracic neoplasia and are frequently supplemented with computed tomography (CT), which gives excellent anatomical definition and allows for accurate localization and staging of the tumour. Histological diagnosis is frequently possible from percutaneous CT-guided biopsy, particularly in cases of peripheral pulmonary and pleural neoplasia. Magnetic resonance imaging (MRI) has a complementary role to CT in selected instances such as in the assessment of superior sulcus tumours and occasionally in the evaluation of the mediastinum.

## Bronchial carcinoma

Bronchial carcinoma is one of the commonest primary cancers with an overall 5-year survival rate of just 10%.[1] It is classified on the basis of histology into small cell carcinoma (approximately 20% of cases) and non-small cell carcinoma (80%). Non-small cell carcinoma may be further divided according to cell type into squamous cell, large cell, adeno- and bronchiolo-alveolar carcinoma. The relative incidence of squamous cell carcinoma appears to be decreasing while that of adenocarcinoma, which is more common in females, is on the increase. Bronchioloalveolar carcinoma is usually considered separately from adenocarcinoma and may account for up to 15% of primary lung cancer.[2,3]

The poor prognosis for most patients with lung cancer compared with the greatly improved survival for those with isolated small peripheral cancers has led to the use of screening programmes using chest radiography for high risk populations. Despite the relative insensitivity of this technique, it detects a significant number of early stage cancers. However, in none of the screening programmes to date has there been any significant reduction in mortality in the screened population as compared to controls.[4,5]

The diagnosis of primary lung cancer is usually suspected from a combination of specific signs and symptoms. These include cough, particularly in association with haemoptysis, dyspnoea, chest pain and persistent pneumonia. The chest radiograph may show direct or indirect signs of carcinoma; the primary tumour may be visible as a pulmonary mass or features such as volume loss and hilar displacement may indicate the presence of an underlying bronchial occlusion.

Appropriate staging of the patient with bronchial carcinoma is important as stage of disease determines the surgical resectability and ultimately the prognosis. Some information can be obtained from the chest radiograph such as tumour size, the presence of gross hilar and mediastinal lymphadenopathy, evidence of pleural effusion and features of haematogenous spread such as rib metastases, but in most cases CT is essential. Staging is based on the TNM classification (Table 4.1) and includes:

1. *Assessment of the primary tumour*: CT is used to assess size and local spread of tumour. The presence of mediastinal and chest wall invasion is important as it determines if the tumour constitutes a T2 (resectable) or T3 (unresectable) lesion. Both CT and MRI detect gross invasion accurately (Fig. 4.1), but are relatively insensitive for lesions which abut but have not obviously extended into the mediastinum or chest wall.

2. *Assessment of nodal spread*: There is some variation in the size of normal nodes depending on their location within the mediastinum; however, they measure less than 1 cm in short axis diameter on CT. Whilst CT depicts nodes accurately it is relatively insensitive for N staging as normal sized nodes may be involved by tumour and a significant proportion of enlarged nodes represent an inflammatory reaction and are not involved by tumour. In this regard, CT and MR have similar sensitivities of 60–70%. Despite these difficulties, CT is invaluable in providing a 'roadmap' for nodal sampling at mediastinoscopy and thereby preventing unnecessary thoracotomies (Fig. 4.2).[6,7]

3. *Assessment of extranodal spread*: A significant proportion of patients will have extrathoracic metastases at initial presentation, the prevalence being greater for adenocarcinoma, and in many cases these metastases are occult.[8] Systemic features such as weight loss are ominous and suggest a poor prognosis.[9] In these cases, evaluation for extrathoracic spread to liver, brain and bone is warranted. Patients with organ-specific clinical findings should also undergo appropriate evaluation for metastatic spread. A high incidence of CNS metastases has been noted in patients with adenocarcinoma and mediastinal node involvement and preoperative evaluation of this group should probably include MRI of the brain.[10]

At our institution, all patients with suspected lung cancer proceed to CT evaluation of the thorax and upper abdomen. This establishes the presence of tumour and evaluates the best approach to biopsy (whether by fibre-

**Table 4.1**  TNM definitions for the International Staging System for Lung Cancer

*Primary tumour (T)*

TX: Tumour proved by the presence of malignant cells in bronchopulmonary secretions but not visualized roentgenographically or bronchoscopically, or any tumour that cannot be assessed as in a retreatment staging.
T0: No evidence of primary tumour.
T1S: Carcinoma *in situ*.
T1*: A tumour that is 3 cm or less in greatest dimension, surrounded by lung or visceral pleura, and without evidence of invasion proximal to a lobar bronchus at bronchoscopy.
T2: A tumour more than 3 cm in greatest dimension, or a tumour of any size that either invades the visceral pleura or has associated atelectasis or obstructive pneumonitis extending to the hilar region. At bronchoscopy the proximal extent of demonstrable tumour must be within a lobar bronchus or at least 2 cm distal to the carina. Any associated atelectasis or obstructive pneumonitis must involve less than an entire lung.
T3: A tumour of any size with direct extension into the chest wall (including superior sulcus tumors), diaphragm, or the mediastinal pleura or pericardium without involving the heart, great vessels, trachea, oesophagus, or vertebral body; or a tumour in the main bronchus within 2 cm of the carina without involving the carina.
T4: A tumour of any size with invasion of the mediastinum or involving the heart, great vessels, trachea, oesophagus, vertebral body, or carina, or presence of malignant pleural effusion.

*Nodal involvement (N)*

N0: No demonstrable metastasis to regional lymph nodes.
N1: Metastasis to lymph nodes in the peribronchial or ipsilateral hilar region, or both, including direct extension.
N2: Metastasis to ipsilateral mediastinal lymph nodes and subcarinal lymph nodes.
N3: Metastasis to contralateral mediastinal lymph nodes, contralateral hilar lymph nodes, ipsilateral or contralateral scalene, or supraclavicular lymph nodes.

*Distant metastasis (M)*

M0: No (known) distant metastasis.
M1: Distant metastasis present – specify sites.

optic bronchoscopy or fine needle biopsy) and assesses both intra- and extra-thoracic spread. (Fig 4.3) Depending on the CT findings, further preoperative evaluation may include biopsy of nodes at mediastinoscopy or mediastinotomy and CT-guided biopsy of likely abdominal metastases.

The following standard CT imaging protocol can be used. Initial 10 mm collimation sections at 10 mm intervals through the thorax are followed by spiral volumetric image acquisition through the mediastinum and central airways (3 mm collimation, table feed of 4.5 mm/s) during intravenous injection of iodinated contrast medium (50 ml of low osmolar, non-ionic contrast medium at a rate of 3–4 ml/s with a delay of 10–12 s).

Further spiral image acquisition through the upper abdomen (8 mm collimation, table feed of 12 mm/s) immediately post contrast medium administration completes the study.

These images allow documentation of tumour size, the size and extent of hilar and mediastinal lymphadenopathy and likely mediastinal and pleural invasion by tumour. Metastases to the liver and adrenals are also visualized (Fig. 4.4). Occasionally, there is uncertainty whether a hepatic or adrenal lesion represents metastatic involvement or an incidental benign lesion; CT-guided percutaneous biopsy of these masses is then required to establish the diagnosis. MRI may also be used to distinguish between an adrenal metastasis and an adenoma. Korobkin *et al*[11] showed that adrenal masses can be characterized as adenomas using chemical shift with a high specificity and acceptable sensitivity by visually comparing the opposed-phase and in-phase gradient echo (GRE) images; only adenomas showed an increase in relative signal intensity ratio on opposed-phase chemical shift images. Krestin *et al*[12] reported that adenomas and non-adenomas have different patterns of gadolinium enhancement on fast GRE images.

## Haemoptysis

Haemoptysis is an important clinical symptom and a common mode of presentation of bronchial carcinoma. It merits full evaluation even though the aetiology is established in only about 50% of cases.[13] Patients with

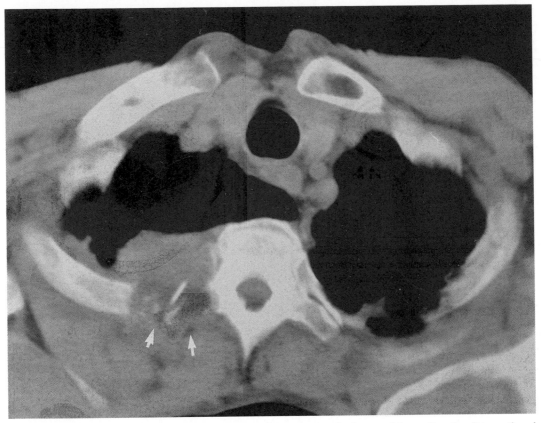

*Figure 4.1* — CT scan shows squamous cell carcinoma in apical segment of right upper lobe eroding the adjacent rib and vertebral body (arrows).

this symptom tend to fall into two categories: those with a normal chest radiogaph and those with radiographic findings suggestive of underlying disease.

Patients with clinical or radiographic findings suggestive of carcinoma require fibre-optic bronchoscopy. CT plays an important role in assessing these patients prior to bronchoscopy as it provides a 'roadmap' for biopsy and also stages the tumour. In patients with a normal chest radiograph, CT has a potentially valuable role in determining which patients should be bronchoscoped. Several studies have emphasized the value of high-resolution CT[14–16] which detects as many as or more tumours than bronchoscopy. In addition, it will demonstrate non-neoplastic processes which may be responsible for haemoptysis (e. g. bronchiectasis which accounts for approximately 15% of cases). A case can be made for using CT as the initial screen for patients with a normal chest radiograph and haemoptysis, reserving bronchoscopy for those with CT evidence of bronchial carcinoma or those with persisting haemoptysis in the face of a negative CT.

## Pleural effusion

Approximately 15% of patients with bronchial carcinoma will have an associated pleural effusion at initial presentation and over 50% of patients with disseminated disease will develop an effusion. The fluid may indicate malignant pleural involvement or be secondary to lymphatic obstruction. Effusions are also found in association with pulmonary atelectasis or pneumonia distal to endobronchial obstruction. The diagnosis of malignant pleural involvement may be established by ultrasound-guided pleural aspiration and biopsy.

## The solitary pulmonary nodule

Determination of the nature of a solitary pulmonary nodule (SPN) is an important and relatively common problem in radiological practice. A SPN is defined as a circumscribed spherical pulmonary opacity < 5 cm in

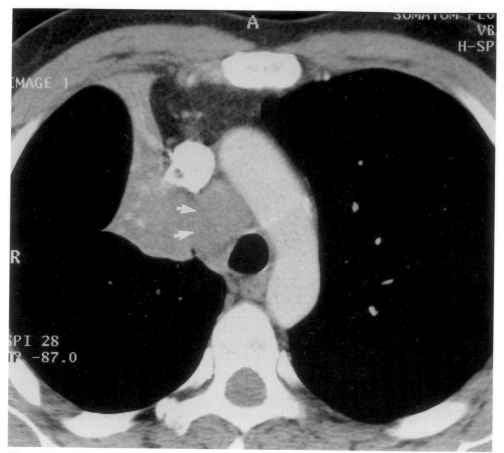

***Figure 4.2*** — CT scan shows collapse of the right upper lobe (due to a bronchoscopically proven carcinoma occluding the right upper lobe bronchus) and enlarged paratracheal nodes which were involved by tumour at mediastinoscopy (arrows).

diameter which is not associated with significant abnormality elsewhere in the thorax. Having established that the lesion is definitely intrapulmonary and not an artefact or innocent chest wall lesion, it is important to determine if it is benign or malignant and in particular whether it represents a primary bronchial carcinoma; 40–60% of bronchial carcinomas present as SPNs but only a number of SPNs are malignant. In the United States, where the prevalence of granulomatous disease is high, only 30% of SPNs are due to primary lung cancer whereas in Europe the likelihood of a SPN being malignant is significantly higher.

The following features are helpful in differentiating benign from malignant lesions:

1. *Past radiographs*: A lesion which has not changed in size over a period of 2 years is likely to be benign.

2. *Computed tomography*: CT is used to assess the size and shape of a nodule and to characterize its architecture.

- *Size*: Clearly visible lesions of less than 1 cm in diameter are more likely to be benign than malignant. Small bronchial carcinomas tend to have ill-defined borders and are difficult to detect on chest radiographs when less than 1 cm in diameter. Benign lesions such as hamartomas and granulomas are denser and more sharply defined and are therefore visible at smaller sizes.

- *Shape*: Malignant lesions tend to be ill-defined and irregular in shape with lobulated or spiculated margins. Benign lesions are more commonly well-defined and circular or oval in shape.

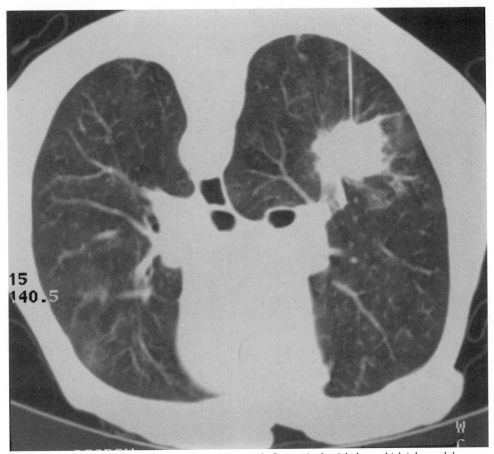

**Figure 4.3** — Percutaneous needle biopsy under CT control of a mass in the right lung which is beyond the range of bronchoscopic vision.

While these generalizations hold true for the majority of SPNs, there are sufficient exceptions to make these assessments of limited value in the individual case. More precise predictive features are:

- *Calcifications*: The determination of the presence or absence of calcification is of great importance. While 5–10% of malignant lesions exhibit evidence of calcification on CT, this is usually granular or sandlike in nature. Laminated calcification or a central nidus of calcification within a lesion is invariably evidence of a benign granulomatous process. 'Popcorn' calcification is a characteristic but uncommon manifestation of a hamartoma. Eccentric calcification may represent a benign granulomatous lesion which has been engulfed by tumour.

- *CT densitometry*: Since its advent, CT has been used to categorize the morphology of SPNs in an attempt bet- ter to distinguish between benign and malignant lesions. CT is clearly of value in defining the presence of calcification and fat; the latter being a good predic- tor of a hamartoma. Absolute assessment of CT atten- uation has also been used. Recently, Swensen *et al*[17] demonstrated the usefulness of CT densitometry fol- lowing intravenous injection of iodinated contrast medium. Enhancement of greater than 20 Hounsfield Units (HU) was found in all malignant lesions, although a proportion of benign lesions also showed significant enhancement. CT densitometry post con- trast medium administration therefore appears to be a sensitive but relatively non-specific test for the differ- entiation of benign from malignant lesions.

## Superior sulcus tumour

Superior sulcus or Pancoast's tumours are apical tumours of any cell type,[18] which invade the chest wall

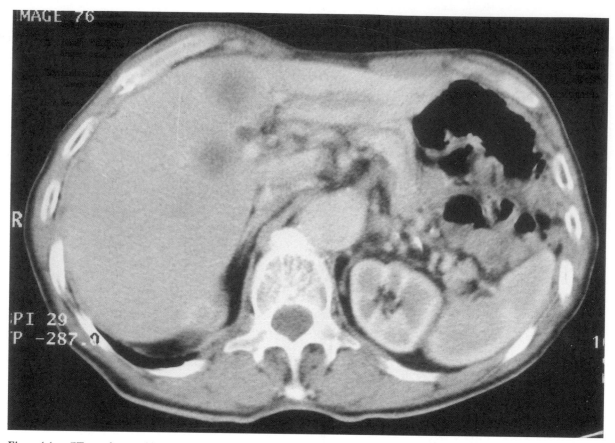

*Figure 4.4* — CT reveals several low attenuation lesions in the liver due to metastases from an adenocarcinoma.

and the lower cords of the brachial plexus and the sympathetic chain to produce the classic complex of pain in the upper limb and Horner's syndrome.

The chest radiograph shows an apical mass in 50–75% of cases and an apical cap resembling pleural thickening in the remainder.[2] The latter tumours may be particularly difficult to diagnose on standard radiographs and CT is valuable in these cases. Bone destruction, involving the adjacent ribs and the spine, is present in approximately one-third of cases.

MRI is currently the imaging modality of choice for further evaluation of superior sulcus tumours. Imaging in both the coronal and sagittal planes allows evaluation of the extrathoracic extent of the tumour and involvement of the brachial plexus and subclavian vessels is optimally visualized. T1-weighted and short T1 inversion recovery (STIR) images in sagittal and coronal planes with 5 mm collimation are recommended.[19–21]

# Pulmonary metastases

The primary tumours which most commonly metastasize to lung arise in the breast, colon, kidney, prostate and head and neck. Metastases may be visible on the chest radiograph as multiple pulmonary nodules which frequently, although not invariably, have well defined margins. CT allows detection of a significantly increased number of nodules partly because of its superior resolution and also because the cross-sectional images of CT are free from overlying structures (Fig. 4.5). Haematogenous metastases are characteristically found in the outer one-third of the lung and CT is superior to the chest radiograph for evaluation of this region. Spiral scanning is the optimal CT technique as continuous volume acquisition during a single breath-hold is advantageous in the detection of small lesions which may be missed or duplicated by incremental CT because of respiratory inconsistencies.[22]

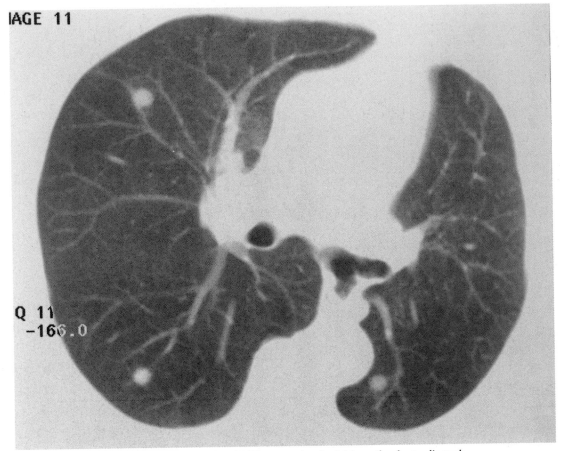

**Figure 4.5** — Lung metastases demonstrated by CT. These were barely visible on the chest radiograph.

## Lymphangitis carcinomatosa

This particular form of metastatic disease is particularly well demonstrated by high resolution CT, which is significantly more sensitive than the chest radiograph and is used when there is a clinical suspicion of lymphangitis in the presence of a normal or equivocal chest radiograph. The CT features of lymphangitis include interlobular septal thickening with bronchial wall thickening and centrilobular micronodules (Fig. 4.6).

## Lymphoma and haematological malignancies

Thoracic involvement is a well recognized feature of the lymphomas. Intrathoracic disease is found in 67–84% of patients with Hodgkin's disease (HD)[23,24] and in 40–50% of those with non-Hodgkin's lymphoma (NHL) at initial presentation and tends to worsen the

prognosis. In North *et al*'s series,[25,26] the 5-year survival for patients with stage I and II disease and mediastinal involvement was 88% versus 98% for those with similar stage disease without mediastinal adenopathy.

The mediastinum is the most frequently involved site. In HD, all nodal groups may be affected but the anterior mediastinal, tracheobronchial and paratracheal nodes are particularly favoured. NHL may have similar appearances but the contiguity of nodes characteristic of HD is frequently absent (Fig. 4.7). Pulmonary involvement by lymphomas is much less common. In HD, it is usually associated with hilar and/or mediastinal disease,[24,27] whereas in NHL, pleural or pulmonary involvement may be found in the absence of mediastinal or hilar adenopathy.

While the chest radiograph is the initial imaging investigation, CT is particularly well suited for displaying both mediastinal and pleuropulmonary involvement and is used routinely in the staging and follow-up of

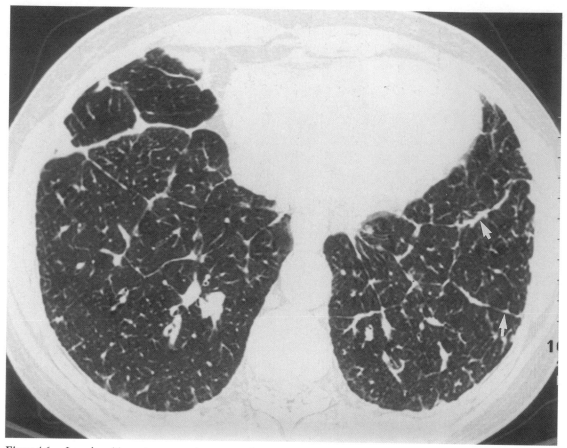

***Figure 4.6*** — Lymphangitis carcinomatosa demonstrated on high resolution CT. The patient complained of dyspnoea and had a normal chest radiograph. The thickening of the interlobular septa (arrows) is characteristic.

lymphoma. The nodal masses usually have a characteristic appearance but there may be difficulties in differentiating focal disease from primary mediastinal tumours such as thymomas and in differentiating multiple symmetrical nodes from sarcoidosis.

When the lungs are involved, CT shows soft tissue opacities surrounding patent bronchi, often mimicking the consolidation of pneumonia. Discrete pulmonary lesions are also seen; they usually take the form of nodules with poorly defined borders. The least common manifestation of pulmonary parenchymal involvement is an interstitial pattern representing disease spread along lymphatic routes.[26]

## AIDS-related lymphoma

Pulmonary lymphoma is the second most common intrathoracic malignancy linked to human immunodeficiency virus (HIV) positivity and while NHL constitutes an AIDS-defining illness, HD does not.[28,29] B cell NHL is the commonest AIDS-related lymphoma and tends to be an aggressive neoplasm with a predilection for extranodal sites including the pulmonary parenchyma.[30,31] Blunt & Padley[32] found the chest to be the major site of involvement in AIDS-related lymphoma in 15 of 116 patients (12%); the pattern of disease tends to be different from lymphoma in the immunocompetent patient with pleural and pulmonary masses, frequently peripheral and cavitating, being the commonest CT finding.

## Treated lymphoma

CT is used to monitor response to chemo- and radiotherapy, for regular follow-up of patients in remission and to detect evidence of relapse. Patients may develop direct complications of their therapy; these are assessed with chest radiography and CT when appropriate.

*Direct complications* include radiation-induced pneumonitis which may progress to pulmonary fibrosis. It classically develops 8–12 weeks after completion of

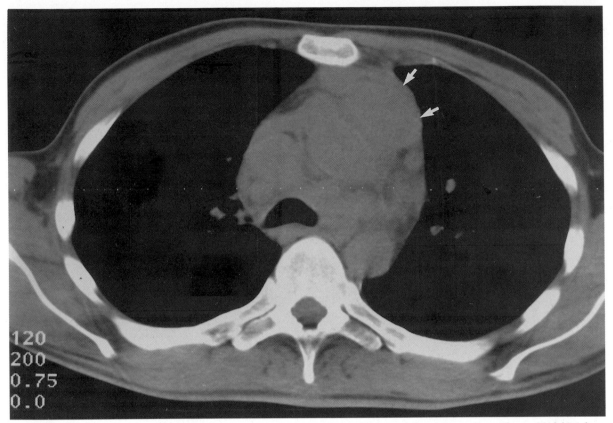

*Figure 4.7* — CT scan reveals multiple enlarged nodes mainly in the anterior mediastinum (arrows) in a patient with non-Hodgkin's lymphoma.

therapy and patients present with cough, dyspnoea and pleuritic chest pain. The chest radiograph may show pulmonary infiltrates which typically lie within the radiation portal. Occasionally, CT will demonstrate changes not visible on the chest radiograph.[33]

The chemotherapeutic agents most frequently associated with pulmonary toxicity in lymphoma patients are bleomycin, methotrexate, chlorambucil and procarbazine. Toxicity is related either to cumulative dosage or to a hypersensitivity reaction and in most cases results in diffuse alveolar damage with interstitial fibrosis. High resolution CT is a much more sensitive technique than the chest radiograph for detection of lung damage and whilst the appearances are seldom diagnostic, they are often characteristic of the disease (Fig. 4.8).

*Indirect complications* of therapy usually result from bone marrow suppression and steroid therapy. Thrombocytopenia may give rise to diffuse pulmonary haemorrhage and increased susceptibility to infection results from neutropenia, lymphopenia and steroid therapy.

Infections encountered in the normal immunocompetent host may occur but these immunocompromized individuals are also susceptible to opportunistic infections of which the most frequently encountered are cytomegalovirus (CMV), *Pneumocystis carinii* pneumonia (PCP), invasive pulmonary aspergillosis and *Candida albicans* pneumonia.

CT has an important role in imaging patients with suspected infection. The CT appearances may be sufficiently characteristic to enable treatment without a tissue diagnosis and this is particularly important in patients who are at risk from bronchoscopic biopsy such as those with a low platelet count. PCP produces patchy ground glass change,[34] whilst invasive aspergillosis typically causes ill-defined nodules with a surrounding halo of haemorrhage; these develop air crescents as the neutrophil count improves.[35] However, it may be difficult on the basis of the imaging findings alone to differentiate drug-induced change and pulmonary parenchymal involvement by lymphoma from infection

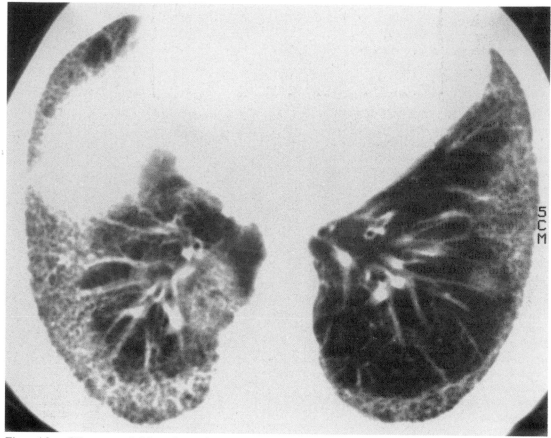

***Figure 4.8*** — CT scan reveals bilateral reticular shadowing at the periphery of both lower lobes which is characteristic of bleomycin toxicity.

and tissue acquired at transbronchial or open lung biopsy is often required for definitive diagnosis

## Mediastinal tumours

Many mediastinal tumors are asymptomatic and symptoms when present are relatively non-specific. Approximately one-third of tumours are malignant. Division of the mediastinum into anterior, middle and posterior compartments is helpful in the differential diagnosis of the lesion. Imaging of mediastinal tumours is with standard chest radiographs, CT and/or MRI.

The chest radiograph determines the position of the lesion within the mediastinum, thus limiting the differential diagnosis, and in a proportion of cases the appearances may suggest a specific diagnosis, as in cases of aortic aneurysm and neurogenic tumours.

Most patients are then evaluated further with CT. MRI may be performed either after or instead of CT. Advan-

tages of MRI include its multiplanar capabilities, its superiority to CT in tissue characterization and its ability to demonstrate spinal canal involvement in neurogenic tumours.

### Anterior mediastinum

*Thymoma* is one of the commonest primary mediastinal tumours and is found in approximately 10% of patients with myasthenia gravis (Fig. 4.9). More frequently, it occurs as an isolated finding in patients with non-specific symptoms. The CT appearances are usually characteristic and the size and extent of the tumour can be assessed as well as the likelihood of local invasion.

*Germ cell tumours* are most commonly found in young adults. There is a variety of histological types, including seminoma and the non-seminomatous germ cell tumours which include teratoma and embryonic cell carcinoma. Whilst the chest radiographic appearances are very similar to thymoma, CT may show diagnostic features such as fat or fat/fluid levels or suggestive fea-

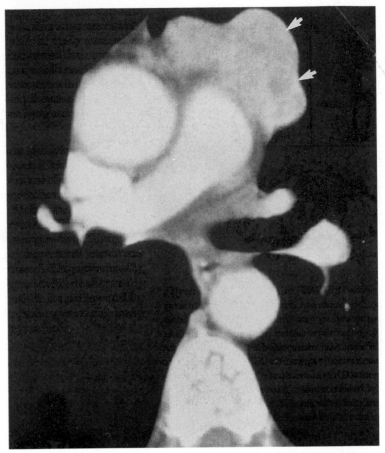

*Figure 4.9* — CT scan of a patient with myasthenia gravis reveals a lobulated thymoma lying anterior to the ascending aorta and main pulmonary artery (arrows).

tures such as cystic components in benign teratoma.

*Thyroid masses* are superior mediastinal lesions with characteristic features, including their paratracheal location, areas of high attenuation on CT representing normal thyroid tissue interspersed with rounded foci of low attenuation and calcification. CT is used to assess the size of the tumour and its secondary effects on the trachea. *Lymphoma* may arise in anterior mediastinal nodes or within the thymus. When this is an isolated finding, the lesion may mimic a thymoma or germ cell tumour.

## Posterior mediastinum

*Neurogenic tumours* account for the large majority of posterior mediastinal lesions and 30% are malignant. They arise from peripheral nerves, sympathetic and parasympathetic ganglia and are usually found in the paravertebral gutter. The chest radiograph may show rib erosion and an increase in the size of the intervertebral foramena but

either CT or MRI are required to define the extent of the tumour. MRI has the advantages of accurate definition of the intraspinal component and of differentiation between neurogenic tumours and lateral meningoceles.

## Pleural malignancy

Pleural malignancy may be due to primary pleural tumour (mesothelioma), metastases from extrapleural sites or direct spread within the thorax.

First described in the North Western Cape Province of South Africa, mesothelioma is the commonest primary pleural malignancy. There is a strong association with occupational asbestos exposure and it is estimated that approximately 6% of asbestos workers will die of diffuse malignant mesothelioma. The incidence of mesothelioma in the United Kingdom continues to increase, reflecting the lack of protection for asbestos workers until relatively recently coupled with the long latent period (usually 20–40 years].

Pleural metastases are the commonest cause of pleural malignancy accounting for 95% of cases and the majority relate to a primary tumour in the breast, bronchus or gastrointestinal tract. Bronchial carcinomas frequently involve the pleura and chest wall by direct extension. Uncommon pleural malignancies include thymoma (which may seed directly within the pleura) and lymphoma.

Pleural malignancy commonly results in a pleural effusion. In most instances, this is well demonstrated on the chest radiograph which may provide further clues to the diagnosis such as the underlying bronchial carcinoma. More frequently, the diagnosis is established by cytological analysis of the pleural aspirate and closed pleural biopsy. When the effusion is small or loculated, ultrasound is invaluable for localization of fluid prior to aspiration and biopsy. CT may also be helpful in patients presenting with effusions by demonstrating the underlying pulmonary disease (bronchial carcinoma, lymphangitis carcinomatosa or pulmonary metastases), pleural tumour masses or chest wall invasion. It is usually reserved for those patients in whom a diagnosis cannot be reached from the chest radiograph and pleural aspiration.

A significant number of patients with pleural malignancy do not develop an effusion. They usually present with chest pain and the chest radiograph may show lobulated pleural masses or diffuse pleural thickening. Rarely, there is evidence of associated rib destruction. CT plays an important role in the further investigation of these patients. Not only does cross-sectional imaging better delineate the disease, it also allows differentiation between benign and malignant pleural thickening with a high degree of sensitivity.[36] Nodular pleural thickening of greater than 1 cm, involving the mediastinal pleura and forming a circumferential sheath with lung encasement, is a feature of malignant pleural disease (Fig 4.10). Finally, CT-guided biopsy is an extremely useful technique in patients with either focal or diffuse pleural thickening when a tissue diagnosis is required.[37] It is carried out under local anaesthesia as an outpatient procedure.

More recently, MRI has been used to differentiate benign from malignant pleural disease. Falaschi et al[38] found malignant lesions to be hyperintense relative to muscle on proton-density and T2-weighted sequences with a sensitivity of 100%, a specificity of 87% and a negative predictive value of 100%. MRI may therefore have a complementary role to CT in the evaluation of pleural thickening.

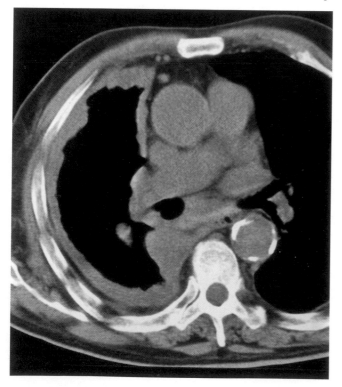

*Figure 4.10* — Mesothelioma encasing the right lung. The tumour has a lobulated outline which is a characteristic feature.

# References

1   Rosado de Christenson M. *Staging of Lung Cancer*. Proceedings of the Armed Forces Institute of Pathology. Washington, DC, Armed Forces Institute of Pathology, April 1994.

2.  Armstrong P. Neoplasms of the lungs, airways and pleura. In: Armstrong P, Wilson AG, Dee P, Hansell DM (eds) *Imaging of Diseases of the Chest*, 2nd edn. St. Louis: Mosby, 1995, pp. 272–368.

3.  Auerbach O, Garfinkel L. The changing pattern of lung carcinoma. *Cancer* 1991; **68**: 1973–1977.

4.  Heelan RT, Flehinger BJ, Melamed MR *et al*. Non-small cell lung cancer. Results of the New York Screening Program. *Radiology* 1984; **151**: 289–293.

5.  Melamed MR, Flehinger BJ, Zaman MB *et al*. Screening for early lung cancer. Results of the Memorial Sloan-Kettering study in New York. *Chest* 1984; **86**: 44–53.

6.  Grover FL. The role of CT and MR in the staging of the mediastinum. *Chest* 1994; **106** (Suppl): 3915–3965.

7.  Webb WR, Jenson BG, Gollitto R *et al*. Bronchogenic carcinoma: Staging with MR compared with CT and surgery. *Radiology* 1985; **156**: 117–124.

8.  Hillers TK, Sauve MD, Guyatt GH. Analysis of published studies on the detection of extrathoracic metastases in patients presumed to have operable non small cell lung cancer. *Thorax* 1994; **49**: 14–19.

9.  Bragg DG. The diagnosis and staging of primary lung cancer. *Radiol Clin North Am* 1994; **32**: 1–14.

10. Gamsu G. Extrathoracic evaluation of suspected pulmonary malignancy. *Proceedings of the Fleischner Society*. 26th Annual Conference on Chest Disease, Vancouver, 1996, pp. 187–191.

11. Korobkin M, Lombardi TJ, Aisen AM *et al*. Characterization of adrenal masses with chemical shift and gadolinium-enhanced MR imaging. *Radiology* 1995; **197**: 411–418.

12. Krestin GP, Steinbrich W, Friedmann G. Adrenal masses: evaluation with fast gradient-echo MR imaging and Gd-DPTA-enhanced dynamic studies. *Radiology* 1989; **171**: 675–680.

13. Müller NL. Hemoptysis: High-resolution CT vs bronchoscopy. *Chest* 1994; **105**: 982–983.

14. Set PAK, Flower CDR, Smith IE *et al*. Hemoptysis: Comparative study of the role of CT and fiberoptic bronchoscopy. *Radiology* 1993; **189**: 677–680.

15. McGuinness G, Beacher JR, Harkin TJ *et al*. Hemoptysis: Prospective high-resolution CT/bronchoscopic correlation. *Radiology* 1993; **189**: 677–680.

16. Naidich DP, Funt S, Ettenger NA *et al*. Haemoptysis: CT-bronchoscopic correlations in 58 cases. *Radiology* 1990; **177**: 357–362.

17. Swensen SJ, Brown LR, Colby TV *et al*. Pulmonary nodules: CT evaluation of enhancement with iodinated contrast material. *Radiology* 1995; **194**: 393–405.

18. Attar S, Miller SE, Sallerfield J *et al*. Pancoast's tumor: irradiation or surgery? *Ann Thorac Surg* 1979; **28**: 578–586.

19. Hamlin DJ, Burgener FA. CT including sagittal and coronal reconstruction in the evaluation of Pancoast tumors. *J Comput Assist Tomogr* 1982; **6**: 35–40.

20. Heelan RT, Demas BE, Caravelli JF *et al*. Superior sulcus tumors: CT and MR imaging. *Radiology* 1989; **170**: 637–641.

21. McLoud TC, Filion RB, Edelman RR *et al*. MR imaging of superior sulcus carcinoma. *J Comput Assist Tomogr* 1989; **13**: 233–239.

22. Touliopoulos P, Costello P. Helical (spiral]) CT of the thorax. *Radiol Clin North Am* 1995; **33**: 843–861.

23. Castellino RA, Blank N, Hoppe RT *et al*. Hodgkin disease: Contributions of chest CT in the initial staging evaluation. *Radiology* 1986; **160**: 603–605.

24. Filly R, Blank N, Castellino RA. Radiographic distribution of intrathoracic disease in previously untreated patients with Hodgkin's disease and non-Hodgkin's lymphoma. *Radiology* 1976; **120**: 277–281.

25. North LB, Fuller LM, Hagemeister FB *et al*. Importance of initial mediastinal adenopathy in Hodgkin disease. *AJR* 1982; **138**: 229–235.

26. North LB, Libshitz HI, Lorrigan JG. Thoracic lymphoma. *Radiol Clin North Am* 1990; **28**: 745–762.

27. Kaplan HS. Contiguity and progression in Hodgkin's disease. *Cancer* 1971; **31**: 1811–1813.

28. Dee P. AIDS and other forms of immunocompromise. In: Armstrong P, Wilson AG, Dee P, Hansell DM (eds). *Imaging of Diseases of the Chest*, 2nd edn. St Louis: Mosby, 1995, pp. 229–271.

29. Boring CC, Brynes RK, Chan WC *et al*. Increase in high grade lymphoma in young men. *Lancet* 1985; **1**: 857–859.

30. Kuhlman JE. Diseases of the Chest in AIDS. *Proceedings of the Fleischner Society – 26th Annual Conference on Chest Disease*, Vancouver, 1996, pp. 57- 71.

31. Sider L, Weiss AJ, Smith MD *et al*. Varied appearance of AIDS-related lymphoma in the chest. *Radiology* 1989; **171**: 629–632.

32. Blunt DM, Padley SPG. Radiographic manifestations of AIDS related lymphoma in the thorax. *Clin Radiol* 1995; **50**: 607–612.

33. Ikezoe J, Takashima S, Morimoto S *et al*. CT appearances of acute radiation-induced injury in the lung. *AJR* 1988; **150**: 765–770.

34. Bergin CJ, Wirth RL, Berry GJ *et al*. *Pneumocystis carinii* pneumonia: CT and HRCT observations. *J Comput Assist Tomogr* 1990; **14**: 756–759.

35. Kuhlman JE, Fishman EK, Burch PA. Invasive pulmonary aspergillosis in acute leukemia: the contribution of CT to early diagnosis and aggressive management *Chest* 1987; **92**: 95–99.

36. Leung AN, Müller NL, Miller RR. CT in differential diagnosis of diffuse pleural disease. *AJR* 1990; **154**: 487–492.

37. Scott EM, Marshall TJ. Flower CDR *et al*. Diffuse pleural thickening: Percutaneous CT-guided cutting needle biopsy. *Radiology* 1995; **194**: 867–870.

38. Falaschi F, Battolla L, Mascalchi M *et al*. Usefulness of MR signal intensity in distinguishing benign from malignant pleural disease. *AJR* 1996; **166**: 963–968.

# 5

# THE BREAST

William E Svensson

**Cancer diagnosis**
**Cancers**
**Imaging following breast cancer diagnosis**
**Imaging follow-up of the breast cancer patient**

Breast cancer is the commonest malignancy affecting women in North America and much of Europe. In the UK 1 in 10 women will develop breast cancer and it is the commonest cause of death in women in the 35–55 year age group. In the US just over half of women in whom breast cancer is detected will die of breast cancer and it is the second commonest cause of cancer mortality in women (17%).

Significant risk factors are age, previous breast cancer, a family history of breast cancer involving a first-degree relative (sisters, mother, aunts or grandmothers). High risk is associated with carriage of the BRCA1 and BRCA2 genes, previous biopsies demonstrating atypia or a typical ductal or lobular hyperplasia. Even higher risk is associated with lobular carcinoma *in situ* and well-differentiated ductal carcinoma *in situ*.

Other factors which are associated with increased risk of breast cancer include a history of fibroadenomas (though fibroadenomas themselves are not premalignant), early menarche, late menopause, no previous pregnancy or late first pregnancy, no breast feeding, post-menopausal obesity, a history of exposure to significant radiation and, possibly, cystic breast disease. The contraceptive pill and hormone replacement therapy have both been implicated in very slight increases of breast cancer but mainly in association with prolonged and/or early usage.

# Cancer diagnosis

## Breast screening

Many studies have shown the benefit of breast screening, particularly in those over 50 years. There is strong evidence for screening between the ages of 40 and 50 but the screening cost per life saved is very high compared with other medical interventions. The age of starting screening and screening interval depend on the relative risk factors of the population being screened and the relative benefits as well as costs. In the general population under the age of 35 the risks to the population as a whole of screening are greater than the risks of not screening (the number of cancers caused by screening is almost certainly greater than the number of lives that would be saved). Between 35 and 40 years the risks are about even. From 40 to 50 the risks of not screening begin to increase over the risks of screening and from 50 onwards the risks of not screening are significantly greater than the risks of screening.

The frequency of screening (screening interval) is determined by cost and the number of cancers which develop or are detected (interval cancers), between screening rounds. Another factor which needs to be considered is one or two views at initial screening and at subsequent screening rounds.

In the UK current practice is two-view screening (oblique lateral and cranial caudal views) mammography at initial screen followed by single views (oblique lateral views) (Fig. 5.1) at follow-up mammography. The female population between the ages of 50 and 65 years is invited for screening at 3-year intervals. Women over the age of 65 are screened at their request. Screening detects approximately one-third of all breast cancers in the breast screening population and the remaining two-thirds are interval cancers which present between screening rounds. (The woman notices a lump within the breast or a lump is detected during a routine examination for some other medical problem.) The arguments for and against more frequent screening are influenced not only by cost but also whether interval cancers are more aggressive cancers and therefore less likely to benefit from more frequent screening. In patients with symptomatic breast problems, recent screening should not be taken to indicate that breast cancer is not present and if a woman presents with a breast problem after recent screening she should still be evaluated in the normal way.

## The symptomatic breast

All breasts are lumpy and the degree of nodularity varies from 'millet seed' to 'dried apricots and figs'. The degree of nodularity for most women is in the 'dried fruit and nuts' range. Large nodules or masses need further evaluation at first presentation. Large nodules or masses which have been previously evaluated and have not changed at all since evaluation may not necessarily need further investigation provided no concerns have been raised previously.

Breast pain is a common presentation and in the under 35s with no risk factors does not require imaging investigation provided there is no asymmetry or variation of nodularity within the breast at the site of pain or elsewhere. If pain is associated with mass or significant thickening, imaging evaluation may well be necessary. As a general rule masses which have been present for less than 1 month should be observed for a complete menstrual cycle to determine whether they are transitory masses associated with the menstrual cycle.

Persisting palpable masses should always be evaluated to obtain a diagnosis which can definitively exclude cancer. Masses that are discovered at well women clin-

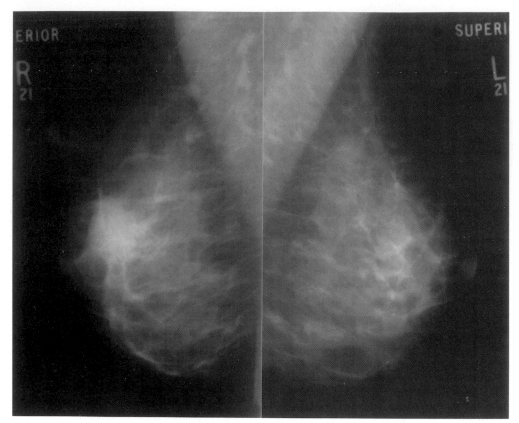

*Figure 5.1* — Oblique lateral views of right and left breasts. In the mid-part of the right breast there is an area of increased density which is somewhat ill defined and merges with the surrounding breast parenchyma. This appearance may be associated with a cyst or, as in this case, a carcinoma. This screening mammography appearance would result in the woman being recalled for further evaluation. Further investigation might include ultrasound and, if there was a palpable mass, also fine needle aspiration cytology (FNAC) or core biopsy if ultrasound showed the mass to be solid rather than a simple cyst.

ics or during a screening examination for another medical problem, are often of no significance if the patient is unable to demonstrate them herself on a subsequent occasion, though there are rare occasions when such lesions are significant. If the patient is aware of a lump or nodule and can regularly demonstrate it, however small and however benign the examining clinician may think it is, it should always be evaluated further as on occasions women detect small cancers before they are obvious to examining clinicians, even experienced breast surgeons. As well as examination by an experienced breast surgeon, evaluation should include imaging and fine needle aspiration cytology (FNAC) or needle for biopsy for histology (triple assessment).

Increasing the number of tests performed improves sensitivity at the cost of worsening specificity. Focused groups of tests can however reduce surgical biopsy rates. FNAC with ultrasonography and mammography is a particularly good combination and is very useful in 'one stop' breast clinics and often allows management decisions to be made the same day. This has a particular advantage for women who are shown to have a benign breast problem as they can be reassured the day of their investigation that they either do not have cancer or almost certainly have a benign problem.

## Breast imaging

### MAMMOGRAPHY

The main imaging modality for the breast is mammography using a dedicated mammography unit. Conventional radiographic equipment does not provide sufficient sensitivity to demonstrate soft tissue differences and does not have the resolution necessary to show the fine soft tissue connective strands and micro-calcifications within the breast. A dedicated mammography X-ray tube contains a molybdenum target which produces lower energy radiation suited to demonstrating the small differences in density of different soft tissues. It has a very fine focal spot to provide high definition. Mammographic films (high detail, single-sided emulsion) and cassettes (carbon fibre) are also designed to give high resolution, good contrast and the Buckey (film cassette holder on the mammography unit) has a high detail moving grid to improve contrast.

For each view the breast is compressed as much as possible to improve tissue differentiation and resolution whilst ensuring as much of the breast as possible is demonstrated on a single view. The compression also reduces the amount of superimposition of tissues making interpretation easier than when a greater thickness of breast is X-rayed.

Two views of each breast are conventionally taken to ensure that the whole of the breast is imaged. Though much of the breast is seen on both views, regions at the edge of the breast may only be seen on one. In particular, the axillary region is seen only on the oblique lateral view and the medial edge only on the craniocaudal view.

Modern equipment helps to reduce the radiation dose to the breast whilst maintaining image quality. The US Mammography Quality Standards Act 1992 requires all mammography facilities to be certified by the FDA. Radiation doses of >300 mrad per exposure require corrective action. The Breast Screening Service of the UK aims to maintain single image radiation doses to at or below 200 mrad.

Mammography should be performed in a specialist mammography unit by a radiographer who has had mammography training under the supervision of a recognized breast screening training centre. Interpretation should be performed by an experienced radiologist with suitable breast imaging training. Best results are obtained in units with a sufficiently high throughput to ensure that expertise is maintained. (The ACR recommends a minimum 40 examinations per month for any unit performing mammography; others suggest double that number. Ideally specialist units should be performing at least these numbers in a week).

Mammography is not recommended in the under 35 year old except in rare individual cases which have been discussed with the radiologist, such as when FNAC or core biopsy and ultrasound have been inconclusive in the evaluation of a suspicious area for which open biopsy is refused or has relative contraindications.

Over the age of 35 mammography is part of the work up in the symptomatic breast (Table 5.1). This may be the evaluation of unexplained recent pain, recently noticed asymmetry, or a mass causing clinical concern. Its main use in the evaluation of palpable lumps is the demonstration of microcalcifications and to evaluate margins and extent of lesions. Mammography is helpful in the staging and evaluation of a known carcinoma at any age and for screening the contralateral breast for an occult second primary. Impalpable mammographic abnormalities can be localized mammographically using stereotaxic mammographic attachments which can be used for FNAC), biopsy or wire localization for surgical excision biopsy. Most current equipment requires the patient to be wedged, sitting erect with the breast compressed in the mammography machine for upwards of 10 min whilst the procedure is performed. Quite frequently the procedure has to be abandoned if the patient experiences a vasovagal attack.

In the absence of a palpable mass, mammography is a screening procedure and the same indications apply as for breast screening. The risks of mammography causing breast cancer are greater in young or large breasts than old or small breasts. Law[1] has estimated, for the UK, that beginning screening at 30–34 years would cause 1 cancer for every 3 detected if two views are

**Table 5.1** Indications for mammography

**Breast screening**

*Over 50* – Indicated: national screening programmes, e.g. U.K.

*Over 40* – Debatable, but there is increasing evidence to suggest that it is indicated.

*Under 40* – Not indicated, but if a first-degree relative developed breast cancer before the menopause, screening may be indicated from the same age at which the relative's cancer was diagnosed.

**The symptomatic breast**

*Over 35*    No recent previous mammogram
and
Palpable mass
or
Evaluation of breast pain, deformity or asymmetry
and/or
Clinical suspicion of carcinoma.

Under 35 ONLY if there is a strong clinical suspicion of malignancy in the presence of *a normal breast ultrasound AND negative needle core biopsy.*

taken for each breast. At age 40–44 it is 1 for every 30 detected while at 50–54 it decreases to 1 for every 90 detected. Mammographic screening, because of the cumulative effect of radiation, is currently not indicated below the age of 40 and between the ages of 40 and 50 the benefits are hotly debated. Over the age of 50 there is a clear benefit from breast screening.

Digital mammographic imaging systems are becoming more accurate with improved image quality and have the additional advantage of quantitative analysis. In due course they will improve on conventional mammography, particularly with the development of more effective computer-aided diagnosis and image interpretation. The major problem is related to image display and resolution. A single 18 cm × 24 cm mammogram with a resolution of 10 line pairs/mm (the minimum required for acceptable detection of microcalcifications and parechymal strands) requires a monitor of 3600 × 4800 pixels for display. The technical problems of image production and display are being overcome but currently remain prohibitively expensive.

### ULTRASOUND

Breast ultrasound has a significant role in the diagnosis of benign and malignant breast masses. Used in conjunction with FNAC it provides high diagnostic accuracy for cancers and reduces the need for diagnostic excision biopsies of benign lesions. It is the examination of choice in patients under the age of 35 and during pregnancy (Table 5.2). Over the age of 35 there is debate as to whether ultrasound or mammography is the first imaging method of choice in aiding the diagnosis of a clinically suspicious mass. In expert hands ultrasound is probably the most suitable. Mammography is still necessary if it has not been performed recently to exclude impalpable abnormality in the remainder of both breasts.

Ultrasound should be performed by an experienced breast radiologist or ultrasonographer using a high-resolution linear array probe (7–10 MHz) on an ultrasound machine, designed for high-resolution, small parts soft tissue imaging, with colour Doppler, if it is to be used to its full potential. Many benign lesions can now be diagnosed ultrasonographically with a high degree of certainty, reducing the need for open biopsy. If FNAC is not performed serial ultrasound measurement, with high definition images, can confirm absence of change in ultrasonically benign lesions. For example, fibroadenomata are now managed conservatively, with FNAC and/or follow-up ultrasound examinations, in many centres.

Table 5.2  Indications for breast ultrasound

**Characterisation of:**
palpable breast masses
impalpable breast masses of uncertain aetiology seen on mammography.

**Primary evaluation of palpable masses:**
In women under 35,
In pregnant or lactating women.

**Evaluation of:**
Asymmetry or distortion on mammography
Lesions seen in only one mammographic projection.

**Guidance for interventional techniques:**
Cyst aspiration
Abscess aspiration
Fine needle aspiration for cytology
Needle core biopsy
Localization for surgery either with skin marker or internal localization wire.

**Imaging of:**
The augmented breast.
The male breast with a suspicious mass or unilateral gynaecomastia
Inflammation
The tender breast
The postoperative breast:
To identify haematoma and seromas
To evaluate new lumps in the scar of patients who have had previous surgery for cancer.

The two imaging methods are now recognized as being complementary rather than competitive. Fine microcalcifications, detected by mammography, are often not associated with any palpable mass in ductal carcinoma *in situ* and are not easily seen with ultrasound. Conversely mammography is often unhelpful in the dense breast and in the evaluation of densities which have moderately well defined margins. As well as evaluating palpable masses, ultrasound may on rare occasions detect impalpable small cancers which are not demonstrated on mammography.

Ultrasound-guided interventions include ultrasound-guided FNAC, needle core biopsy and localization for open excision biopsy, are all simple procedures. Localization for open excision biopsy may just involve marking the overlying skin with the patient positioned as she would be in the operating theatre or using a localization wire. As well as managing ultrasound abnormalities, breast ultrasound is frequently very useful for identifying and localizing the impalpable mammographic mass for FNAC, biopsy or localization. As interventions are performed with the patient lying in a comfortable supine position, vasovagal attacks are very rare and if they occur are unlikely to result in abandonment of the procedure. The ultrasound-guided techniques are more acceptable to the patient and preferred by experienced operators who have experience with both ultrasound- and mammographic-guided interventions. Ultrasound is real-time imaging and always allows optimum placement of needle tips under direct vision.

Using ultrasound to screen for occult breast cancer is less sensitive than mammography because it does not detect much of the microcalcification associated with ductal carcinoma *in situ* (DCIS). The other major disadvantage of ultrasound breast screening is the expense, which is much greater than that of mammographic breast screening, because it requires a lot of time from experienced breast ultrasonographers. Breast ultrasound is safe, because it does not use ionizing radiation; unfortunately its lower sensitivity and cost make it unsuitable for screening at present.

OTHER IMAGING MODALITIES

Other imaging modalities are second-line diagnostic methods which are used in complex cases or potential first-line imaging methods which are currently too expensive and/or are under evaluation.

*Nuclear medicine*

Nuclear medicine methods for imaging breast cancer include $^{99m}$Tc-methyoxy-iso-butyl-isonitrile (MIBI), which is selectively taken up by both the primary carcinomas and lymph node metastases (Fig. 5.2). $^{201}$Thallium also is taken up by breast cancers, presumably due to the increased metabolism within them. Radiolabelled monoclonal antibodies are also under evaluation. Positron emission tomography (PET) using $^{18}$fluorine-labelled FDG is showing promise in the diagnosis of of primary breast cancer and breast cancer recurrences, detecting tumour foci as small as 0.4 cm in diameter. Lymphoscintigraphy, which used only to be of help in the evaluation of lymphoedema (an important complication of breast cancer treatment), is now important as a staging investigation using technetium-labelled microaggregated albumin or sulphur colloid.

*Magnetic resonance imaging*

Magnetic resonance imaging (MRI) alone has not lived up to early expectations as a method of breast imaging (Fig. 5.3). MRI, with intravenous gadolinium contrast agents to show vascularity, is a rapidly

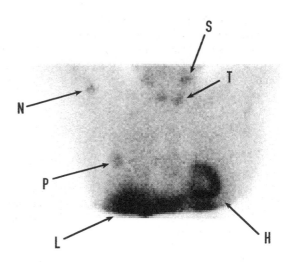

*Figure 5.2* — A MIBI scintigram of a patient with a right breast carcinoma. P is the primary tumour in the breast, N an axillary lymph node containing tumour, H the heart which takes up MIBI (which is also used for cardiac scintigraphy), L the liver, S the left submandibular gland and T the left lobe of the thyroid. In this case the MIBI demonstrated a large lymph node deposit high in the lateral side of the right axilla as well as the known primary.

expanding area of research (Fig. 5.4). Gadolinium-DTPA dynamic enhancement profiles are helping to differentiate malignant tumours from benign lesions with the aid of digital subtraction techniques. Interpretation, however, often requires a large number of images to be examined. Gadolinium-containing melanin polymers coupled to monoclonal antibodies specific for breast carcinoma are being synthesized for targeted MRI.

Despite a wide variety of imaging sequences and techniques, even with dedicated coils and IV contrast agents, the current indications for MRI are still mainly restricted to:

- imaging breasts with silicone implants to demonstrate adjacent malignancy or implant defects (leakage);

- differentiation of scarring from malignancy;

- detection of malignancy in dense breast tissue (including the diagnosis of multifocal disease in the presence of a known malignancy);

- monitoring the response to chemotherapy.

- Cost and availability of equipment in many countries are important additional considerations.

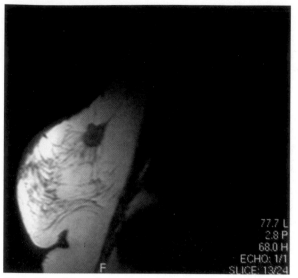

**Figure 5.3** — Magnetic resonance sectional image of a carcinoma in the upper part of the right breast. Note the irregular margin and radiating strands particularly in the area beneath the tumour.

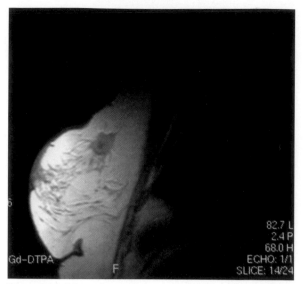

**Figure 5.4** — Magnetic resonance sectional image following intravenous enhancement with gadolinium DTPA. Note how the signal is stronger from within the tumour (the tumour is brighter than on the unenhanced image in Fig. 5.3).

### Ductography

Ductography, classically, is the demonstration of a duct by injection of X-ray contrast after cannulation of the duct. Indications are continuing discharge after previous surgery and suspicion of ductal abnormality despite a normal ultrasound examination. However, intraductal lesions of sufficient size, such as intraductal papillomata, are demonstrated on ultrasound. Smaller lesions can be demonstrated with ultrasound ductography (saline is injected into the duct and duct wall irregularity can be easily demonstrated).

### Research modalities

Thermography, like transillumination, does not have sufficient specificity or sensitivity to be recommended as a routine examination. Research into the use of light for breast cancer diagnosis is concentrating on infrared and near infrared light, i.e. that part of the electromagnetic spectrum that humans feel as heat. Modern infrared cameras can detect temperature variations of <0.1°C at 1 m. Of greater interest is the use of near infrared light spectroscopy in which the breast is transilluminated with laser light; fibreoptic detectors detect small changes of frequency when the light is reflected by moving red cells. Spectral mapping of the changes may allow the increased and altered vascularity associated with breast tumours to be detected.

## Cancers

### Invasive ductal carcinoma

Invasive ductal carcinoma is the most common type of breast cancer (approximately 75% of all breast cancers). Clinically the woman usually presents with a palpable mass which may be associated with distortion or skin retraction, particularly with larger tumours. The mammographic appearance most commonly is that of a spiculated mass (Fig. 5.5), often associated with local architectural distortion and skin thickening if the tumour is close enough to the skin surface. It may on occasions present as a more rounded, well-defined or partially-defined mass with a more benign appearance (Fig. 5.6). Though this appearance is also commonly associated with the rarer breast cancers, because invasive ductal carcinoma is so common, it is the commonest cause for this mammographic presentation. There may be associated malignant microcalcifications if there is a combination of invasive ductal carcinoma and ductal carcinoma *in situ* (see below).

The ultrasound appearance is also most commonly that of a spiculated mass with distortion of the surrounding parenchyma. It usually shows loss of echogenicity centrally with quite marked posterior shadowing (Fig. 5.7). Invasive ductal carcinoma can also present as a more defined lesion of low, fairly

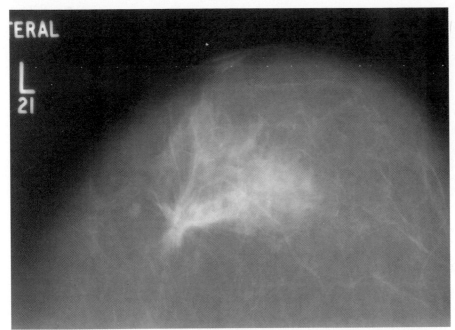

*Figure 5.5* — A small mass in the left breast with a stellate shape. Note the strands radiating from it and the way in which it distorts the adjacent fairly homogeneous breast parenchyma. This is a typical appearance of a small invasive ductal carcinoma.

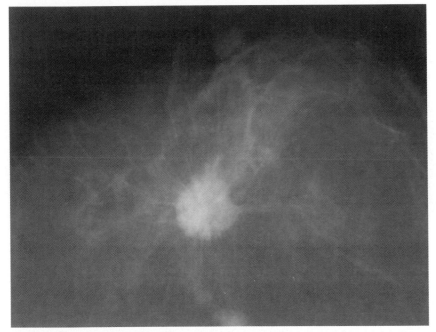

*Figure 5.6* — A more rounded tumour which has a more defined shape. Its edges are slightly irregular with a 'brush border' appearance. There are also stellate radiating strands into the adjacent breast similar to the small carcinoma in Fig. 5.5. This is also an invasive ductal carcinoma but the more rounded definition might also occur in one of the rare breast cancers such as a medullary or mucinous carcinoma.

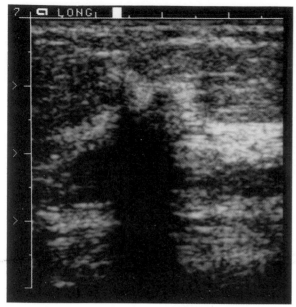

**Figure 5.7** — A typical ultrasound appearance of an irregular stellate carcinoma with absorption of the sound centrally resulting in a central anechoic area with posterior shadowing. Like the stellate carcinoma on a mammogram it has strands extending into the surrounding normal tissues.

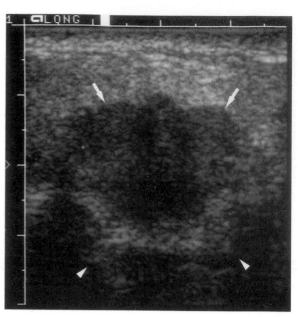

**Figure 5.8** — A carcinoma with a lobulated shape and slightly reduced heterogenous internal echogenicity (arrows). There is some 'bright up' with higher echogenicity in the tissues deep to it (arrow heads).

homogeneous internal echogenicity with good through transmission of sound and a posterior increased echogenicity, 'bright up' (Fig. 5.8).

## Invasive lobular carcinoma

Invasive lobular carcinoma is the cause of approximately 10% of all breast cancers. It is often bilateral with a reported incidence in some series as high as 28%. It can be difficult to diagnose as a discrete mass, may not be palpable and mammographically may be associated with very subtle diffuse changes. Only half present as a focal mass (usually spiculated) and in the other half parenchymal asymmetry and architectural distortion are the only signs. This is also the finding on ultrasound, although when there is distortion there is often quite marked posterior shadowing which if focal can be helpful in diagnosis.

## Ductal carcinoma in situ

A quarter to almost a half of all breast cancers diagnosed mammographically are ductal carcinoma *in situ* (DCIS). Many patients are asymptomatic as the majority of these cancers are impalpable and the apparent rise in incidence of DCIS is attributed to high-quality mam-

mographic screening. Just under one-third of biopsy-proven DCIS progress to invasive disease. The treatment of DCIS is controversial and is being evaluated in a number of trials.

Mammographically, DCIS has microcalcifications orientated in the line of the ducts, often with branching microcalcifications (Fig. 5.9). These may be seen on ultrasound as very bright echoes, occasionally with shadowing. Less commonly, DCIS is associated with well-defined mammographic or ultrasound masses which may not have the associated malignant type calcifications.

## Rare breast cancers

The remaining rarer types of carcinoma, which have a better prognosis, are mainly detected on screening and in the most part rarely present clinically.

LOBULAR CARCINOMA IN SITU

This is most commonly an incidental finding in breast biopsies performed in premenopausal women carried out for other reasons. Approximately 30% of these women go on to develop invasive carcinoma, which may be either ductal or lobular, over the following 20 years. It is often bilateral and multifocal and there is

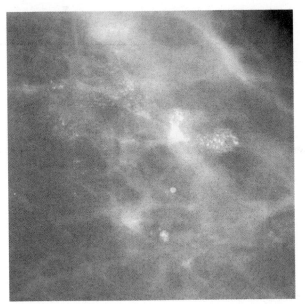

*Figure 5.9* — Fine microcalcifications in the breast associated with extensive ductal carcinoma in situ (DCIS). On examination this patient's breasts felt quite normal and there was no mass. She had a routine screening mammogram because of a family history of breast carcinoma. In this magnified image, multiple irregular small flecks of microcalcification can be seen. Some are linear in shape and are arranged in rows, some of which are branching. The calcifications are associated with carcinoma extending along the duct lumen. The branching of the microcalcifications occurs when the ducts branch. At operation, this patient was found to have DCIS and invasive ductal carcinoma.

great debate as to whether it represents a true carcinoma. This debate extends to the management of these women, ranging from observation to prophylactic bilateral mastectomy. There is no mammographic or ultrasound abnormality in these patients until the development of the invasive carcinoma, which is more easily detected if it is ductal than lobular (see above).

### TUBULAR CARCINOMA

In its pure form, tubular carcinoma occurs in <2% of breast cancers. It is multicentric in over a quarter of patients and may be bilateral in a similar number. It presents as a small spiculated lesion on mammography and may be difficult to differentiate from radial scars.

### MEDULLARY CARCINOMA

Approximately 5% of breast cancers are medullary carcinoma. It is commoner in young women. Both on mammography and ultrasound it presents as a round-ed mass with not particularly well defined borders (Fig. 5.6). On the ultrasound it shows reduced echogenicity. It is often locally quite aggressive but the prognosis is often better than with infiltrating ductal carcinomas.

### MUCINOUS CARCINOMA

Approximately 2% of breast cancers are mucinous carcinomas. They are more common in older women and have a good short-term prognosis, although systemic recurrences more than 10 years after initial treatment have been reported. Again mammographically they tend to be lobulated or rounded, moderately well-defined masses (Fig. 5.1). On ultrasound they are quite well defined with reduced echogenicity which has a heterogeneous echo pattern and increased echogenicity posteriorly (Fig. 5.8). On colour Doppler they show a marked increased blood flow within them.

### PAPILLARY CARCINOMA

Papillary carcinomas account for approximately 1–2% of all breast cancers. They usually occur in older patients presenting with a clinical history of nipple discharge or nipple retraction. They are often large, lobulated, palpable masses in the subareolar region. They appear as quite well-defined masses on mammography. On ultrasound they may be complex cystic masses with internal echogenicity or may be mainly solid.

### PAGET'S DISEASE

Between 1 and 5% of all breast carcinomas present as Paget's disease and approximately half show a palpable mass. On mammography, if there is no significant mass, the only signs may be nipple and areolar thickening or nipple calcifications and in many patients mammography may be normal.

### MALE BREAST CANCER

Approximately 1 in 200 breast cancers occur in males. The mean age of 64 is older than that for female breast cancers. It usually presents as a painless hard mass. It should always be excluded in patients who are otherwise thought to have gynaecomastia. The majority (85%) are infiltrating ductal carcinomas with the remainder divided between intraductal or papillary carcinomas. Lobular carcinoma is extremely rare. On mammography, male breast cancers can range from well circumscribed (Fig. 5.10) to spiculated masses and microcalcifications occur in up to one third of patients. Similarly, ultrasound appearances are those of well-defined circumscribed (Fig. 5.11) to spiculated masses

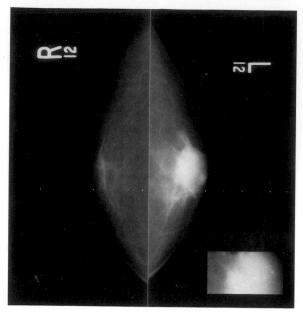

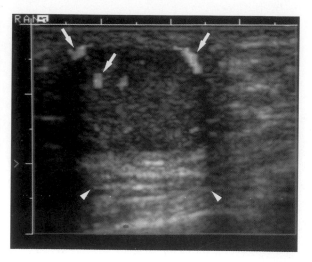

*Figure 5.10* — Craniocaudal views of the right and left breast of a 63-year-old male with unilateral enlargement of the left breast area. This was thought to be gynaecomastia by the referring physician. The mammogram shows a non-specific increase in density which is asymetric behind the left nipple. Careful examination (see inset of magnified view of mass) shows there are abnormal small calcifications within the mass which means it cannot be benign gynaecomastia. This was an invasive ductal carcinoma in a male.

*Figure 5.11* — Ultrasound of the male breast carcinoma shown in Fig. 5.10. The mass is moderately well defined with fairly heterogenous internal echoes. It has increased abnormal vascularity (colour Doppler positive), the vessels are both around the edge and within the tumour (arrows) and there is quite prominent posterior 'bright up' deep to the tumour (arrow heads).

which have a different appearance from the breast tissue development associated with gynaecomastia.

# Imaging following breast cancer diagnosis

## Staging of breast tumours

Final staging of breast tumours is done postsurgically for accurate assessment of tumour size and determination of nodal status, because micrometastases in nodes cannot be imaged before surgery. Because of the low pick up rate of metastatic disease in node negative T0 and Tl, some centres do not routinely search for metastatic disease at presentation. Staging for metastatic disease is often left until operative staging is completed, particularly if the initial tumour is T0 (impalpable) or Tl (<2 cm). Larger tumours, however, benefit from preoperative staging as the stage often determines the extent of the initial surgery and many centres also stage

before surgery for smaller tumours. Imaging plays an important part in both these situations.

## Mammography and ultrasound

If the diagnosis is made prior to mammography, mammography is still indicated to exclude multifocal or bilateral carcinoma. It is often helpful in assessing the size of the tumour. Breast ultrasound is also useful for assessing tumour size and the two imaging techniques are often complementary in this situation as the tumour may be better evaluated with one rather than the other.

Ultrasound evaluation of axillary lymph nodes is useful in staging of breast cancer. High-resolution ultrasound, with careful examination, is sensitive for detecting macroscopic involvement of lymph nodes. Irregular and/or enlarged nodes if supported by an increase in vascularity are very suspicious of malignant infiltration. Micrometastases may not cause any significant architectural change in lymph nodes or any increase in blood flow.

Abdominal ultrasound, particularly of the liver, is a sensitive means of detecting metastatic disease within the liver. Well-defined target lesions are pathognomonic of liver metastases (Fig. 5.12). More diffuse metastatic disease associated with diffuse heterogenecity of the liver can be difficult initially to differentiate from focal fatty change which is associated with factors such as previous hepatitis, significant alcohol intake, obesity and some drug therapies as well as adjuvant chemotherapy treatment. These changes are not only seen with the more toxic chemotherapeutic agents but also with hormonal therapeutic agents such as tamoxifen.

## Nuclear medicine

### BONE SCINTIGRAPHY

$Tc^{99m}$ MDP bone scintigraphy is the most sensitive method for detecting bony metastatic disease (Fig. 5.13). It detects bony metastatic disease up to 6 months before there is sufficient bony destruction for demonstration on plain film radiography. It may require plain film radiography of increased activity to exclude other causes of 'hot spots' such as degenerative change or osteoporotic collapse. It can be helpful in assessing response to treatment, although the flare response of increased activity which occurs in the first 3 months of response to chemotherapy can be confusing to those unfamiliar with the use of bone scintigraphy in the treatment of metastatic disease.

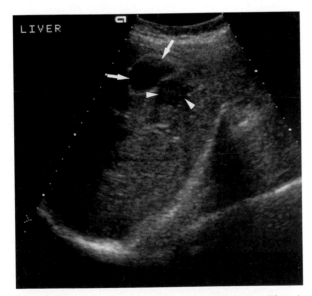

**Figure 5.12** — Ultrasound of the liver in sagittal section. There is a metastasis (arrow heads) just deep to the gallbladder (arrows). Note the low echo rim of the metastasis with the brighter central echoes, the so-called 'target lesion' appearance.

### BREAST LYMPHOSCINTIGRAPHY

Ultrasound of axillary nodes can be helpful in confirming nodal involvement, but as already mentioned is less helpful for excluding it. Breast lymphoscintigraphy following the injection of radiolabelled colloid into the breast primary allows identification of lymph node drainage from the tumour and can be used to demonstrate the site of the sentinel node, biopsy of which is a good predictor of nodal involvement. Accurate sampling of the drainage lymph nodes also allows greater accuracy in determining routes of lymph node drainage, thus reducing the need for more extensive lymph node sampling with its increased risk of postoperative arm swelling (lymphoedema). Dye injections just prior to surgery provide similar information but do not show as easily the site of the sentinel node, which can be used for histology to determine the likelihood of microscopic disease.

## Imaging in primary treatment

Ultrasound is particularly useful for patients with large tumours who are treated with primary chemotherapy and radiotherapy to reduce the bulk of the primary and allow less radical surgery with a better cosmetic result. Follow-up with ultrasound can be used to confirm response. Colour Doppler flow changes in response to therapy (an increase in vascularity is associated with increasing tumour size while decreasing vascularity is associated with decrease in size) can occur up to 4 weeks before clinical or ultrasound measured changes in many patients.

# Imaging follow-up of the breast cancer patient

Mammography should be performed annually for the first 5 years following breast cancer treatment. Thereafter patients should be screened every 2 years because of the increased risk of a second cancer developing in the contralateral breast. Recurrence at the sight of previous surgery may often be masked by changes due to the surgery and radiotherapy so that the first postoperative mammograms are often less helpful in the diagnosis of local recurrence than subsequent mammograms.

Ultrasound is helpful in detecting breast cancer recurrence at the site of previous surgery by demonstrating regions of reduced echogenicity. While ultrasound does not detect the microcalcifications associated with recurrence, it often detects local recurrences which may not be demonstrated on mammography. Thus the two techniques are complementary in this important problem. Ultrasound is less helpful in early recurrence where the only change is distortion of tissue with no obvious mass deposits. The usefulness of colour Doppler in diagnosing early recurrence in areas which have an appearance of disruption due to scar formation is uncertain but is under investigation in conjunction with ultrasound contrast media.

Bone scintigraphy is the most sensitive method for determining early bone metastases. Plain film radiography is useful to exclude other causes of increased activity but is not indicated, however, in the routine follow-up of patients with breast cancer. Abdominal ultrasound is the first examination for the detection of liver metastases. In equivocal cases computed tomography (CT) may be indicated to demonstrate the occasional metastases which are not shown by ultrasound. Very occasionally, [18]fluorine FDG PET scanning is useful in diagnosing tumour or tumour recurrence which is not diagnosed by any other method (Fig. 5.14) and the expense of this very sensitive test for tumour can be justified.

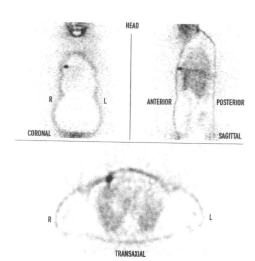

*Figure 5.14* — A [18]fluorine FDG PET whole body scan of a patient who has had a bilateral mastectomy for previous bilateral carcinoma. The sites of the bilateral mastectomy were scarred and nodular. Previous fine needle aspiration cytology (FNAC) of some of the nodules had not revealed any evidence of recurrence of carcinoma. The PET scan was performed to see if there was any evidence of local or distant recurrence. The three sectional images (coronal anterior, transaxial mid-thorax and right sagittal) show that there is a small area of increased activity at the medial end of the right mastectomy scar. Subsequent biopsy confirmed that this was an area of local recurrence.

# References

1.  Law J. Variations in individual radiation dose in a breast screening programme and consquences for the balance between associated risk and the benefit. *Br J Radiol* 1993; **66**: 394–397.

2.  Adler DD, Wahl RL. New methods for imaging the breast: techniques, findings, and potential. *AJR* 1995; **164**: 19–30.

3.  Buscombe JR, Cwikla JB, Thakrar DS, Hilson AJW. Scintigraphic imaging of breast cancer: A review. *Nuclear Med Commun* 1997; **18**: 698–709.

4.  Gardenosa G (ed). *Breast Imaging Companion*. Philadelphia: Lippincott-Raven, 1997.

5.  Jack D. Hot spots inside the body. *Lancet* 1997; **350**: 790.

6.  Khalkali I, Mena I, Diggles L. Review of imaging techniques for the diagnosis of breast cancer: a new role of prone scintimammography using technetium-99m sestamibi. *Eur J Nuclear Med* 1994; **81**: 357–362.

7.  Sabel M, Aichinger H. Recent developements in breast imaging. *Phys Med Biol* 1996; **41**: 315–368.

8.  Scheidhauer K, Scharl A, Pietrzyk U *et al.* Qualitative (18F)FDG positron emission tomography in primary breast cancer: clinical relevance and practibility. *Eur J Nuclear Med* 1996; **23**: 618–623.

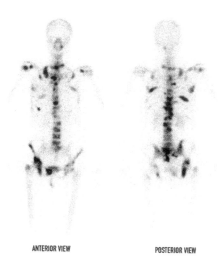

*Figure 5.13* — Anterior and posterior views of an MDP 99mTc bone scintigram of a patient with multiple bone metastases from a breast carcinoma primary. Note the multiple areas of increased activity in thoracic and lumbar vertebrae, ribs, both shoulders, pelvis and upper femora. The patient has had a previous right mastectomy. The anterior ends of the left ribs are not as clearly seen as on the right because the thickness of the left breast tissue attenuates the photons which arise in the ribs on the left.

9.  Svensson WE. A review of the current status of breast ultrasound. *Eur J Ultrasound* 1997; **6**: 77–101.

10. Tuck AK (ed) *Textbook of Mammography*. Edinburgh: Churchill Livingstone, 1993.

11. Tohno E, Cosgrove DO, Sloane JP (eds). *Ultrasound Diagnosis of Breast Diseases*. Edinburgh: Churchill Livingstone, 1994.

12. Veronesi U, Paganelli G, Galimberti V *et al*. Sentinel-node biopsy to avoid axillary dissection in breast cancer with clinically negative lymph-nodes. *Lancet* 1997; **349**: 1864–1867.

# Acknowledgements

The author thanks Helen Young for the PET images, Nandita De Souza for the MR images, Muhammad Mubashar for the MIBI image and Damien Sell and Graham Reed for preparation of all the figures.

# 6

# THE OESOPHAGUS, STOMACH, DUODENUM AND SMALL INTESTINE

Daniel J Nolan

**Oesophagus**
**Stomach**
**Duodenum**
**Small Intestine**

# Oesophagus

Oesophageal carcinoma is fairly common and accounts for about 2.5% of all malignancies and for almost all primary oesophageal malignant neoplasms.[1] Rare primary oesophageal malignancies include adenosquamous carcinoma, carcinosarcoma, pseudosarcomas, oat cell carcinomas and melanomas.

## Carcinoma

### CLINICAL ASPECTS

Oesophageal carcinoma has a poor prognosis with a 5-year survival of less than 10%.[2] Numerous factors can predispose to oesophageal carcinoma but in Western Europe and North America smoking and alcohol, particularly a combination of the two, are by far the most important. Previously squamous carcinoma accounted for about 90% of carcinomas while most of the rest were adenocarcinomas; currently there is an increase in the incidence of adenocarcinoma. Squamous carcinomas are distributed throughout the oesophagus, although involvement of the oesophagogastric junction is unusual. Adenocarcinomas arise in the lower third of the oesophagus on a background of columnar metaplasia, probably induced by gastroesophageal reflux.[3]

Most patients present with dysphagia. Unfortunately this usually indicates that the neoplasm has reached an advanced stage at the time of presentation. Some patients locate the dysphagia accurately to the site of the lesion, while in others the perceived site of food sticking does not correspond to the location of the carcinoma. Anorexia, weight loss, chest pain and anaemia are other, less frequently encountered, symptoms.

In many cases the carcinoma has spread beyond the oesophagus so that it is inoperable at the time of diagnosis. Lack of serosa around the oesophagus and the thin nature of the oesophageal wall encourage early spread of carcinoma. Spread of oesophageal carcinoma is by direct extension, lymphatic permeation and blood-borne metastases. Direct extension is mostly to adjacent mediastinal structures such as the trachea, bronchi, lung parenchyma, aorta and pericardium. Bronchoesophageal fistulae and occasionally aortoesophageal fistulae may develop. Spread to the fundus of the stomach is frequently seen in patients with adenocarcinoma of the lower end of the oesophagus. In such cases it may be impossible to establish whether the adenocarcinoma originated in the oesophagus or fundus of the stomach. Lymphatic spread is mostly to the peri-oesophageal lymph nodes and nodes in the mediastinum and neck.[4,5]

Spread to lymph nodes below the diaphragm with involvement of the paracardial, gastric lesser curve and coeliac lymph nodes can occur. Blood-borne metastatic spread is mostly to liver, lung, adrenals, kidneys, pancreas and peritoneum and bones.[2]

### RADIOLOGICAL DIAGNOSIS

The barium swallow remains an extremely efficient initial investigation for suspected oesophageal malignancy. The examination takes 10–15 minutes to perform, requires no sedation, the patient does not need to be accompanied and normal activities, such as work, can be resumed afterwards. The only requirement is that the patient should be fasting for 6 hours. A barium swallow should be performed as a matter of urgency on any patient who presents with dysphagia. Views of the whole length of the oesophagus, fully distended by the barium suspension, should be obtained and these should be supplemented by air-contrast views. When an oesophageal stricture is present the upper limit is normally well shown but the lower limit may be difficult to define. It is important, however, to demonstrate the lower limit and thus the full extent of the lesion, whenever possible. Double-contrast views are obtained by getting the patient to hold the nostrils closed while swallowing barium suspension in the upright position. Double-contrast views are best for showing early oesophageal carcinoma, mucosal abnormalities and small polypoid lesions.

Early oesophageal carcinoma is shown on double-contrast views as a small sessile intraluminal filling defect or a plaque-like lesion of abnormal mucosa.[6] Most patients, however, develop dysphagia when the lumen of the oesophagus is considerably narrowed by the carcinoma and characteristic appearances are then seen on barium swallow. Oesophageal carcinomas are frequently shown as an irregular stricture with shouldering of the margins (Figs. 6.1 and 6.2). Others are shown as a polypoid mass (Fig. 6.3) and occasionally an infiltrating neoplasm produces a tapering stricture (Fig. 6.4). Adenocarcinoma may be indistinguishable from squamous carcinoma – involvement of the gastric fundus makes adenocarcinoma much more likely.

### STAGING

Staging of oesophageal carcinoma is necessary to define the extent of spread as many carcinomas are inoperable at the time of presentation. A chest radiograph is normally taken at the time of diagnosis to establish whether there is evidence of advanced disease in the mediastinum or chest. Computed tomography (CT) is cur-

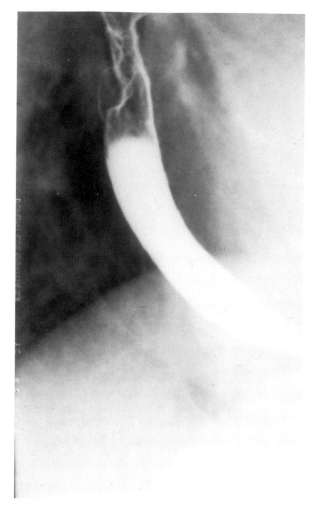

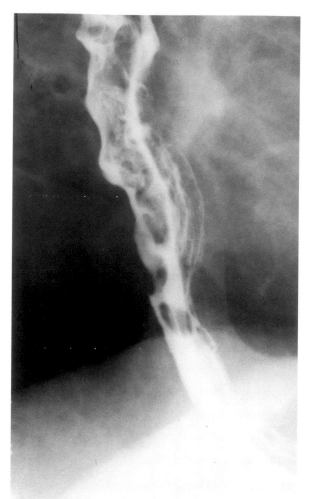

*Figure 6.1* — Carcinoma of the oesophagus: barium swallow shows an irregular stricture with mucosal destruction and well-defined margins in the lower oesophagus.

*Figure 6.2* — Carcinoma of the oesophagus: barium swallow shows an irregular stricture, with some polypoid filling defects near its lower end, occupying much of the lower third of the oesophagus.

rently the most widely used technique for staging oesophageal carcinoma (Fig. 6.5). CT has the ability to demonstrate the extent of mediastinal involvement and thus help to decide whether or not an attempt at curative surgical resection may be made. Spread outside the oesophagus is assessed on CT by showing whether there is evidence of spread to adjacent mediastinal structures as shown by loss of the fat planes between the oesophagus and adjacent structures, enlargement of lymph nodes (Fig. 6.5) and the presence of hepatic, pulmonary or abdominal metastases.[7] A paucity of mediastinal fat can make interpretation of the CT examination difficult.[8] Normally, there is no fat plane separating the oesophagus from the trachea or left main bronchus, which can make airway invasion difficult to

diagnose. Aortic invasion may also be difficult to assess as many patients do not have a fat plane separating the oesophagus from the aortic arch or descending thoracic aorta. There can be difficulty deciding whether there is evidence of spread to lymph nodes as involved perioesophageal lymph nodes are frequently of normal size, even though they are engulfed by tumour.[8] Despite these limitations, CT remains the most useful technique for staging oesophageal carcinoma. Evidence of mediastinal invasion, liver metastases and abdominal adenopathy, as demonstrated on CT, predict a shortened survival time regardless of the type of treatment.[9]

Endoscopic ultrasound is a new technique using high frequency, high resolution, real-time ultrasound

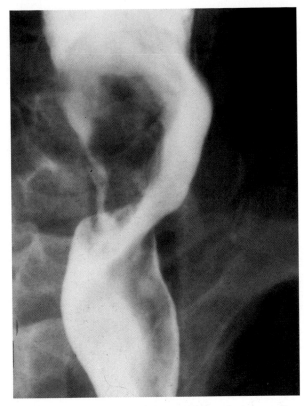

*Figure 6.3* — Carcinoma of the oesophagus: barium swallow shows a large irregular polypoid mass on the right side of the cervical oesophagus. (Reproduced from Phillips and Nolan 1995[89] with permission).

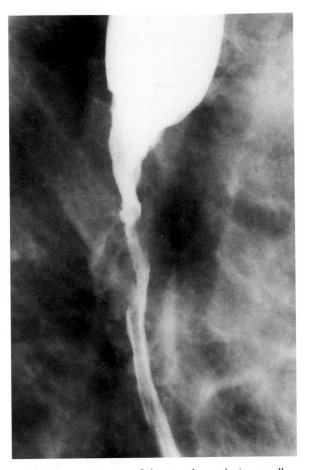

*Figure 6.4* — Carcinoma of the oesophagus: barium swallow shows a tight infiltrating stricture with slightly irregular margins in the mid oesophagus. The marked obstruction caused by the stricture makes it difficult to identify its lower margin.

images obtained from within the oesophagus by an ultrasound probe incorporated into the tip of a fibreoptic endoscope.[10] The depth of oesophageal invasion is shown by identifying the layers of the oesophageal wall that are involved by tumour (Fig. 6.6). Metastatic involvement of peri-oesophageal lymph nodes can also be identified. Involved lymph nodes are usually >10 mm in diameter and are frequently spherical.[11] Endoscopic ultrasound can also make it possible to determine whether the neoplasm has infiltrated adjacent structures.

## Other primary malignancies

Leiomyosarcomas are rare and may be polypoid or infiltrating or show a combination of these features. They may be indistinguishable radiologically from carcinoma.

Pseudosarcomas and carcinosarcomas may represent carcinomas that have undergone metaplasia, giving rise

to sarcomatous elements.[12] These neoplasms consist predominantly of malignant-looking spindle cells with a small localised component of carcinomatous material usually in the margin of the neoplasm or superficially invading the mass.[1] They have a more favourable prognosis than carcinoma when treated surgically. These rare oesophageal neoplasms are characteristically seen on barium swallow as large polypoid masses.

## Secondary neoplasms

Oesophageal involvement is not unusual in patients in the late stages of other malignancies.[13] Secondary neoplastic involvement of the oesophagus frequently occurs by direct spread from a neoplasm in an adjacent organ such as the pharynx, thyroid, bronchus or stom-

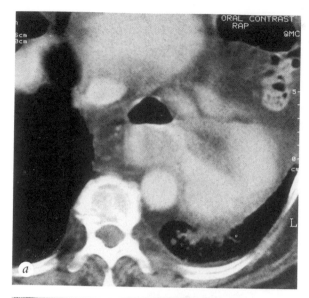

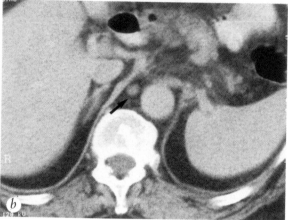

*Figure 6.5* — Carcinoma of the oesophagus: (a) CT shows a mass (arrow) involving the posterior and lateral walls of the oesophagus. The anterior wall is spared. (b) Involvement of a retrocrural lymph node (arrow) is seen on another section. (*Courtesy of Dr Niall Moore*).

ach. Radiologically, most of these are seen as extrinsic compression or invasion of the oesophageal wall or lumen and may simulate a primary oesophageal carcinoma. Usually, however, an associated extrinsic mass allows the correct diagnosis to be identified. Lymph node metastases may develop and the resulting enlarged adjacent lymph nodes may produce radiological evidence of extrinsic compression with a mass pressing and protruding into the oesophageal lumen. Blood-borne metastases may be from lung or breast, although

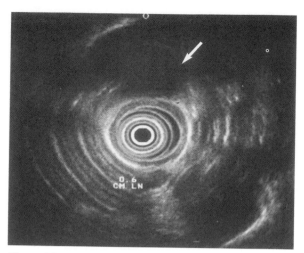

*Figure 6.6* — Carcinoma of the oesophagus: endosonography showing the extent of carcinoma in the wall of the oesophagus (arrow). (*Courtesy of Dr James Virjee*).

metastases from the kidneys, bladder, pancreas and cervix have been described.[1]

# Stomach

Carcinoma is by far the most common primary malignant neoplasm of the stomach. Lymphoma, although much less common, is occasionally seen and may be difficult to differentiate from carcinoma. Other primary malignant neoplasms that are occasionally encountered include carcinoid tumours and leiomyosarcoma.

## Carcinoma

The incidence of carcinoma of the stomach has declined in recent years, although there is an increasing incidence of carcinoma of the cardia. Previously, carcinoma of the stomach was more common in males but the male: female ratio is now about 1: 1.[14] The incidence of carcinoma of the stomach varies in different geographical locations; this is due to environmental factors rather than genetic predisposition. A number of conditions predispose to gastric carcinoma and these include pernicious anaemia, gastric atrophy, adenomatous gastric polyps and partial gastrectomy.

Gastric carcinoma is nearly always adenocarcinoma, although squamous carcinoma and adenosquamous carcinoma are occasionally encountered. In the great majority of cases gastric carcinoma is at a late stage when the diagnosis is made and as a result the prognosis is poor with a 5-year survival rate of less than 20%.

This is because symptoms are absent or are trivial in the early stages. In Japan, where the incidence of gastric carcinoma is high, screening programmes using endoscopy or barium studies enable gastric carcinoma to be diagnosed at an early stage. This has led to the concept of 'early gastric cancer' with a more favourable prognosis and a 5-year survival rate of over 90%. Early gastric cancer is defined as being localised to the mucosa or submucosa regardless of the presence or absence of lymph node involvement and may be seen as a depressed, protuberant or flat lesion.[15] Because of the low incidence of carcinoma of the stomach in Western countries screening programmes are not justified. Gastric cancer detected at an early stage in the West similar to the Japanese early gastric cancer has a prognosis of nearly 70% 5-year survival.[16,17]

Presenting symptoms of gastric carcinoma include anorexia, weight loss, anaemia and epigastric pain. Symptoms are frequently late developing and are often vague. As a result most carcinomas are diagnosed when they have reached an advanced stage.

Gastric carcinoma spreads by direct extension, lymphatic permeation and blood-borne metastases. Direct spread from the gastric wall occurs early and extends to involve adjacent structures. Transperitoneal dissemination is common once the neoplasm has broken through the gastric serosa. Peritoneal metastases can spread to other organs such as the ovaries giving rise to a Krukenburg tumour. Direct extension across the gastroesophageal junction is common with carcinoma of the cardia and these neoplasms may present with dysphagia. In the past, extension across the pylorus to the duodenum was considered unusual but in a recent study transpyloric spread occurred in 25% of adenocarcinomas of the gastric antrum.[18]

Spread to lymph nodes is common. The most frequently involved are the perigastric lesser curve nodes followed by greater curve nodes, and the coeliac and porta hepatis groups. Spread to supradiaphragmatic lymph nodes, including the supraclavicular and mediastinal groups, is well recognised. Lymphangitis carcinomatosis may develop secondary to mediastinal lymph node involvement. Metastatic spread to the liver is common but may also occur to the lungs, skin, ovaries, adrenals and bone.

RADIOLOGICAL DIAGNOSIS

Gastric carcinoma is well demonstrated on barium studies. Most carcinomas are seen as a nodular or polypoid intraluminal mass (Fig. 6.7). The lesions have an irregular surface and the margins are usually well-

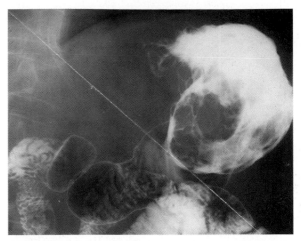

*Figure 6.7* — Carcinoma of the stomach: barium examination shows a large irregular polypoid mass occupying the upper half of the stomach.

defined. An ulcer crater is the predominant feature of ulcerating carcinomas. Malignant ulcers tend to be greater in width than depth, often with nodularity of the floor and the edge of the ulcer may show a nodular appearance. Radiating mucosal folds may be tapered, clubbed, fused or terminate abruptly. Gastric ulcers should preferably be biopsied endoscopically to firmly establish whether the lesion is benign or malignant. The linitis plastica appearance is seen in scirrhous carcinoma when there is extensive submucosal infiltration by the neoplasm. On barium examination the gastric lumen is markedly narrowed with nodularity and distortion of the mucosal fold pattern. The limited ability of the stomach to distend is confirmed by using large quantities of an effervescent agent (Fig. 6.8). Endoscopic biopsies are frequently negative in patients with linitis plastica. and as a result the diagnosis may be missed at endoscopy. If there is any suspicion of linitis plastica at endoscopy further evaluation by barium examination or CT is indicated.

On CT polypoid carcinoma is seen as a mass protruding into the lumen of the stomach. Ulcerating carcinoma can be difficult to detect on CT if there is not much thickening of the gastric wall. Linitis plastica shows marked gastric wall thickening on CT (Fig. 6.9).

STAGING

A number of imaging modalities may be used to stage gastric carcinoma and assess whether the neoplasm is resectable. A chest radiograph is useful for detecting the presence of pulmonary or mediastinal lymph node spread or the presence of lymphangitis carcinomatosis.

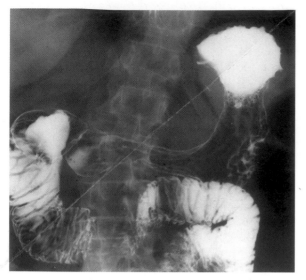

*Figure 6.8* — Carcinoma of the stomach: the typical features of linitis plastica are shown on a barium study in this patient with an infiltrating carcinoma. There is only slight mucosal irregularity. During the examination the stomach failed to distend.

Ultrasound is widely used to detect hepatic metastases. Ultrasound may also show subdiaphragmatic lymph node enlargement and demonstrate ascites. The characteristic ultrasound appearances of gastric carcinoma have been described.[19,20] Although ultrasound is not frequently used for staging gastric carcinoma it is

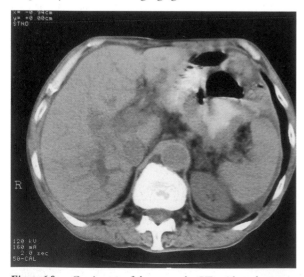

*Figure 6.9* — Carcinoma of the stomach: CT, with oral contrast medium, shows marked irregular thickening of the wall of the stomach. Small volume lymph node metastases and 'mucky' peritoneal fat is seen between the stomach and aorta. (*Courtesy of Dr Fergus Gleeson*).

important for those performing abdominal ultrasound to recognise gastric wall thickening or a mass lesion so that further investigation can be directed towards the stomach in patients referred for ultrasound with non-specific upper abdominal symptoms due to underlying gastric carcinoma.

At the present time CT is the technique of choice for staging carcinoma of the stomach. CT is able to demonstrate gastric wall thickening, extension into adjacent viscera, nodal involvement, hepatic and adrenal metastases and ascites.[21,22] It has been shown that the CT findings correlate well with the surgical and pathological findings and the high accuracy rate of CT can help to avoid unnecessary laparotomy in many patients.[22]

## Other primary neoplasms

The stomach is the most frequent site of gastrointestinal lymphoma and accounts for 2–5% of all gastric malignancy.[23,24] The great majority of gastrointestinal tract lymphomas are non-Hodgkins in type. Symptoms are similar to those of gastric carcinoma.

The antrum and body of the stomach are the most frequent sites of involvement. Lymphoma tends to occur in a submucosal or intramucosal location and gives rise to diffuse thickening of the gastric wall with a lobulated surface and thickening of the mucosal folds. The surfaces of these thickened mucosal folds are relatively smooth in contrast to the irregularity seen in widespread carcinoma. The volume of the stomach is preserved, unlike in carcinoma and the lymphomatous stomach retains its distensibility.[25] Gastric lymphoma may manifest itself as ulceration and these ulcers may be large and can be multiple and may be associated with a mass lesion. Single or multiple polypoid lesions are occasionally seen, usually on a background of thickened mucosal folds. Lymphoma may infiltrate across the gastro-oesophageal junction. Spread of lymphoma across the pylorus into the duodenum is fairly common in patients with antral involvement and was seen in 50% of the patients reviewed by Cho and colleagues.[18]

Primary carcinoid tumours of the stomach are recognised but are rare. They are usually seen as a small intramural lesion protruding into the lumen and are usually about 2cm in diameter with ulceration in about 40%.[26] Rarely gastric carcinoids may be seen as multiple small sessile polyps occurring throughout the stomach or in clusters.[27] Radiologically they are similar to multiple polyposis and as biopsy is superficial polypectomy is necessary to achieve a definitive diagnosis. Rarely carcinoid tumours are seen as large polypoid masses or large malignant ulcers radiologically indistinguishable from primary carcinoma.[26] The primary neoplasm and secondary deposits grow slowly and long survival may be achieved by surgical resection of the primary lesion and the metastases.

## Secondary neoplasms

The stomach may be involved by direct spread from carcinomas in adjacent structures such as oesophagus, pancreas, transverse colon, left kidney and left adrenal. Spread of adenocarcinoma from the lower oesophagus is not uncommon, although it is unusual for squamous oesophageal carcinoma to spread to the stomach. Carcinoma of the transverse colon can spread along the greater omentum to the stomach.

The most common blood-borne metastases to the stomach are from malignant melanoma and carcinoma of the breast. Metastatic melanoma is characteristically seen in the submucosa and produces an intraluminal polypoid mass which frequently shows central ulceration, giving it the characteristic 'bull's eye' appearance.[28] The most frequent manifestation of metastatic breast carcinoma is diffuse infiltration producing a linitis plastica-type appearance (Fig. 6.10).[29] The gastric mucosa usually remains intact, although it may develop a serrated or nodular configuration. Metastases from other organs have been described.[30]

# Duodenum

Primary malignant neoplasms of the duodenum are uncommon. Carcinoma is the most frequently encountered and accounts for 80–90% of primary duodenal malignancies.[31] Leiomyosarcoma[32] and lymphoma are seen much less frequently. Other neoplasms that rarely involve the duodenum include carcinoid tumour, Kaposi's sarcoma, malignant schwannoma, lymphangiosarcoma and plasmocytoma.[33] Secondary neoplastic involvement of the duodenum occurs as a result of direct spread from an adjacent organ or as metastases.

## Primary Neoplasms

About half of all small intestinal carcinomas arise in the duodenum while most of the remainder develop in the jejunum.[34] Carcinoma of the duodenum can be classified into carcinoma of the papilla of Vater and true carcinoma of the duodenum.[35] Patients with carcinoma of the ampulla of Vater usually present with obstructive jaundice. Carcinoma of the ampulla is shown on barium studies as irregular enlargement of the papilla, sometimes with spiculation and ulceration.[36]

Non-papillary duodenal carcinoma mostly presents clinically with symptoms of duodenal obstruction, mostly abdominal pain, nausea and vomiting. Other presenting symptoms are varied and can mimic peptic ulceration, hiatus hernia and pancreatic or biliary disease.[37] Barium examination shows the carcinoma as an annular lesion with shouldered margins (Fig. 6.11), as a polypoid mass or as an ulcerative lesion. The appearances are similar to carcinomas elsewhere in the gastrointestinal tract. CT shows duodenal carcinoma as asymmetrical thickening of the duodenal wall or as a

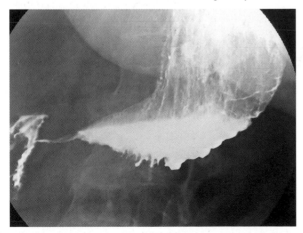

*Figure 6.10* — Secondary carcinoma of the stomach: marked narrowing and irregularity of the gastric antrum is seen, resulting from infiltration by metastatic breast carcinoma.

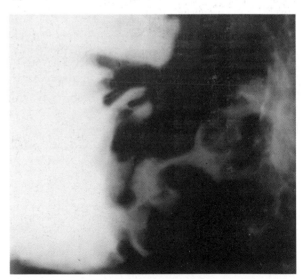

*Figure 6.11* — Carcinoma of the duodenum: an irregular polypoid stricture with mucosal destruction is shown on a barium study obstructing the third part of the duodenum.

polypoid mass.[33] It may be difficult to differentiate duodenal carcinoma from pancreatic carcinoma invading the duodenum.[33]

Leiomyosarcomas are very uncommon, but may develop in the duodenum. Clinical presenting symptoms include gastrointestinal bleeding, abdominal pain, obstructive jaundice or a palpable mass.[38] Leiomyosarcomas are usually large and are mostly shown on barium studies as a large cavitating mass with much of the tumour extending extraluminally. There is frequently compression of adjacent organs but leiomyosarcomas do not usually invade them.[33] CT shows leiomyosarcoma as a large lobulated cavitating mass with inhomogeneous attenuation and varying contrast enhancement, often with hypervascular liver metastases.[39] Characteristically no evidence of lymphadenopathy is seen.

Primary duodenal lymphoma is rare. Most lymphomas involve the duodenum either from transpyloric spread of gastric lymphoma or secondary encasement by paraduodenal lymph nodes.[33] Primary duodenal lymphoma may be an infiltrative lesion of the duodenal wall or as a cavitating mass indistinguishable from leiomyosarcoma.

## Secondary Neoplasms

The duodenum may be invaded by malignant neoplasms from adjacent organs or it may be the site of blood-borne metastatic deposits.

The most common neoplasms to invade the duodenum are gastric carcinoma and gastric lymphoma extending across the pylorus. In a recent series transpyloric spread occurred in 40% of lymphomas and 25% of adenocarcinomas of the gastric antrum, demonstrating contour deformities and nodular filling defects in the duodenum.[18]

Carcinoma of the head of the pancreas may cause a double contour, irregularity of the inner border (Fig. 6.12) and sometimes stricturing of the second part of the duodenum. The reversed '3' sign of Frostberg is a well recognised but infrequent finding.[40] It is not unusual for carcinoma of the body of the pancreas to invade the fourth part of the duodenum (Fig. 6.13) resulting in obstruction or bleeding.

Other carcinomas that may invade the duodenum include carcinoma of the colon, kidney, gallbladder or common bile duct. Colon carcinoma, particularly lesions in the hepatic flexure may distort and invade the duodenal loop (Fig. 6.14).[41] Occasionally carcinoma of

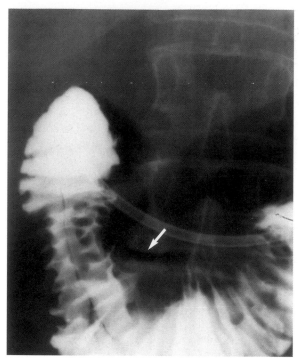

***Figure 6.12*** — Carcinoma of the pancreas involving the duodenum: barium examination shows narrowing of the lumen and distortion of the mucosal folds of the mid second part of the duodenum. A double contour is seen on the medial aspect at the junction of the second and third part of the duodenum (arrow). A spiculated appearance is seen on the inner border of the duodenum and this most marked in the third part of the duodenum.

the left kidney spreads through the lymphatics to the fourth part of the duodenum.[33]

Barium studies are excellent for showing the luminal changes in the duodenum caused by neoplasms invading from adjacent organs. CT is ideal for demonstrating the full extent of the primary neoplasm.

Blood-borne metastases to the duodenum are uncommon. Metastatic melanoma is the one that most frequently metastasises to the duodenum. Other primary carcinomas that metastasise to the duodenum include colon, kidney, lung, uterus, breast and testis (Fig. 6.15). The radiological appearances of metastases to the duodenum are similar to those seen in the jejunum and ileum and will be described in the following section.

## Small intestine

Malignant neoplasms are uncommon in the small intestine and account for less than 2% of all primary

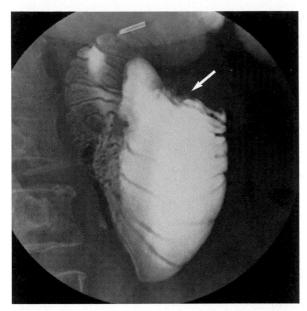

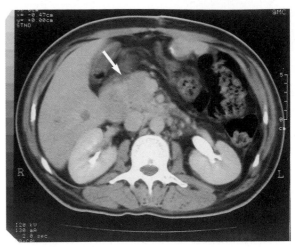

**Figure 6.15** — Duodenal metastasis: CT shows a large irregular duodenal mass (arrow). This proved to be metastatic teratoma of the testis. Note the metastatic deposits in the liver. (*Courtesy of Dr Fergus Gleeson*).

**Figure 6.13** — Carcinoma of the pancreas involving the duodenum: a barium study shows complete obstruction to the fourth part of the duodenum (arrow). Carcinoma of the body of the pancreas was subsequently confirmed.

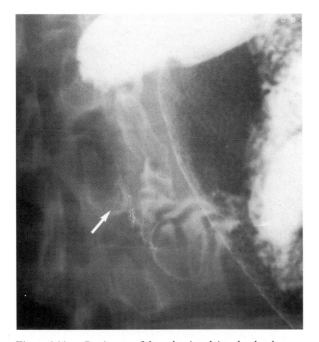

**Figure 6.14** — Carcinoma of the colon involving the duodenum: barium examination shows a fairly tight stricture of the second part of the duodenum is seen (arrow) resulting from invasion of the duodenum by carcinoma of the colon.

malignancies of the gastrointestinal tract.[42–45] The diagnosis of small intestinal neoplasms is difficult. Most patients present with insidious symptoms and vague, mild non-specific complaints that are often overlooked and easily dismissed.[45] In the series of 153 cases reviewed by Hancock[46] more than half were initially considered to be neurotic. Delay in diagnosis is due to a combination of factors; patients are reluctant to seek early medical attention because of the mild symptoms, physicians frequently do not recognise the importance of the presenting symptoms, resulting in a delay requesting the relevant imaging investigations. Further delay in diagnosis is often because of inadequate or incorrect interpretation of radiological examinations.

## Radiological investigation

The small intestine is the longest and most inaccessible part of the gastrointestinal tract. As yet endoscopy is not a practical procedure for routinely examining the small intestine and the barium examination remains the method of choice for demonstrating changes in the lumen of the jejunum and ileum.

Each barium examination is a challenge to the radiologist. This is because of the length of the intestine and difficulty manipulating the barium suspension so that all segments are clearly visualised.[47] A number of barium techniques are available and are based on the small intestinal follow-through, using orally administered barium or enteroclysis (small bowel enema). The barium follow-through is the most widely used technique, although enteroclysis is being introduced in an increasing number of centres

During enteroclysis the barium suspension is introduced directly into the small intestine through a tube.[48,49] Enteroclysis is superior to the follow-through because the intestine is well distended by the barium suspension, providing optimum visualisation of the jejunum and ileum. There is sometimes a reluctance to perform enteroclysis because it is necessary to intubate the duodenum. Duodenal intubation can be performed easily, quickly and with only minor patient discomfort, using one of the newer 10 French tubes.[50] The enteroclysis technique is easy to learn and the radiologist and quickly become more skilled using this examination than the time-consuming repeated fluoroscopy required for the barium follow-through.[51]

The available evidence indicates that enteroclysis is superior to the barium follow-through for detecting and demonstrating morphological abnormalities in the intestine.[52] Keats and Sakai[53] reported 84 cases of primary small intestinal neoplasms and found that on the barium follow-through neoplasms were reported in 50%, another 9% were described as abnormal and in the remaining 41% the report was negative. A retrospective study of 71 patients with histologically proven primary malignant neoplasms were reported by Bessette and colleagues.[54] Fourteen had been examined by the follow-through, 16 by enteroclysis and 4 by both techniques. Eleven of the 18 follow-throughs were abnormal and the actual neoplasm was shown in 6 of the 18. Nineteen of the 20 enteroclysis examinations were abnormal and the neoplasm was shown in 18 out of 20. My own experience would indicate that enteroclysis provides excellent visualisation of carcinomas,[55] lymphoma,[56] carcinoid tumours[57] and secondary neoplasms.[58]

CT plays an important role in the evaluation of neoplastic disorders of the small intestine. Unsuspected disorders may be seen at CT and localised to the small intestine in patients referred for unusual or nonspecific abdominal complaints.[59] Mural and extraluminal components of neoplasms can be evaluated by CT, including changes in the lymph nodes, mesenteric surfaces and peritoneal reflections.[59,60]

Ultrasound has a limited role in evaluating intestinal neoplasms. Like CT unsuspected abnormalities may be detected by ultrasound and require further evaluation by other imaging modalities. Intestinal neoplasms may be diagnosed using a dedicated ultrasound technique.[61,62]

Angiography is frequently used in the investigation of obscure gastrointestinal bleeding and may occasionally detect a malignant neoplasm as the cause of the bleeding. Otherwise angiography has a very limited role in the evaluation of small intestinal malignancy. Different neoplasms show specific features at angiography.[63]

Nuclear medicine imaging does not have a significant role in small intestinal malignancy although the development of tumour specific imaging agents may, in the future, lead to an increasing use of nuclear medicine studies in the diagnosis, management and therapy of functioning small intestinal neoplasms.[64]

## Primary neoplasms

The most frequently encountered primary malignant small intestinal neoplasms are adenocarcinoma, lymphoma, carcinoid tumours and leiomyosarcoma

### CARCINOMA

Adenocarcinoma of the small intestine is uncommon and represents approximately 0.6% of all primary gastrointestinal malignancies.[65] Despite its rarity and even when lesions in the duodenum are excluded, adenocarcinoma is probably the most common primary neoplasm of the small intestine, with a peak incidence in the 6th and 7th decades.[66] Adenocarcinomas are mostly located in the duodenum and proximal jejunum. Most patients present with abdominal pain, which can be vague, intestinal obstruction or chronic blood loss. The prognosis for adenocarcinoma is poor with a five-year survival of 15–28%.[67,68]

Barium studies are more reliable than CT or ultrasound for detecting primary adenocarcinoma[69] and enteroclysis is excellent for demonstrating the neoplasm.[55] Adenocarcinomas are mostly located in the jejunum, particularly the proximal jejunum. The appearances on enteroclysis are similar to those of adenocarcinoma elsewhere in the gastrointestinal tract. Most are infiltrating and are shown as short, well-demarcated, symmetrical, constricting lesions with mucosal destruction and shouldered margins (Fig. 6.16). There is frequently a degree of intestinal obstruction and pre-stenotic dilatation may be present. Polypoid adenocarcinomas are less common and are shown as an irregular filling defect or an irregular polypoid mass with mucosal destruction. Ulceration is seen in most adenocarcinomas, particularly in infiltrating lesions. The ulcers are usually small, although occasionally adenocarcinoma presents as a large cavitating mass.

### LYMPHOMA

Lymphoma is one of the more common neoplasms encountered in the small intestine. The majority are

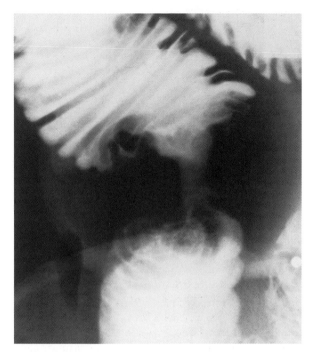

*Figure 6.16* — Carcinoma of the jejunum: an irregular stricture with mucosal destruction and shoulderer margins is shown at an enteroclysis examination.

non-Hodgkins lymphoma. Lymphoma arises in the small intestine either as a primary neoplasm, arising focally from lymphoid tissue[70] or as part of a more widespread disease process.[71] Intestinal lymphoma is considered to be primary if the predominant lesion is in the intestine, the initial presenting symptoms are related to intestinal involvement and there is no evidence of a generalised or intestinal predisposing factor.[56] Disorders that predispose to lymphoma are coeliac disease, chronic lymphatic leukaemia, previous extra-intestinal lymphoma, immunoproliferative small intestinal (α chain) disease and immunological dysfunction, including acquired immunodeficiency syndrome (AIDS).[66] Most primary intestinal lymphomas are in the ileum, where lymphoid follicles are most numerous, with the jejunum the site of involvement in a small percentage of cases.

Abdominal pain, diarrhoea, weight loss and blood loss are the most frequent presenting symptoms. Patients occasionally present acutely with perforation. Intestinal lymphoma has a poor prognosis with an overall 5-year survival of 36% .[56,72]

A broad spectrum of radiological signs is demonstrated by enteroclysis. Characteristic features include luminal narrowing with stricturing, broad-based ulceration, cavitation, thickening of the valvulae conniventes, discrete intraluminal filling defects and an extraluminal mass.[56,66] A large cavitating mass is highly characteristic (Fig. 6.17), although similar lesions may be seen in leiomyosarcoma and metastases. Rarely, the characteristic 'aneurysmal' dilatation may be seen. The lesions are multifocal in up to 40% of patients.[56] Occasionally, small lesions or polyps may be distributed throughout the intestine.

A variety of appearances are exhibited by CT in patients with intestinal lymphoma. These include bulky masses with central cavitation, nodules, aneurysmal dilatation and irregular fold thickening.[59] Lesions in the intestinal wall are relatively homogeneous and there is less contrast enhancement in lymphoma than that seen in leiomyosarcoma or epithelial neoplasms. Evidence of mesenteric lymph node enlargement may be seen and the characteristic 'sandwich' appearance may be seen when the enlarged lymph nodes surround the mesenteric vessels.[73]

CARCINOID

Carcinoid tumours are mostly located in the ileum, particularly in the terminal ileum and are multifocal in about one-third of cases. Small intestinal carcinoids are

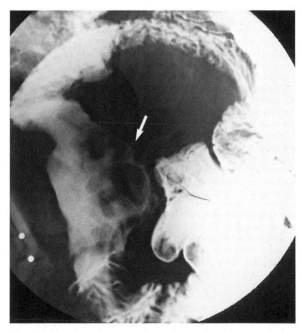

*Figure 6.17* — Lymphoma of the small intestine: a large cavitating mass (arrow) is seen in the ileum in an elderly patient who presented with an episode of acute gastrointestinal bleeding.

considered to be of low grade malignancy with a likelihood to metastasise. The primary lesion may be small and frequently patients present with the carcinoid syndrome in which the characteristic cutaneous flushing and diarrhoea are the dominant symptoms, occurring in the presence of extensive hepatic metastases. The primary tumour, although usually small, may cause abdominal pain which may be non-specific or colicky, characteristic of intestinal obstruction that may be due to recurrent intussusception. A large mass resulting from local invasion and fibrosis may be palpable at the time of presentation. The prognosis is related to tumour size and resectability and prolonged survival is not uncommon with a 5-year survival rate of up to 75% for localised or operable cases.

The radiological signs shown on enteroclysis may be those of the primary lesion itself, those of a secondary mesenteric mass, or those developing from interference with the ileal blood supply.[57,66] Primary ileal carcinoids are seen as sharply defined intramural or intraluminal filling defects with regular margins in the ileum, particularly the distal ileum (Fig. 6.18). Multiple lesions may be present.[74] Narrowing of the lumen with stricture formation is sometimes seen. Hypertrophy of muscle tissue occurs as a result of tumour infiltration with radiologically evident thickening of the valvulae conniventes. In patients with extensive mesenteric fibrosis adjacent loops of ileum are separated, and compressed, making it impossible to identify the primary tumour.

Sharp angulation or kinking of one or more intestinal loops may be seen.

CT shows the intestine, mesentery, lymph nodes and liver in a single investigation and is ideal for staging carcinoid tumours. In patients with extensive mesenteric fibrosis CT demonstrates displacement, kinking or angulation of adjacent loops and the characteristic stellate radiation of mesenteric neurovascular bundles (Fig. 6.19).[75]

LEIOMYOSARCOMA

Leiomyosarcoma is encountered less frequently than adenocarcinoma, lymphoma and carcinoid tumour. Most leiomyosarcomas attain a large size and much of the mass grows extraluminally. Acute bleeding is a common clinical presentation, although occasionally patients present with perforation. Leiomyosarcoma is seen radiologically as a cavitating mass outlined with barium. On CT the rim of the neoplasm around the cavity enhances markedly following intravenous contrast medium.[76]

KAPOSI'S SARCOMA

Kaposi's sarcoma may be seen in the small intestine in association with AIDS and in many cases is asymptomatic. The radiological appearances cover a wide spectrum, including thickened valvulae conniventes, mural thickening, submucosal nodularity, polypoid filling defects and plaque-like lesions.[66]

OTHER PRIMARY MALIGNANT NEOPLASMS

A variety of other extremely rare malignant neoplasms have been reported in the small intestine. They include

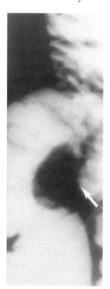

*Figure 6.18* — Small intestinal carcinoid tumour: enteroclysis shows a well-defined intraluminal filling defect (arrow) in the ileum in a patient who was shown to have multiple ileal carcinoids.

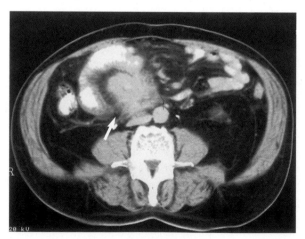

*Figure 6.19* — Carcinoid tumour of the small intestine: CT shows a mass (arrow) with the characteristic stellate radiation of mesenteric neourvascular bundles and thickening of the walls of the adjacent ileum.

angiosarcomas, fibrosarcomas, liposarcomas, malignant schwannomas, lymphangiosarcomas and malignant mesotheliomas[66] The clinical features and radiological appearances do not differ significantly from those of other small intestinal malignancies.

## Secondary Neoplasms

Malignant neoplasms can spread to the small intestine by direct invasion from adjacent structures, by lymphatic extension, by intraperitoneal seeding and by embolic blood-borne metastases.[28,30,77] In some patients more than one mechanism of spread occurs; a combination of direct spread and intraperitoneal seeding is the combination most often seen.[78]

### DIRECT EXTENSION

Direct invasion of the small intestine from carcinomas of the colon, ovary, uterus and kidney may occur and this indicates that an aggressive malignant neoplasm has broken through fascial planes.[28] Intestinal obstruction is the most frequent indication that there is invasion of the small intestine by recurrent colon carcinoma (Fig. 6.20) or gynaecological malignancy, particularly ovarian carcinoma.[79] It is important to distinguish secondary involvement by gynaecological malignancy from chronic radiation enteritis. Chronic radiation enteritis has characteristic appearances, including thickening of the valvulae conniventes, stenosis, mural thickening, mucosal tacking, effacement of the mucosal pattern and adhesions.[80] On CT characteristic appearances of peritoneal metastases are seen and these include omental caking, infiltration of mesenteric lesions and soft tissue attenuation along loops of intestine.[59,81,82]

### LYMPHATIC SPREAD

Lymphatic extension plays a minor role in the spread of neoplasm to the small intestine. A characteristic example is spread of caecal carcinoma to the terminal ileum with resulting stricture formation.[83,84] The first manifestation of caecal carcinoma may be when the patient presents with intestinal obstruction. from ileal stenosis (Fig. 6.21). Narrowing of the lumen with effacement of the mucosal pattern is the characteristic appearances seen at enteroclysis (Fig. 6.21).[79]

### INTRAPERITONEAL SEEDING

Intraperitoneal seeding of abdominal neoplasms to the small intestine occurs as a result of spread via ascitic fluid. Primary neoplasms and even intraperitoneal lymph nodes metastases can shed malignant cells into the ascitic fluid when they break through the peritoneal

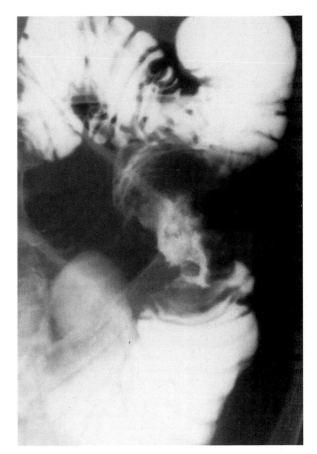

***Figure 6.20*** — Small intestinal invasion by colonic carcinoma: enteroclysis shows a constricting lesion with mucosal destruction, an irregular ulcerating lumen and a degree of shouldering of the margins in the proximal jejunum. At operation this proved to be direct invasion from recurrent carcinoma of the colon. (Reproduced from Nolan 1997[79] with permission).

cavity, although it is not necessary to have much ascites for the transport and deposit of maligant cells.[77] In the peritoneal cavity ascitic fluid flows preferentially along the small intestinal mesentery towards the right lower quadrant. Forty per cent of intraperitoneal seeding is localised in the right lower quadrant and at the lower end of the small intestinal mesentery.[85]

Radiological examination shows characteristic changes in the terminal ileum. These include separation of adjacent loops, often with parallel configuration, multiple scalloped deflections, sometimes with gross mass deflections and distorted, tethered mucosal folds on the mesenteric border. Angulation, fixation and separation of distal ileal loops can occur, particularly in gastric, colonic, pancreatic and ovarian carcinoma.[85]

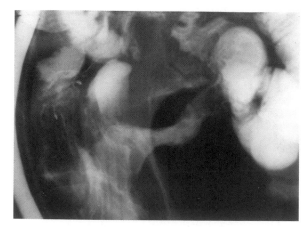

*Figure 6.21* — Secondary involvement of ileum from carcinoma of the caecum: on enteroclysis a stricture with mucosal destruction and shouldered margins is seen at the terminal ileum. At operation this proved to be a caecal carcinoma that had spread via the lymphatics to the terminal ileum.

### EMBOLIC METASTASES

The small intestine is an uncommon site for embolic blood-borne metastases from primary neoplasms at other sites.[28,30] Embolic metastases are frequently multiple and tend to be submucosal. Gastrointestinal bleeding is a common presentation from the central ulceration that develops as the metastases outgrow their blood supply. Other clinical presentations include obstruction, often due to intussusception, and occasionally perforation. Melanoma is one of the most common neoplasms to metastasise to the small intestine.

On barium studies melanoma metastases are mostly seen as multiple filling defects with central ulcers or

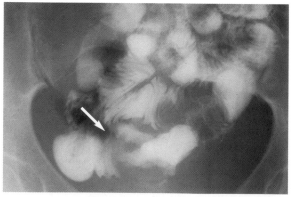

*Figure 6.22* — Metastatic melanoma of the small intestine: on enteroclysis a cavitating mass is demonstrated in the ileum (arrow). The patient, a middle-aged female who had previously had a malignant melanoma resected, presented with acute gastrointestinal bleeding.

cavities outlined with barium. They may be solitary and be seen as a large cavitating mass on barium examination[86] (Fig. 6.22) or CT (Fig. 6.23).

Breast carcinoma occasionally spreads to the small intestine. Metastatic breast carcinoma is mostly seen as an infiltrating lesion that results in stricture formation and obstruction.[28,87] There may be long segment of intestinal narrowing (Fig. 6.24) similar to the infiltrating linitis plastica appearance of breast carcinoma metastatic to the stomach.[79]

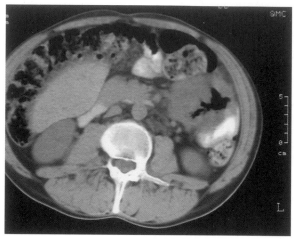

*Figure 6.23* — Metastatic melanoma of the small intestine: a large cavitating mass is shown on the left side of the abdomen on CT. (Coutesy of Dr Fergus Gleeson)

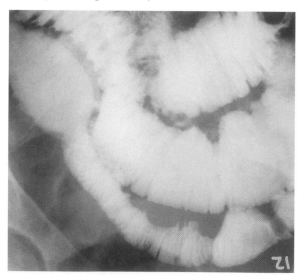

*Figure 6.24* — Metastatic breast carcinoma: a long segment of narrowing is seen in a segment of ileum with effacement of the mucosa on the upper border of the narrowed segment. (Reproduced from Nolan 1997[79] with permission).

Carcinoma of the lung and kidney metastasise on rare occasions to the small intestine. Metastatic lung carcinoma may present as perforation, bleeding or obstruction and is shown radiologically as a large mesenteric mass with infiltration of the intestinal wall.[28] Metastatic renal carcinoma is usually seen as a solitary, bulky intramural mass.[28,88]

# References

1. Cadman PJ, Nolan DJ. The oesophagus, stomach and small intestine. In: Johnson RJ, Eddleston B and Hunter RD, eds. *Radiology in the Management of Cancer*. Edinburgh: Churchill Livingstone, 1990; 151–180.

2. Levine MS, Halvorsen RA. Esophageal carcinoma. In: Gore RM, Levine MS and Laufer I, eds. *Textbook of Gastrointestinal Radiology*. Philadelphia: WB Saunders, 1994; 446–478.

3. Poleyard GD, Marty AT, Birhaun WB, O'Reilly RR. Adenocarcinoma in columnar lined oesophagus. *Arch Surg* 1977; **112**: 997–1000.

4. Mandard AM, Chasle J, Marnay J, et al. Autopsy findings in 111 cases of esophageal cancer. *Cancer* 1981; **48**: 329–335.

5. Sannohe Y, Hiratsuka R, Doki K. Lymph node metastases in cancer of the thoracic esophagus. *Am J Surg* 1981; **141**: 216–218.

6. Levine MS, Dillon EC, Saul SH, et al. Early esophageal cancer. *AJR* 1986; **146**: 507–512.

7. Moss AA, Schnyder P, Theoni RF, Margulis AR. Esophageal carcinoma: pretherapy staging by computed tomography. *AJR* 1981; **136**: 1051–1056.

8. Thompson WM, Halvorsen RA, Foster WL, Williford ME, Postlethwait RW, Korobkin M. Computed tomography for staging esophageal and gastroesophageal cancer: re-evaluation. *AJR* 1983; **141**: 951–958.

9. Halvorsen RA, Magruder-Habib K, Foster WL, Roberts L, Postlethwait RW, Thompson WM. Esophageal cancer staging by CT – long term follow-up. *Radiology* 1986; **161**: 147–151.

10. Shorvon PJ, Lees WR, Frost RA, Cotton PB. Upper gastrointestinal endoscopic ultrasonography in gastroenterology. *Br J Radiol* 1987; **60**: 429–438.

11. Murata Y, Muroi M, Yoshida M, Ide H, Hanyu F. Endoscopic ultrasonography in the diagnosis of esophageal carcinoma. *Surg Endosc* 1987; **1**: 11–16.

12. Mitros FA. Pathology of the oesophagus, stomach and duodenum. In: Appleton HD, ed. *Pathology of the oesophagus, stomach and duodenum*. Edinburgh: Churchill Livingstone, 1984; 1–35.

13. Toreson WE. Secondary carcinoma of the esophagus as a cause of dysphagia. *Arch Path* 1944; **38**: 82–84.

14. Antonioli DA. Gastric cancer. In: Appleman HD, ed. *Pathology of Oesophagus, Stomach and Duodenum* Edinburgh: Churchill Livingstone, 1984; 121–144.

15. Shirakabe H. Early gastric carcinoma. In: Marshak RH, Lindner AE, Maclansky D, eds. *Radiology of the Stomach*. Philadelphia: WB Saunders, 1983; 147–171.

16. Fielding WL, Ellis DJ, Jones BG et al. Natural history of 'early' gastric cancer: results of a ten year regional survey. *Br Med J* 1980; **281**: 965–968.

17. Green PHR, O'Toole KM, Weinberg LM, Goldfarb J. Early gastric cancer. *Gastroenterology* 1981; **81**: 247–256.

18. Cho KC, Baker SR, Alterman DD, Fusco JM, Cho S. Transpyloric spread of gastric tumors: comparison of adenocarcinoma and lymphoma. *AJR* 1996; **167**: 467–469.

19. Yek H-C, Rabinowitz JE. Ultrasound and computed tomography of gastric wall lesions. *Radiology* 1981; **141**: 147–155.

20. Derchi LE, Biggi E, Rolland GA, Cicio GR, Neumaier CE. Sonographic staging of gastric cancer. *AJR* 1983; **140**: 273–276.

21. Lee KR, Levine E, Moffat RE, Bigongiari LR, Hermreck AS. Computed tomographic staging of malignant gastric neoplasms. *Radiology* 1979; **133**: 151–155.

22. Moss AA, Schnyder P, Marks W, Margulis AR. Gastric adenocarcinoma: a comparison of the accuracy and economics of staging by computerized tomography and surgery. *Gastroenterology* 1981; **80**: 45–50.

23. Brady LW, Asbell SO. Malignant lymphoma of the gastrointestinal tract. *Radiology* 1980; **137**: 291–298.

24. Herrmann R, Panahorn AM, Barcos MP, Walsh D, Stutzman L. Gastrointestinal involvement in non-Hodgkin's lymphoma. *Cancer* 1980; **46**: 215–222.

25. Sherrick DW, Hodgson JR, Docherty MB. The roentgenological diagnosis of primary gastric lymphoma. *Radiology* 1965; **84**: 925–932.

26. Pochaczevsky R, Sherman RS. The roentgen appearance of gastric argentaffinoma. *Radiology* 1959; **72**: 330–337.

27. Balthazar EJ. Carcinoid tumours. In: Marshak RH, Lindner AE and Maclansky D, eds. *Radiology of the Stomach*. Philadelphia: WB Saunders, 1983; 205–215.

28. Meyers MA, McSweeney J. Secondary neoplasms of the bowel. *Radiology* 1972; **105**: 1–11.

29. Jaffe N. Metastatic involvement of the stomach secondary to breast carcinoma. *AJR* 1987; **123**: 512–521.

30. Willis RA. *The spread of tumours in the human body*. 3rd edn. London: Butterworth, 1973.

31. Cortese AF, Cornell GN. Carcinoma of the duodenum. *Cancer* 1972; **29**: 1010–1015.

32. Kanematsu M, Imaeda T, Iinuma G et al. Leiomyosarcoma of the Duodenum. *Gastrointest Radiol* 1991; **16**: 109–112.

33. Cho KC. Neoplasms of the duodenum. In: Gourtsoyiannis NC and Nolan DJ, eds. *Imaging of Small Intestinal Tumours*. Amsterdam: Elsevier, 1997; 249–282.

34. Shillito JG, Barlet WC, Graves JW. Tumours of the duodenum. *Am J Surg* 1959; **25**: 91–99.

35. Nolan DJ. The duodenum. In: Grainger RG and Allison DJ, eds. *Diagnostic Radiology – A Textbook of Medical Imaging*. 3rd edn. New York: Churchill Livingstone, 1997; 973–983.

36. Nix GAJJ. Early carcinoma of the ampulla and papilla of Vater. *Clin Radiol* 1980; **31**: 95–100.

37. Craig O. Duodenal carcinoma. *Br J Surg* 1969; **56**: 39–44.

38. Kanematsu M, Imaeda T, Iinuma G, Mon S, Yamawaki Y, Doli H, Takao H. Leiomyosarcoma of the duodenum. *Gastrointest Radiol* 1991; **16**: 109–112.

39. Megibow AJ, Balthazar EJ, Hulnick DH, Naidich DP, Bosniak MA. CT evaluation of gastrointestinal leiomyomas and leiomyosarcomas *AJR* 1985; **144:** 727–731.

40. Frostberg N. Characteristic duodenal deformity in cases of different kinds of peri-varterial enlargement of the pancreas. *Acta Radiol* 1938; **19:** 164–173.

41. Treitel H, Meyers MA, Maze V. Changes in the duodenal loop secondary to carcinoma of the hepatic flexure of the colon. *Br J Radiol* 1970; **43:** 209–213.

42. Treadwell TA, White RR. Primary malignant tumors of the small bowel. *Am J Surg* 1975; **130:** 749–755.

43. Goel IP, Didolkar MS, Elias EG. Primary malignant tumors of the small intestine. *Surg Gynecol Obstet* 1976; **143:** 717–719.

44. Barclay THC, Schapira DV. Malignant tumor of the small intestine. *Cancer* 1983; **51:** 878–881.

45. Gourtsoyiannis NC. General considerations. In: Gourtsoyiannis NC and Nolan DJ, eds. *Imaging of Small Intestinal Tumours.* Amsterdam: Elsevier, 1997; 3–14.

46. Hancock RJ. An 11 years review of primary tumors of the small bowel including duodenum. *Canad Med Assoc* J 1970; **103:** 1177–1179.

47. Nolan DJ, Traill ZC. Review: the current role of the barium examination of the small intestine. *Clin Radiol* 1997; **52:** 809–820.

48. Nolan DJ, Cadman PJ. The small bowel enema made easy. *Clin Radiol* 1987; **38:** 295–301.

49. Nolan DJ. Radiological examination of the small intestine. In: Gourtsoyiannis NC and Nolan DJ, eds. *Imaging of Small Intestinal Tumours.* Amsterdam: Elsevier, 1997; 17–27.

50. Traill ZC, Nolan DJ. Technical note: intubation fluoroscopy times using a new enteroclysis tube. *Clin Radiol* 1995; **50:** 339–340.

51. Theoni RF. Radiography of the small bowel and enteroclysis: a perspective. *Invest Radiol* 1987; **22:** 930–936.

52. Nolan DJ. The true yield of the small-intestinal barium study. *Endoscopy* 1997; **29:** 447–453.

53. Keates TE, Sakai HR. An evaluation of the sources of error in the roentgenologic diagnosis of neoplasms of the small intestine. *Gastroenterology* 1955; **29:** 554–562.

54. Bessette JR, Maglinte DDT, Kelvin FM et al. Primary malignant tumors in the small bowel: a comparison of the small bowel enema and conventional follow-through examination. *AJR* 1989; **153:** 741–744.

55. Papadopoulos VD, Nolan DJ. Carcinoma of the small intestine. *Clin Radiol* 1985; **36:** 409–413.

56. Gourtsoyiannis NC, Nolan DJ. Lymphoma of the small intestine: radiological appearances. *Clin Radiol* 1988; **39:** 639–645.

57. Jeffree MA, Barter SJ, Hemingway AP, Nolan DJ. Primary carcinoid tumours of the ileum: the radiological appearances. *Clin Radiol* 1984; **35:** 451–455.

58. Nolan DJ. Secondary neoplasms. In: Gourtsoyiannis NC and Nolan DJ, eds. *Imaging of Small Intestinal Tumours.* Amsterdam: Elsevier, 1997; 191–211.

59. Megibow AJ. Computed tomography. In: Gourtsoyiannis NC and Nolan DJ, eds. *Imaging of Small Intestinal Tumours.* Amsterdam: Elsevier, 1997; 347–371.

60. Coscina WF, Arger PH, Levine MS, et al. Gastrointestinal tract focal mass lesions: role of CT and barium evaluations. *Radiology* 1986; **158:** 581–587

61. Bin W, Jianguo L, Baowei D. The sonographic appearences of small bowel tumours. *Clin Radiol* 1992; **46:** 30–33.

62. Bin W. Ultrasonography In: Gourtsoyiannis NC and Nolan DJ, eds. *Imaging of Small IntestinalTumours.* Amsterdam: Elsevier, 1997; 323–343.

63. Athanasoulis CA. Angiography. In: Gourtsoyiannis NC and Nolan DJ, eds. *Imaging of Small Intestinal Tumours.* Amsterdam: Elsevier, 1997; 283–308.

64. Vivian G. Nuclear medicine studies. In: Gourtsoyiannis NC and Nolan DJ, eds. *Imaging of Small Intestinal Tumours.* Amsterdam: Elsevier, 1997; 309–321.

65. Williamson RCN, Welch CE, Malt RA. Adenocarcinoma and lymphoma of the small intestine. *Ann Surg* 1983; **197:** 172–178.

66. Gourtsoyiannis NC. Primary malignant neoplasms. In: Gourtsoyiannis NC and Nolan DJ, eds. *Imaging of Small Intestinal Tumours.* Amsterdam: Elsevier, 1997; 105–189.

67. Bridge MF, Perzin KH. Primary adenocarcinoma of the jejunum and ileum. *Cancer* 1975; **36:** 1876–1887.

68. Adler SN, Lyon DT, Sullivan PD. Adenocarcinoma of the small bowel. Clinical features, similarity to regional enteritis and analysis of 338 documented cases. *Am J Gastroenterol* 1982; **77:** 326–330.

69. Kusomoto H, Takahashi I, Yoshida M, et al. Primary malignant tumours of the small intestine: analysis of 40 patients. *J Surg Oncol* 1992; **50:** 139–143.

70. Cooper BT, Read AE. Small intestinal lymphoma. *World J Surg* 1985; **9:** 930–937.

71. Gray GM, Rosenberg SA, Cooper AD, Gregory PB, Stein DT, Herzenberg H. Lymphomas involving the gastrointestinal tract. *Gastroenterology* 1982; **82:** 143–152.

72. Makepeace AR, Fermont DC, Bennett MH. Gastrointestinal non-Hodgkin's lymphoma. *Clin Radiol* 1987; **38:** 609–614.

73. Mueller PR, Ferrucci JT, Harbin WP, Kirkpatrick RH, Simeone JF, Wittenberg J. Appearance of lymphomatous involvement of the mesentery by ultrasound and body computed tomography. The 'sandwich' sign. *Radiology* 1980; **134:** 467–473.

74. Jeffree MA, Nolan DJ. Multiple ileal carcinoid tumors. *Br J Radiol* 1987; **60:** 402–403.

75. Gould M, Johnson RJ. Computed tomography of abdominal carcinoid tumour. *Br J Radiol* 1986; **59:** 881–885.

76. Price J, McGuire LJ, Chan MSY. Case of the month. Multiple mystifying melaenas. *Br J Radiol* 1988; **61:** 521–522.

77. Meyers MA. Intraperitoneal spread of malignancies and its effect on the bowel. *Clin Radiol* 1981; **32:** 129–146.

78. Meyers MA. *Dynamic Radiology of the abdomen: Normal and Pathologic Anatomy.* New York; Springer Verlag, 1976.

79. Nolan DJ. Secondary neoplasms. In: Gourtsoyiannis NC, Nolan DJ, eds. *Imaging of Small Intestinal Tumours.* Amsterdam: Elsevier, 1997; 193–211.

80. Mendelson RM, Nolan DJ. The radiological features of chronic radiation enteritis. *Clin Radiol* 1985; **36:** 141–148.

81. Levitt RG, Sagel SS, Stanley RJ. Detection of neoplastic involvement of the mesentery and omentum by computed tomography. *AJR* 1978; **131:** 835–838.

82. Walkey MM, Friedman AC, Sohotra P, Radecki PD. CT manifestations of peritoneal carcinomatosis. *AJR* 1988; **150:** 1035–1041.

83. Grinnell IR. Lymphatic block with atypical and retrograde lymphatic metastases and spread in carcinoma of the colon and rectum. *Ann Surg* 1966; **163:** 272–280.

84. Moffat RE, Gourley WK. Ileal lymph node metastases from cecal carcinoma. *Radiology* 1980; **135:** 55–58.

85. Meyers MA. Mesenteric seeding along the small bowel mesentery. *AJR* 1975; **123:** 67–73.

86. Pomerantz H, Margolin HN. Metastases to the gastrointestinal tract from malignant melanoma. *AJR* 1962; **88:** 712–717.

87. Rees BI, Okwonga W, Jenkins IL. Ileal metastases from carcinoma of the breast. *Clin Oncol* 1976; **2:** 113–119.

88. Khilmani MT, Wolf BS. Late involvement of the alimentary tract by carcinoma of the kidney. *Am J Dig Dis* 1960; **5:** 529–540.

89. Phillips AJ, Nolan DJ. Radiology of oesophageal dysphagia. *Br J Hosp Med* 1995; **53:** 458–466.

# 7

# THE COLON AND RECTUM

Clive I Bartram

**Colorectal cancer**
**Carcinoid tumours**
**Lymphoma**
**Kaposi sarcoma**
**Leiomyosarcoma**

Malignant tumours of the colorectum may be considered as being of epithelial origin or from some other component of the bowel wall, but those of epithelial origin are by far the most important. Colorectal cancer (CRC) is now the second commonest cancer in England and Wales, with about 28 000 new cases and 19 000 related deaths annually. Some 20% present with metastases and the 5-year survival rate of 40% has remained unchanged for some years.

In the non-colitic population, CRC arises from changes in adenomatous tissue described as the adenoma-cancer sequence. An adenoma is a circumscribed elevation of intraepithelial neoplasia. Dysplasia within adenomas may be graded as mild, moderate or severe. Severe dysplasia is more frequent in large or villous type adenomas. Penetration of dysplastic cells into the submucosa defines cancer.

The level of lymphatic supply to the mucous membrane of the gastrointestinal tract varies. Dysplastic cells must be able to enter the lymphatic circulation for the tumour to behave as a cancer. There is no lymphatic tissue in the mucosa of the colon and rectum, only relatively few lymphatics in the muscularis mucosa, but a rich plexus in the submucosa. As a result lymphatic spread occurs in colorectal tumours only when dysplastic cells have crossed the muscularis mucosa layer into the submucosa. This is the basis for the definition of CRC and why 'carcinoma in situ' is not recommended as a term to describe severe dysplasia that does not penetrate beyond the muscularis mucosa.

The meticulous analysis of resected rectal cancer specimens by Dukes demonstrated a clear relationship between the extent of tumour invasion of the rectal wall, lymph node involvement and survival. The Dukes classification (Table 7.1) has been widely modified, but remains the basis for staging CRC. Tumour permeation into the submucosal veins seems to have little effect on prognosis, but once the extramural thick-walled veins become affected, there is a significant reduction in survival due to metastatic disease, which is independent of the Dukes stage. Metastases may involve the liver (75%), lungs (15%), bones (5%) and brain (5%). Tumour penetration of the visceral peritoneum results in transcoelomic spread. Malignant cells may be implanted at anastomotic, abdominal wall incision or colostomy sites, but locoregional recurrence implies continued growth of residual malignant tissue from inadequate resection.

Imaging has several roles in CRC: diagnosis of the precursor of CRC, the adenomatous polyp, and of overt cancer and staging of that cancer. Interventional imaging-based techniques may play an increasing role in the management of advanced cancer. Treated patients require follow-up and first-degree relatives should be investigated to exclude polyps.

# Colorectal cancer

## Diagnosis

Although the number of barium enemas is falling due to increasing primary referral to colonoscopy, the barium enema and in particular the double contrast barium enema (DCBE) remains an important method for polyp and cancer detection. Compared to colonoscopy, the DCBE is cheaper and considerably safer with a mortality of <1 in 50 000[1] and should always demonstrate the proximal colon. Total colonoscopy is difficult in about 25% where diverticular disease is present or in females with long transverse colons.[2] Colonoscopic localization of tumours is difficult. This rarely causes problems with standard surgical resection, but if laparoscopic resection is planned, DCBE is useful to confirm the site of the tumour, as resection of a tumour in the transverse colon is not feasible technically.

Size, shape, surface texture and number should be used to define polyps (Fig. 7.1). The risk of cancer is negligi-

Table 7.1 Dukes staging for colorectal cancer.

| Stage | Description | 5-year survival (rectal: colonic) |
| --- | --- | --- |
| A | Muscularis propria not breached | 80: 85% |
| B | Muscularis propria breached but no nodal involvement | 55: 67% |
| C | Regional nodes involved | 32: 37% |

NB This staging is based on histological examination of the resected specimen. Stage C has been divided into C1 where the apical node is not involved and C2 where it is. Stage D may be used to indicate the presence of distant metastases, but was not part of the original description by Dukes.

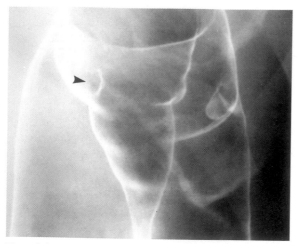

*Figure 7.1* — Two sessile polyps on a DCBE. One shows a meniscus around the base of the polyp only (arrowhead), the other a meniscus around the base and a coating over the surface to form the classical "hat sign".

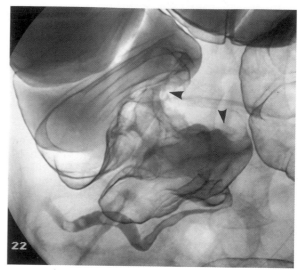

*Figure 7.2* — Carcinoma adjacent to the ileo-caecal valve, presenting as a irregular mass (arrowheads).

ble (<1%) in polyps <1 cm in diameter, increasing to >20% for polyps of >2 cm. Most series relating the incidence of cancer to polyp size are based on endoscopic measurement. There is considerable magnification during DCBE, so that a polyp measuring 1 cm may be only 7 mm endoscopically. A radiological size of <1 cm is therefore conservative. Polyps that are pedunculated are often considered benign, but this is a misconception. The incidence of cancer in the head of the polyp is similar to that for a sessile lesion. However, even if the head of the polyp is malignant, the risk of spread into the bowel wall is negligible providing the stalk is intact. Once this is invaded, the lesion reverts to a sessile appearance.

The natural history of adenomas remains unclear, but recent work suggests that small polyps (<1 cm) frequently undergo spontaneous regression.[3] Larger polyps may have mutated oncogenes that make further growth with malignant transformation more likely.

Cancers are typically either polypoid or annular, depending on invasive growth within the bowel wall. Flat, plaque-like lesions represent an early stage of annular growth and are the most difficult to image on DCBE (Fig. 7.2). The detection rate for CRC by DCBE is 85–9%.[4] Perceptive error is the commonest reason for missing a lesion and highlights the value of double reading examinations.[5]

Flexible sigmoidoscopy followed by DCBE detects all significant colorectal neoplasia[6] and may be used in

cancer screening where flexible sigmoidoscopy is negative to exclude proximal disease (Fig. 7.3).

Cancers may be picked up on routine transabdominal US. Filling the colon with water has been used to improve detection and staging.[7] In elderly, infirm patients, where bowel preparation would be difficult, an unprepared CT is a useful alternative to DCBE or colonoscopy.[8] Helical CT and fast MR sequences enable large volumes of data to be acquired in a single breath hold, and has increased the utility of these techniques for examining the bowel. However, the data sets obtained are too large to review in a standard fashion. Advances in computer processing and 3D software developments have allowed volume rendering and cine

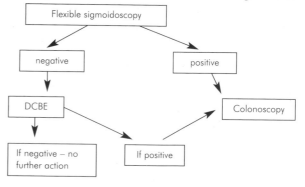

DCBE = double contrast barium enema

*Figure 7.3* — Algorithm for CRC detection based on initial flexible sigmoidoscopy[6]

loop techniques to be applied. CT colography can resolve 70% of polyps of 5 mm in diameter.[9] IV contrast enhancement highlights any neoplastic lesion as both adenomas and cancers are highly vascular, which helps define the tumour. Although 3D reconstructions are currently time consuming, this technology holds great promise and may soon find a place in routine investigation.

If a distal cancer has been diagnosed, total colonic examination is still indicated to exclude further neoplasia that may be impalpable at operation. Synchronous lesions are present in 4–5%. Colonoscopy may be difficult as the tumour inhibits manipulation of the endoscope. Bowel preparation is often poor, so that visualization of the proximal colon is not ideal. The same restriction also applies to a DCBE, but a complete examination should usually be possible and sufficient to exclude a further carcinoma or large polyp.[11]

## Staging

Dukes classification is a pathological one. For cross-sectional imaging, the TNM system[12] is more relevant (Table 7.2).

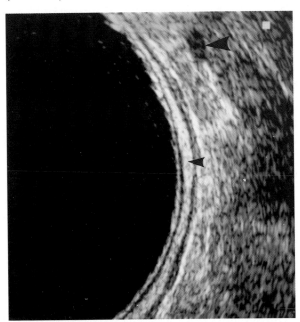

***Figure 7.4*** — Normal rectal wall on endosonography. The submucosa is a prominent central reflective layer (small arrowhead). Outside this is the muscularis propria, divided into two layers by a thin reflective fascia. Inside the submucosa is the low reflective layer of the deep mucosa and then the first interfac e reflection with the surface of the mucosa. A small benign lymph node (large arrowhead) is noted.

Table 7.2   TNM Classification of CRC.[12]

| Description |  |
| --- | --- |
| **T Stage** | |
| T1 | Tumour invades submucosa |
| T2 | Tumour invades muscularis propria |
| T3 | Tumour invades through muscularis propria into subserosa or non-peritonealized pericolonic or perirectal tissues |
| T4 | Visceral peritoneum or adjacent structure invaded |
| **N Stage** | |
| N0 | No regional node metastasis |
| N1 | 1–3 pericolic or perirectal nodes involved |
| N2 | >3 pericolic or perirectal nodes involved |
| N3 | Involved nodes along any named vascular trunk |
| **M Stage** | |
| M0 | No distant metastasis |
| M1 | Distant metastases |

### THE PRIMARY TUMOUR (T STAGING)

'T' staging describes how far the tumour has penetrated the bowel wall and related structures. CT and MRI are limited to showing if a lesion is intramural (i.e. T1 or T2) or extramural (i.e. T3 or T4). The only modality capable of defining the various wall layers is endosonography and this is the most accurate method for staging rectal cancers.

The normal rectal wall has a five-layer sonographic pattern (Fig. 7.4), which is made up of interface reflections as well as reflections from actual tissue layers. Interface reflections occur at junctions between tissue layers of different acoustic impedance. The thickness of the reflection depends on the axial resolution of the transducer. The five layers are as follows:

1. The first inner layer is a narrow bright interface between the water-filled balloon and mucosal surface.

2. Deep to this is a narrow band of low reflectivity from the deep mucosa. The muscularis mucosae is not visualized as a separate layer and is thought to be part of an interface reflection merging into the submucosa.

3. The submucosa is a prominent central reflective band. This appears wider sonographically than it is histologically, as the interface reflection with the muscularis propria extends down into the muscle layer, making this appear narrower and the submucosa wider.[13]

4. The muscularis propria is of low reflectivity. A thin reflective fascial plane divides the inner circular layer from the outer longitudinal layer. This may be detected using high resolution probes of 10 MHz or more.

5. At the outer border of the muscle layer is the fifth outer layer, which is another interface reflection with the fascia and perirectal fat.

A disposable enema is required to cleanse the rectum. Rigid probes may be inserted blind into the distal rectum, but higher insertion necessitates passing the probe through a short sigmoidoscope to negotiate the rectal folds. A water-filled balloon system maintains acoustic contact with the rectal wall.

Rectal endosonography (RES) requires experience. It is important to view the entire lesion at right angles to the wall to obtain proper staging. This is difficult with lesions on the posterior wall of the ampulla and is a significant cause of incorrect staging.[14] Most systems for RES use axial imaging. This is one instance where a linear probe is helpful. Artefacts during RES are common.[15] A typical problem is air, either in the balloon or between the balloon and the lesion, causing acoustic shadowing.

Cancers are of low reflectivity and easy to distinguish from normal bowel wall (Fig. 7.5). A peritumoural reaction composed of inflammatory cells, oedema and fibrosis is usually present and is the most likely explanation as to why the T2 tumours are most frequently overstaged. Maier et al[16] suggest that this layer may be

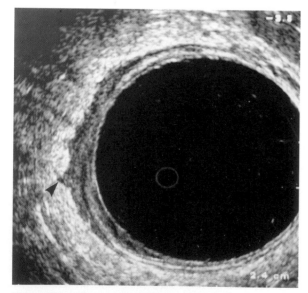

***Figure 7.5*** — T3 cancer showing tumour extending outside the muscle layer (arrowhead) into the perirectal fat.

recognized as a rim of reduced reflectivity around the lesion. Excluding this layer from the staging process increased accuracy from 70% to 95%.

Endoscopic sonography[17] allows a tumour in any part of the colon to be staged. However, this facility is not widely available. Colonic hydrosonography, where a water-filled colon is scanned by transabdominal US, may be used instead with 70% accuracy and a claimed 100% sensitivity for infiltration of adjacent structures.[18] Endoscopic staging could be important in the resection of malignant polyps to exclude deep infiltration of the bowel wall or lymph node involvement.

CT is more accurate than MRI in staging rectal cancer for >T3 (74 vs 58%),[19] but has about the same accuracy for colon cancers (62 vs 64%).

The majority of cancers are resected regardless of stage and preoperative knowledge of the tumour stage is required in relatively few situations:

1. Large rectal tumours that seem fixed on clinical examination require imaging to confirm invasion of adjacent structures. CT pre- and post-radiotherapy indicated.

2. Small rectal tumours that are mobile and suitable for local excision transanally should be examined sonographically. The lesions should be T2, N0, of low grade malignancy and <3.5 cm in diameter for a local excision.

3. Malignant change in large villous adenomas is difficult to detect clinically but contraindicates submucosal resection. RES is indicated preoperatively.

4. Adjuvant chemotherapy (5 flurouracil ± levamisole or folinic acid) may be recommended for more advanced cancers (<T2). Developments in adjuvant chemotherapy are potentially the most important indication for preoperative staging.

5. If laser therapy is planned, it is important to know the thickness of a tumour and proximity of structures such as the bladder.

LYMPH NODE INVOLVEMENT (N STAGING)

Infiltration of the lymphatic system is a highly significant factor in survival, as indicated by the Dukes classification, where lymphatic involvement places the tumour into grade C regardless of the depth of bowel wall infiltration.

*In vitro* sonography of perirectal and pericolic lymph nodes suggests that benign nodes are typically ovoid, heterogeneous in reflectivity and <5 mm in diameter, whereas malignant nodes are rounded, homogeneous in reflectivity and >5 mm in diameter. Nodal enlargement may be due to tumour infiltration or non-specific inflammatory change. Tumour replacement of the internal nodal architecture should produce a homogeneous echopattern of low reflectivity. The internal architecture is maintained with non-specific changes and typically these nodes show increased reflectivity. However, there is considerable overlap and some 60% of nodes cannot be differentiated on sonographic images.[20] Only about half the nodes present in an operative specimen can be seen during *in vitro* scanning and during *in vivo* endosonography it is impossible to scan a field equivalent to that of the surgical specimen with a rigid rectal probe. It is therefore not surprising that endosonography is relatively inaccurate in determining N stage. From pooled data a kappa of only 0.58 is reported.[21]

CT and MRI have a lower sensitivity than endosonography, of about 45% for detecting malignant adenopathy. This is based on visualizing a node of any size in a position where nodes are not normally seen, i.e. the perirectal fat, or demonstrating nodes >1 cm anywhere.

Overall the imaging of nodal involvement is very disappointing. The fundamental problem lies in the nature of metastases to lymph nodes. Micrometastases within an otherwise normal node will not be detected, and nodes involved by micrometastases may be very small. In one study metastases were present in 32% of nodes of 5 mm or less and in 8% of nodes of 2 mm or less along the superior rectal artery chain.[22] Clearance of involved perirectal nodes is essential to prevent local recurrence. Tumour rests may be found in the mesorectum for up to 3 cm distal to the primary tumour. Lymph node clearance up to 5 cm is therefore recommended for tumours in the mid and lower rectum and is achieved by total mesorectal (perirectal fascia) excision.[23] Incomplete clearance is considered to be the cause of high local recurrence rates (>10%). Internal iliac nodes are involved in 30% and are always secondary to mesorectal node involvement.

Advances in immunoscintography may improve imaging in this field, but the problem of micrometastases is still a limiting factor.

METASTASIS (M STAGING)

About 20% of patients presenting with CRC have metastatic spread and >50% will develop hepatic metastases during the course of the disease. There are two main pathways for haematogenous spread depending on the site of the primary tumour. Tumour cells from rectal cancers may enter the systemic circulation as the rectal venous plexi drain via the middle and inferior rectal veins into the hypogastric veins and inferior vena cava. Only the portal circulation is involved in colonic tumours, with drainage via the superior and inferior mesenteric veins. Pulmonary metastases may develop without hepatic involvement in rectal cancers, whereas these are always secondary to hepatic spread in colonic lesions.

Documentation of hepatic metastases has become important as hepatic resection is now a practical therapeutic option. Imaging has a vital role in patient selection. Criteria for resection are the presence of <5 liver metastases and the absence of systemic spread or hepatic nodal involvement. At least 30% of normal liver must remain following resection to avoid liver failure. About 12% of CRC cases have metastases confined to the liver and some 25–50% of these may be suitable for surgical resection. Successful resection significantly improves 5-year survival.

It is probable that many tumour cells enter the portal circulation. Metastases are more common in the right lobe, not only because this is larger, but also a lamella flow may direct dependent tumour emboli into the right portal branch. Most of these perish in the endothelial lining of the sinusoids without implantation. It is possible that some pass directly through into the hepatic veins and pulmonary circulation, but most pulmonary metastases, with the exception of rectal cancer, arise from cells shed by hepatic metastases. An alternative route for metastatic emboli to reach the pulmonary bed is via the lymphatic system. Tumour cells may escape from the nodal chain into the thoracic duct and so into the systemic venous system.

Pulmonary and bony metastases are seen in about 5% at the time of diagnosis. A chest radiograph is part of routine preoperative screening and is adequate in most cases. Skeletal investigation with nuclear medicine scanning is undertaken only for symptomatic disease.

There are two particular situations where metastatic disease detection is poor: hepatic lymph node involvement and small volume deposits on the peritoneal surface. There is early spread from liver metastases via lymphatics into the hepatic nodes. These are located deep to the common duct surrounding the first part of the duodenum and are extremely difficult to image. Peritoneal seeding of <0.5 cm in size is also not detectable even with a meticulous CT technique.[24]

## Imaging techniques for liver metastasis

Transabdominal US has the advantages of being a simple, rapid and readily available technique ideally suited for screening, though it is less accurate, especially for smaller metastases, than other cross-sectional modalities. The reflectivity of metastases may be equal, increased or decreased relative to normal parenchyma. There is often a surrounding low reflective halo of compressed tissue that helps outline the lesion. Cystic change is not seen with CRC metastases, though larger metastases may undergo necrosis. Punctate calcification is diagnostic of a metastasis from a mucinous secreting adenocarcinoma (Fig. 7.6). Diffuse disorganization of the hepatic parenchyma is a subtle pattern to recognize. A mass effect from the metastasis alters the contour of superficially placed lesions or compresses central tubular structures.

In one series the overall detection of focal liver lesions was 68% for CT, 63% for MRI and 53% for US.[25] Only 20% of lesions of <1 cm in diameter were detected by US, compared to 49% by CT. Reports[26–28] suggest that Doppler measurement of the ratio of hepatic artery to the portal vein blood flow, termed the Doppler perfusion index (DPI), is a highly sensitive index for metastatic disease. Of those 80 consecutive cases whose DPI was normal, 97% were disease-free after 2 years, compared to recurrent disease in 78% of those with elevated DPI.[26] It is suggested that an abnormal DPI is a significant risk factor for metastatic disease, sufficient to warrant chemotherapy (28). Intraoperative US is capable of detecting lesions of ≤ 5 mm in diameter and is considered more accurate than CT arteriography.[27] However, follow-up of patients with negative intraoperative US[29] has shown that 16% develop liver metastases, proving that a significant proportion of metastases escape all attempts to be imaged.

Metastases receive their blood supply mainly from the hepatic artery, with only a little from the portal venous circulation. Intravascular contrast may be used to enhance contrast between tumour and normal parenchyma to improve tumour conspicuity.[30] Intra-arterial injection into the hepatic or superior mesenteric artery has been used to maximize filling of tumour circulation when the parenchymal background will only be minimally enhanced as during the arterial phase there will be no contrast in the portal circulation. This will be most beneficial with hypervascular tumours. CRC metastases are generally hypovascular, nevertheless CT arteriography of the liver has been considered the most accurate method for the preoperative detection of CRC metastases.

CT arteriography will be impractical for most UK departments. Scanning in the portal venous phase after IV contrast is essential to maximize tumour detection (Fig. 7.7). Injection of 100 ml of contrast agent at a rate of 3 ml/s using a pump, with 5 mm slices is recommended after a 45 s delay. If the patient is given a bowel preparation, gas insufflation of the colon with IV buscopan to prevent bowel motility, may be used to visualize the primary lesion. If the tumour is known to be in the pelvis, this should be scanned at 5 mm slices, otherwise 10 mm for the abdomen (Fig. 7.8). An entire

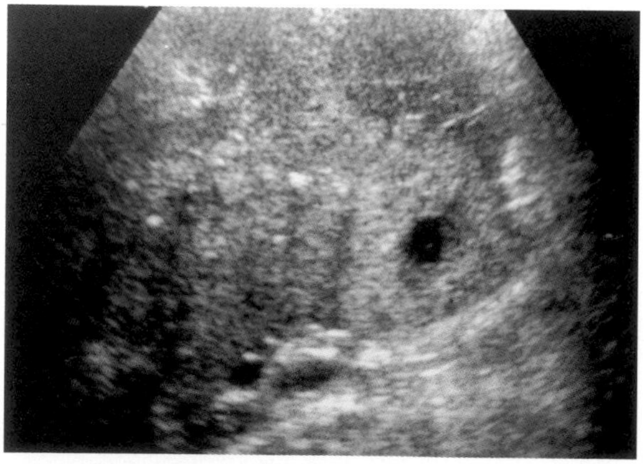

*Figure 7.6* — US of the liver showing a large diffuse metastasis with some scattered bright foci. These were due to microcalcification from a mucinous secreting adenocarcinoma. A small area of necrosis is noted in part of the metastasis.

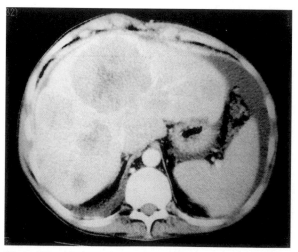

*Figure 7.7* — Enhanced CT scan of the liver during the portal phase revealing a number of metastases of varying size. Some ascites is present.

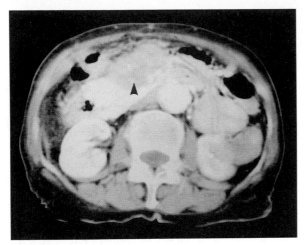

*Figure 7.8* — CT scan just below the liver revealing a large peritoneal deposit (arrowhead).

assessment of the primary tumour and intra-abdominal or hepatic spread may therefore be made during one study.[10]

## Follow-up

Within a year of surgery, a 'clean' colon, i.e. one without any polyp, should be established. Colonoscopy is preferred for this as a polyp of any size may be significant. After this baseline examination, DCBE or colonoscopy may be recommended at 3–5 yearly inter-

vals until the age of 70, although there is no evidence that this increases survival. Repeat liver scanning is recommended for the first 2 years to detect any potentially resectable metastasis. With a high grade rectal tumour and low anterior resection, repeat rectal endosonography is indicated[31] to pick up recurrent disease early and at a resectable stage. Locoregional recurrence is about 10%. A rising CEA titre is a useful marker for recurrent disease and warrants repeat CT, chest X-ray and possibly bone scan.

There is a problem differentiating scar tissue from recurrence on CT. Where applicable, needle biopsy provides histological confirmation. PET scanning and MRI may also be helpful.[32]

The family history is important in CRC and the patient's relatives must also be considered. The risk of CRC in first-degree relatives is 2–4 times that of the general population. Two genetically determined conditions place relatives at a much greater risk. Familial adenomatous polyposis accounts for 1% of CRC in the UK and should be picked up by the presence of numerous adenomas throughout the colon and rectum. All members of the family will need screening and a Polyposis Registry conducts this most effectively. Hereditary non-polyposis colorectal cancer (HNPCC) is more common, accounting for about 5% of CRC. In the Lynch Type I variant (hereditary site-specific colon cancer) flat adenomas may be present, there is a greater incidence of right-sided cancers and the risk of syn-

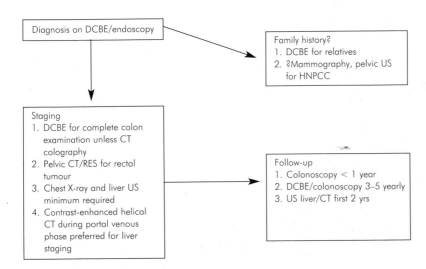

DCBE = double contrast barium enema; HNPCC = hereditary non-polyposis colorectal cancer; RES = rectal endosonography.

*Figure 7.9* — Algorithm for CRC management

chronous tumours is very high, estimated at 3% annually. In the Type II (or cancer family syndrome) cancers may be found at other sites, notably uterus, breast, ovary, stomach and pancreas. HNPCC patients require more intensive screening of the colon and in Type II cancers other sites must also be screened with mammography and pelvic US.

## Carcinoid tumours

Carcinoid tumours arise from the enterochromaffin cells belonging to the Amine Precursor Uptake and Decarboxylation (APUD)-cell system. Overall, they account for about 6% of all malignant epithelial lesions in the colon and rectum. A small (<1 cm) submucosal nodule in the rectum is a common presentation. Large polypoid lesions may develop in the colon. Ulceration suggests the lesion has metastasized. Size is a good indication of the risk of metastasis, with 15% of those <1 cm metastasizing, rising to >75% for tumours of >2 cm in size. As liver metastases are hypervascular they are best seen in the hepatic arterial phase of biphasic helical CT,[30] and tend to be well defined and bright on US. The carcinoid syndrome is relatively rare with colorectal tumours, but when present implies diffuse metastatic disease.

## Lymphoma

Primary lymphoma of the colon represents <1% of all malignant colorectal tumours. It is commonest in the caecum or rectum at the sites where lymphoid tissue is most abundant. The tumour may be annular, polypoid or ulcerated, and is frequently larger than CRC. Aneurysmal dilatation may occur. Another rare presentation is diffuse polyposis, with multiple small submucosal nodules that are typically umbilicated. The differential diagnosis for this is malignant melanoma or metastatic carcinoma. Lymphoid polyposis should not be confused with familial adenomatous polyposis or lymphoid hyperplasia, where the lesions are not umbilicated in adults, <2 mm in size and usually limited to part of the colon.

The primary lesion may be diagnosed on DCBE, but CT will be required for staging nodal and extranodal involvement.

## Kaposi sarcoma

Kaposi sarcoma is a systemic multifocal tumour of the reticuloendothelial system that is common in AIDS patients. The process starts with diffuse submucosal nodules, which coalesce to form a narrowed segment with irregular folds. Typical changes are seen on DCBE. CT will demonstrate surrounding inflammatory change in the mesentery and local lymph node enlargement.

## Leiomyosarcoma

Now classified as being neurogenic in origin, these tumours are of low grade malignancy, with local recurrence and the capability to metastasize. They are most commonly situated in the rectum and only the intraluminal part is visible on DCBE. CT or TRUS reveal the mural and extramural components.

## Conclusion

Micrometastases in lymph nodes and the liver limits the accuracy of current imaging techniques. Developments in radiolabelled monoclonal antibody using a hand held detector during surgery might provide a way forward,[33] but there is still a major role for imaging during the oncological management of colorectal neoplasia.

## References

1. Blakeborough A, Sheridan MB, Chapman AH. Complications of barium enema examination: a survey of UK consultant radiologists 1992–4. *Clin Radiol* 1997; **52**: 142–148.

2. Saunders BP, Fukumoto M, Halligan S *et al*. Why is colonoscopy more difficult in women? *Gastrointest Endosc* 1996; **43**: 124–126.

3. Hofstad B, Vatn MH, Andersen SN *et al*. Growth of colorectal polyps: redetection and evaluation of unresected polyps for a period of three years. *Gut* 1996; **39**: 449–456.

4. Stevenson G. Screening for colorectal cancer and suspected lower gastrointestinal bleeding. *Abdom Imag* 1995; **20**: 381–383.

5. Brady AP, Stevenson GW, Stevenson I. Colorectal cancer overlooked at barium enema examination and colonoscopy: a continuing perceptual problem. *Radiology* 1994; **192**: 373–378.

6. Hough DM, Malone DE, Rawlinson J *et al*. Colon cancer detection: an algorithm using endoscopy and barium enema. *Clin Radiol* 1994; **49**: 170–175.

7. Hernandez-Socorro CR, Guerra C, Hernandez-Romero J, Rey A, Lopez-Facal P, Alvarez-Santullano V. Colorectal carcinomas: diagnosis and preoperative staging by hydrocolonic sonography. *Surgery* 1995; **117**: 609–615.

8. Dixon AK, Freeman AH, Coni NK. CT of the colon in frail elderly patients. *Semin Ultrasound CT MR* 1995; **16**: 165–172.

9. Hara AK, Johnson CD, Reed JE *et al*. Detection of colorectal polyps by computed tomographic colography: feasibility of a novel technique. *Gastroenterology* 1996; **110**: 284–290.

10. Amin Z, Boulos PB, Lees WR. Technical report: spiral CT pneumocolon for suspected colonic neoplasms. *Clin Radiol* 1996; **5**: 56–61.

11. Isabel-Martinez L, Chapman AH, Hall RI. The value of a barium enema in the investigation of patients with rectal carcinoma. *Clin Radiol* 1988; 39: 531–533.

12. Spiessl B, Beahrs OH, Hermanek P *et al. UICC TNM Atlas*. New York, Berlin: Springer-Verlag, 1992.

13. Kimmey MB, Martin RW, Haggitt RC, Wang KY, Franklin DW, Silverstein FE. Histologic correlates of gastrointestinal ultrasound images. *Gastroenterology* 1989; **96**: 433–441.

14. Herzog U, von Flue M, Tondelli P, Schuppisser JP. How accurate is endorectal ultrasound in the preoperative staging of rectal cancer? *Dis Colon Rectum* 1993; **36**: 127–34.

15. Hulsmans FH, Castelijns JA, Reeders JW, Tytgat GN. Review of artifacts associated with transrectal ultrasound: understanding, recognition, and prevention of misinterpretation. *J Clin Ultrasound* 1995; **23**: 483–494.

16. Maier AG, Barton PP, Neuhold NR, Herbst F, Teleky BK, Lechner GL. Peritumoral tissue reaction at transrectal US as a possible cause of overstaging in rectal cancer: histopathologic correlation. *Radiology* 1997; **203**: 785–9.

17. Yoshida M, Tsukamoto Y, Niwa Y *et al*. Endoscopic assessment of invasion of colorectal tumors with a new high-frequency ultrasound probe. *Gastrointest Endosc* 1995; **41**: 587–592.

18. Dux M, Roeren T, Kuntz C, Richter GM, Kauffmann GW. TNM staging of gastrointestinal tumors by hydrosonography: results of a histopathologically controlled study in 60 patients. *Abdom Imag* 1997; **22**: 24–34.

19. Zerhouni EA, Rutter C, Hamilton SR *et al*. CT and MR imaging in the staging of colorectal carcinoma: report of the Radiology Diagnostic Oncology Group II. *Radiology* 1996; **200**: 443–451.

20. Nielsen MB, Qvitzau S, Pedersen JF. Detection of pericolonic lymph nodes in patients with colorectal cancer: an *in vitro* and *in vivo* study of the efficacy of endosonography. *Am J Roentgenol* 1993; **161**: 57–60.

21. Solomon MJ, McLeod RS. Endoluminal transrectal ultrasonography: accuracy, reliability, and validity. *Dis Colon Rectum* 1993; **36**: 200–205.

22. Dworak O. Number and size of lymph nodes and node metastases in rectal carcinomas. *Surg Endosc* 1989; **3**: 96–99.

23. Heald RJ, Ryall RD. Recurrence and survival after total mesorectal excision for rectal cancer. *Lancet* 1986; **1**: 1479–1482.

24. Sugarbaker PH. Surgical decision making for large bowel cancer metastatic to the liver. *Radiology* 1990; **174**: 621–626.

25. Wernecke K, Rummeny E, Bongartz G *et al*. Detection of hepatic masses in patients with carcinoma: comparative sensitivities of sonography, CT and MR imaging. *Am J Roentgenol* 1991; **157**: 731–739.

26. Leen E, Angerson WG, Cooke TG, McArdle CS. Prognostic power of Doppler perfusion index in colorectal cancer. Correlation with survival. *Ann Surg* 1996; **223**: 199–203.

27. Solomon MJ, Stephen MS, Gallinger S, White GH. Does intraoperative hepatic ultrasonography change surgical decision making during liver resection? *Am J Surg* 1994; **168**: 307–310.

28. Leen E, Goldberg JA, Robertson J *et al*. Early detection of occult colorectal hepatic metastases using duplex colour Doppler sonography. *Br J Surg* 1993; 80: 1249–1251.

29. Paul MA, Blomjous JG, Cuesta MA, Meijer S. Prognostic value of negative intraoperative ultrasonography in primary colorectal cancer. *Br J Surg* 1996; **83**: 1741–1743.

30. Oliver III JH, Baron JH. Helical biphasic contrast-enhanced CT of the liver: technique,indications, interpretation, and pitfalls. *Radiology* 1996; **201**: 1–14.

31. Ramirez JM, Mortensen NJ, Takeuchi N, Humphreys MM. Endoluminal ultrasonography in the follow-up of patients with rectal cancer. *Br J Surg* 1994; **81**: 692–694.

32. Ito K, Kato T, Tadokoro M *et al*. Recurrent rectal cancer and scar: differentiation with PET and MR imaging. *Radiology* 1992; **182**: 549–552.

33. Cote RJ, Houchens DP, Hitchcock CL *et al*. Intraoperative detection of occult colon cancer micrometastases using 125 I-radiolabled monoclonal antibody CC49. *Cancer* 1996; **77**: 613–620.

# 8

# THE LIVER, BILIARY SYSTEM AND PANCREAS

Michel Lafortune and Luigi Lepanto

**Hepatic tumours**
**Bile duct tumours**
**Pancreatic neoplasms**

This chapter describes the imaging methods used in the investigation of tumours of the liver, bile ducts and pancreas. The algorithms used may vary from centre to centre, depending on available modalities and expertise. Knowledge of the strengths and weaknesses of each examination allows the physician to select appropriate screening and to understand the logical order of further tests.

# Hepatic tumours

Presenting symptoms in patients with liver tumours are often non-specific. Symptoms reflect the primary disease in patients with metastases or cirrhosis, or may be due to increased liver size. Clinical signs include jaundice and a right upper quadrant mass. Most liver tumours are incidental findings at sonography or CT performed for other reasons. Table 8.1 shows the pathologic classification of liver tumours.[1,2] The commonest tumours in clinical practice are discussed.

**Table 8.1** Pathologic classification of liver tumours.

*Benign tumours*

*hepatocellular:*
simple cyst
focal nodular hyperplasia
adenoma
nodular regenerative hyperplasia

*mesenchymal:*
haemangioma
lymphangiomatosis
angiomyolipoma
lipoma

*epithelial and mesenchymal*
teratoma

**Malignant tumours**
*Primary*
*hepatocellular:*
hepatoblastoma
hepatocellular carcinoma
fibrolamellar carcinoma

*vascular:*
angiosarcoma
haemangioendothelioma epithelioid

*muscle tissue:*
leiomyosarcoma
rhabdomyosarcoma

*Secondary:*
metastasis

## Benign tumours

SIMPLE CYSTS

One of the most frequent masses of the liver (up to 20%), cysts are usually incidental findings at sonography performed for other reasons. Single or multiple, they are lined by a single layer of cuboidal epithelium. The differential diagnosis includes biliary cysts and echinococcal infections; the latter usually results in multilocular cysts. When multiple (as in association with polycystic kidneys), they may cause liver enlargement. Rarely they cause pain and jaundice by compression of bile ducts and surgical treatment is needed.[3] The diagnosis of a simple cyst is straightforward at sonography and complementary tests are rarely required. When first seen with CT, sonography may be used to confirm the diagnosis.

HAEMANGIOMA

This is the most frequent benign mesenchymal tumour of the liver and occurs in 0.7–7% of the general population, with a peak incidence at age of 30–50 years. Haemangiomas are thought to represent hamartomatous lesions, a consequence of an acquired hepatic arteriolar malformation. Because haemangiomas occur more frequently in women than in men, a possible relationship with oestrogen or progesterone has been suggested. Haemangiomas are usually found incidentally at sonography or CT. Haemangiomas of >4 cm may manifest as right upper quadrant pain, hepatomegaly or as an abdominal mass.[4] This lesion is not pre-malignant. Bleeding after trauma or biopsy is a rare but potentially serious complication. The tumours are well demarcated, ranging in size from a few millimetres to more than 20 cm. They are composed of blood-filled spaces of varying size. The centre of the lesion, especially when large, is mucinous or fibrous.

On *sonography* the majority (+ 70%) of haemangiomas are hyperechogenic and show acoustic enhancement. They are usually smaller than 3 cm. Some lesions are atypical (hypoechogenic, isoechogenic or heterogenous) especially when greater than 3 cm in diameter or when the lesion occurs in a fatty liver. Very large haemangiomas (>5 cm) usually have a hyperechogenic external rim and a hypoechogenic centre. When compressed, haemangiomas may 'disappear', being suddenly isoechogenic with the rest of the parenchyma. This phenomenon is easily observed in the operating room where compression of the haemangioma by the transducer is easy. No blood flow is detected with Doppler sonography.[5]

On CT, lesions are classically hypodense before injection of contrast medium and the periphery of the lesion enhances rapidly after injection. The centre becomes progressively filled with contrast on delayed sequences (3–60 min after the injection).[6] This description is true in 55–80% of haemangiomas. Small lesions, multiple lesions or lesions with fibrosis tend to be more difficult to categorize with CT. Rarely, metastatic lesions may mimic haemangiomas on CT studies.

MRI is sensitive and specific, both over 90%, in the diagnosis of haemangiomas (Fig. 8.1). The lesion is hypointense on T1-weighted images and hyperintense on T2-weighted images. The latter persist even on images with longer TE. Haemangiomas are homogenous, well circumscribed, often with polylobulated contours. Specificity and sensitivity of MRI for the diagnosis of hemangiomas is over 90%. Cysts may look like haemangiomas at MRI, but are readily characterized with sonography. The injection of paramagnetic agents serves as a diagnostic tool for giant hemangiomas. The sequences of enhancement from the periphery to the centre of the lesion is similar to that seen with CT.

Haemangiomas, especially when large (>2 cm), can be readily diagnosed with red blood cell scintigraphy. The combination of a photopenic lesion on HIDA or colloid scans, decreased perfusion on the flow study and increased activity within the lesion on the blood pool study is characteristic of haemangiomas. The sensitivity and specificity of radionuclide scintigraphy is between 80 and 90%.

Biopsy of haemangiomas is rarely performed because of the danger of haemorrhage, which may be fatal. However, haemorrhage after biopsy is very rare, especially when the lesion is surrounded by normal liver parenchyma which tends to contain any haemorrhage. Biopsy of peripheral lesions should be avoided.

*What should be done in practice?* If a lesion is thought to be a haemangioma at sonography. and if the patient is asymptomatic, with normal liver tests, no other test is necessary. A follow-up study is performed 6 and 12 months later. Haemangiomas usually have not grown on subsequent exams.[7] If the patient is cirrhotic or if the patient has cancer, MRI is performed. If the lesion is more than 3 cm in diameter, MRI is still the best tool, but CT and scintigraphy can be used.

## FOCAL NODULAR HYPERPLASIA

Focal nodular hyperplasia (FNH) is a benign lesion of unknown origin; it may represent a hamartoma or a response to a vascular malformation.[8] It affects all ages and is more common in women. Anovulant therapy may stimulate growth of FNH. FNH is usually asympto-

matic (75%) and is usually an incidental finding on CT or ultrasound. FNH is a well-demarcated, non-encapsulated nodule, often solitary, measuring less than 5 cm in diameter. Characteristically there is a central scar with radiating vascular structures encased in fibrous septa. Between the septa are hyperplastic nodules composed of normal hepatocytes. The lesion usually projects from the surface of the liver and is often pedunculated.

On sonography FNH is usually a homogenous lesion, isoechogenic with the surrounding liver. It lacks a capsule and may therefore be difficult to detect. A bulge on the surface of the liver may be the initial manifestation. Sometimes a central scar is seen. Doppler sonography (Fig. 8.2) may be quite characteristic: a feeding artery is seen in the centre of the lesion which gives rise to arteries which radiate in a spoke-wheel fashion. Contrary to malignant tumours, venous signals are rarely seen within FNH.[9]

On MRI FNH is typically an isointense lesion on all pulse sequences. A central scar is present in 70–85% of lesions: it is hypointense on T1-weighted images and hyperintense on T2 weighted images. FNH is enhanced by contrast injection. No capsule is seen. When all these features are present, the MRI diagnosis is specific.

With Technetium 99m colloid scintigraphy, FNH shows three patterns of uptake: iso-, hypo- or hyperfixation. Iso- and hyper-fixation are the most frequent and the most characteristic.

FNH is iso- or hypo-dense on pre-contrast CT examinations. Soon after bolus injection of contrast medium, there is contrast enhancement of the lesion. During the portal phase, the lesion becomes isodense. The central scar is visible in only 15–45% of patients.

*What should be done in practice?* FNH is a benign lesion and there is no reason for excision, except for the rare situation where the lesion causes symptoms (abdominal pain due to torsion or compression). If FNH is suspected at Doppler sonography, and MRI confirms the diagnosis, the investigation can stop there. Annual follow-up of the lesion with Doppler sonography may be undertaken.

## ADENOMA

This rare tumour bleeds readily and occurs mainly in women (male:female = 1:9), between the ages of 15 and 45 years. It is related to the use of oral contraceptives: the incidence increases 20–100 fold after 5 years and 500-fold after 7 years of anovulant therapy. Regression of adenomas has been reported after with-

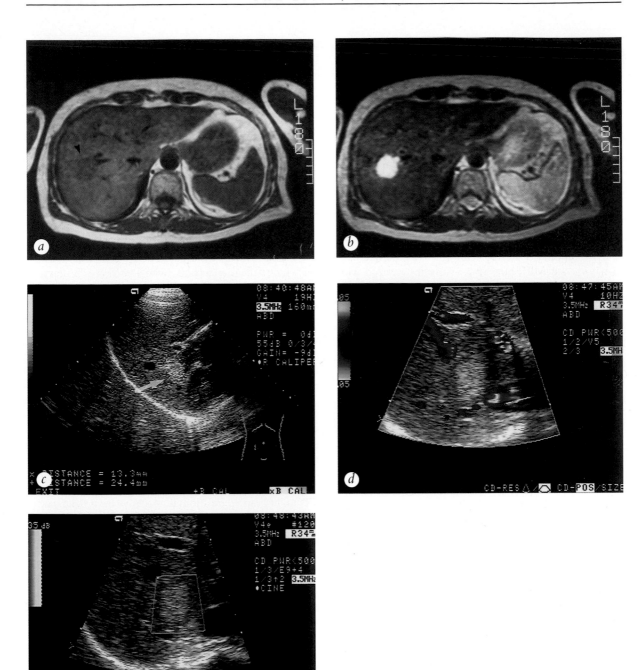

***Figure 8.1*** — Haemangiomas. MRI of the liver: a) T1-weighted image shows a 2 cm hypointense mass in the right lobe. b) The lesion becomes hyperintense on T2- weighted image. c) Sonographic examination (another example): a uniformly hyper-echogenic mass is outlined. d) No Doppler signals are identified with colour or e) power mode.

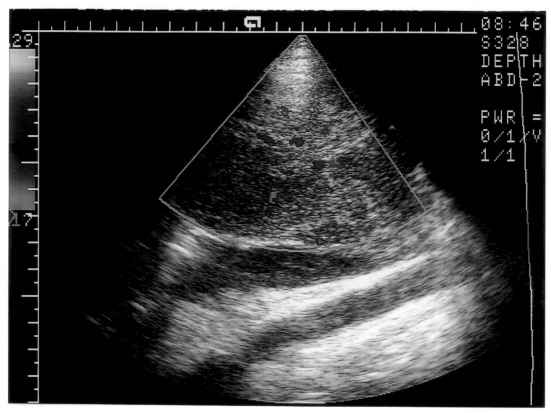

***Figure 8.2*** — Focal nodular hyperplasia: Colour Doppler sonography shows vessels radiating from the centre of a mass towards the periphery. This is a classic appearance of a FNH at Doppler sonography.

drawal of oral contraceptives. Since 1990, the incidence of adenoma has declined, probably because the dose of oestrogen in anovulants has been greatly reduced. Patients with glycogenosis (type I and III) and males treated with androgenic steroids also have a higher incidence of adenomas, and their risk of malignant transformation is higher than in women taking oral contraceptives. The patient with an adenoma may be asymptomatic or may present with an abdominal mass or chronic abdominal pain. When bleeding occurs in the mass or the peritoneum, patients may have acute abdominal pain. Serum α-fetoprotein levels are normal. Adenomas are well demarcated, occasionally encapsulated, solitary tumours, that can be quite large (5–30 cm). At histology, adenomas are composed of hepatocytes slightly larger than normal, which frequently have a pale cytoplasm because of glycogen or fat accumulation. Infarction and haemorrhage are frequently present and are followed by fibrosis. Unlike normal liver parenchyma, adenomas do not have portal or central veins, nor bile ducts. They are vascularized by large arteries entering from the periphery of the mass.

On sonography adenomas usually have the same echogenicity as the surrounding liver. However, they are often heterogeneous with hypoechogenic (necrotic) areas. They can be well demarcated with a hypoechogenic rim. The surrounding vessels are compressed, but not invaded. The hepatic artery feeding the lesion is usually dilated. Peripheral vessels are well visualized with colour Doppler sonography and identified as arteries or veins with pulsed Doppler. The centre of the mass usually contains vessels with venous flow. Sonographic surveillance of the lesion is indicated when surgery is contraindicated.

Adenomas usually present as photopenic lesions on sulphur colloid scintigraphy.

Adenomas differ from FNH in their heterogeneous architecture. On T1-weighted MR images, adenomas are usually hypo- or iso-intense. In 30%, a hypointense rim is present. Haemorrhagic areas or fat within the mass are seen as hyperintense signals. On T2-weighted images, hypointense bands of tissue are seen and represent necrosis or haemorrhage.[10]

Haemorrhagic areas are usually clearly seen with unenhanced CT. After contrast injection the lesion is seen as a heterogeneous mass. No central scar is identified.

As the treatment is often surgical, adenomas are rarely biopsied. If doubt exists as to the exact mature of an adenoma, excision is indicated, since the distinction between adenoma and hepatocarcinoma may be impossible to make with imaging methods.

*What should be done in practice?* When MRI with or without CT indicates that the lesion is not FNH or if doubt persists, the diagnosis of adenoma is likely but must be distinguished from hepatocarcinoma. Surgery may be necessary. The role of biopsy (guided with sonography or CT) is still uncertain.

## Malignant tumours

### HEPATOCARCINOMA

Hepatocarcinoma (HCC) usually occurs in association with chronic liver disease, especially cirrhosis. There is a higher incidence of HCC where viral hepatitis is common, especially in Asia and sub-Saharan Africa, and where there is exposure to various hepatocarcinogens (e.g. aflatoxine). HCC is rare in the western hemisphere. Non-alcoholic postnecrotic cirrhosis is more frequently associated with HCC than alcoholic cirrhosis. HCC has an earlier age of onset in countries with a high incidence of hepatitis (third decade rather than seventh to eighth decade). HCC occurs more frequently in men than in women. In countries with a low incidence of HCC, the onset of symptoms is insidious and includes malaise, anorexia, fever and abdominal pain. Jaundice is rare. In regions with a high incidence of HCC, the clinical symptoms may be more dramatic and include abdominal distension and spontaneous tumour rupture, with massive haemoperitoneum. The α-fetoprotein levels are often elevated in patients with HCC. Several classifications exist, based on the gross appearance of HCC. Eggel's (1901) is still much in use and serves as the basis for newer classifications. There are three types:

1) Massive: there is a single large mass (with or without satellite nodules);

2) Nodular: there are multiple small nodules;

3) Diffuse: multiple, indistinct nodules are seen throughout the liver.

Tumour masses tend to necrose and bleed. Capsules are frequent and tend to become thicker as tumour size increases. They are composed of fibrous tissue and compressed vessels and bile ducts.[11] HCC tends to invade portal veins and, more rarely, hepatic veins, the inferior vena cava and bile ducts.[11] Metastatic seeding tends to occur via the portal veins within the liver. Extrahepatic spread of tumour occurs late in the course of the disease.

The sonographic appearance of HCC is variable. In Asia, HCC may have a high fat content (fatty metamorphosis) and the lesion may present as an echogenic mass. Elsewhere, HCCs are usually hypoechogenic, sometimes heterogeneous (especially if >3 cm), with a surrounding hypoechogenic rim. The chaotic intratumoural vascularization can be outlined with colour and pulsed Doppler sonography. A network of neovasculature with abnormal blood flow is often detected with Doppler sonography: high systolic Doppler shifts are outlined, as well as evidence of arteriovenous shunting. This is the result of angiogenesis stimulated by the tumour. Such Doppler shifts are detectable at the periphery of a number of malignant tumours within the abdomen. Tumour thrombi within the portal veins may contain arterial blood flow, detected with pulsed Doppler (Fig. 8.3); this is characteristic of tumour thrombus. The sensitivity of sonography in the diagnosis of HCC is good (around 90%). It tends to be less sensitive in eastern countries, probably because HCC grows in cirrhotic livers, where small tumours blend into the nodular liver architecture. Tumours are difficult to detect until they reach 2–3 cm in diameter. The same is true of HCC complicating metabolic diseases in children (e.g. tyrosinaemia and glycogenosis).

HCCs are photopenic at sulphur colloid scintigraphy. There is an accumulation of gallium in 90% of masses.

The appearance on T1-weighted MR images is variable (low-, iso-, high- or mixed-intensity). They are hyperintense on T2-weighted images. Fat content and the surrounding pseudocapsule are hyperintense on T1-weighted images. Invasion of vessels by HCC is clearly shown with MRI.

On unenhanced CT, HCCs are usually hypodense. On dynamic CT the mass enhances rapidly during the arterial phase but becomes iso- or hypo-dense in the portal phase. The capsule usually enhances and necrosis within the tumour is seen as an hypodense area. Haemoperitoneum and invasion of portal and hepatic veins and of the inferior vena cava can be detected with CT. Because HCCs trap the contrast agent Lipiodol that is injected into the hepatic artery, the tumours become highly visible on CT and remain so for several weeks. Small seeding tumours, which are otherwise difficult to detect, become readily visible with this technique.

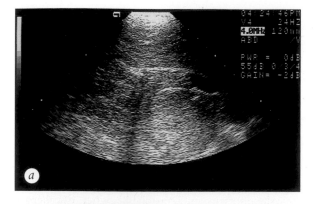

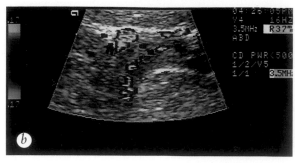

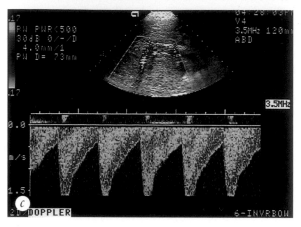

*Figure 8.3* — Hepatocarcinma: vascularized tumour thrombus. a) The sonographic examination of the left lobe of the liver shows thrombus extending into the lumen of the left portal vein. b) Colour Doppler shows signals originating from the thrombus. c) At pulsed Doppler, these are identified as high velocity signals, characteristic of flow in tumour vessels.

HCC is a vascular tumour that is seen on arteriography The hepatic arteries are usually enlarged, with neovascularization, arteriovenous shunts and vascular invasion. Arteriography is rarely performed for diagnostic purposes, but rather as a therapeutic gesture or for the study of the extension of HCC using Lipiodol.

Chronic liver disease carries an increased risk of HCC and any nodule within the already heterogeneous cirrhotic liver may be an HCC. If α-fetoprotein levels are high, a nodule is most probably an HCC. If levels are low, a nodule could still be an HCC, but could also represent a metastasis or a regenerative nodule. A nodule in a cirrhotic patient is more likely to be an HCC than any other focal lesion. If excision or embolization is planned, guided biopsy is performed. If liver transplantation is planned, biopsy is avoided because of the possible recurrence of HCC along the path of the biopsy.

*What should be done in practice?* Routine screening for HCC is performed with sonography.[12] The majority of HCCs are clearly seen on sonography, as long as the lesion diameter is at least 2 cm and technical factors are optimal. Where clinical doubt exists and the α-fetoprotein level is elevated, other imaging methods are useful in detecting the HCC, especially CT following intraarterial Lipiodol injection. Doppler sonography, CT and MRI are good tools to evaluate the portal and hepatic veins and possible invasion by the tumour.

METASTASIS

Common primary sites of liver metastasis include the lung, colon, breast and pancreas. As many as 50% of patients dying of cancer have hepatic metastases. In western countries, metastases are the commonest liver tumour. HCC is relatively more frequent in Asia. Symptoms from metastases relate to their number, the primary cancer site and the hepatic reserve. At times a patient may present with liver metastases when no primary site is known. Patients may be asymptomatic for a long time before hepatic insufficiency occurs. Jaundice and ascites are late events. When metastases are found the patient is referred for the optimum specific treatment. Surgical removal of liver metastases from a colon cancer in patients who have undergone resection of the primary tumour and regional lymphadenectomy and who have no evidence of extrahepatic metastatic disease gives a 5-year survival of 25%.[13]

On sonography metastases are visualized as nodules of various echogenicity. Most are hypoechogenic and surrounded by a poorly defined halo. Their size and architecture are unrelated to the primary tumour. Many studies have compared the rate of detection of metastasis with sonography to other imaging techniques and have shown that the sensitivity of sonography is at best equal to CT and MRI. The experience of the operator, the time taken to perform the study and the quality of the ultrasound machine are important factors in determining the precision of the sonographic examination. Intraoperative sonography is more sensitive and highly useful in guiding excision. Ultrasound contrast agents are used in clinical practice in some centres in Europe and are used experimentally in North America. These agents improve contrast between lesions and liver parenchyma and enhance the detection of tumour vascularity.

Single-photon-emission CT is more sensitive than conventional planar scintigraphy. Scintigraphy is less sensitive than CT or ultrasound, and for this reason, is not used as the primary screening method for metastatic disease.

On CT the typical appearance of a liver metastasis is that of a focal, round lesion that is less dense than the normal surrounding parenchyma. Other patterns may also be seen: heterogeneous architecture, hyper- or isodense or diffuse invasion. The use of intravenous contrast agents increases contrast between the focal lesion and the normal liver. On dynamic CT there may be mild enhancement of the periphery of the lesion; conversely, the entire lesion may be less dense than the contrast-enhanced parenchyma. On delayed CT, metastatic adenocarcinoma may display a distinct pattern: the centre is dense and the periphery has low uptake of contrast. CT arterial portography is the most sensitive tool for detecting liver metastases.

Most metastatic lesions are homogeneous and less intense than normal liver on T1-weighted MR images and inhomogeneous and hyperintense on T2-weighted images.

Biopsy of a possible metastasis is performed before specific treatment. It can be performed with CT or ultrasound guidance to confirm that the lesion is linked to the known primary cancer.

*What should be done in practice?* In screening for hepatic metastasis the sensitivity and specificity of the imaging method should be high and the examination cost effective. In experienced hands, sonography is quite sensitive

and specific, low in cost and widely available. CT and MRI are complementary tests. CT arterial portography is helpful in certain circumstances such as before a segmental hepatectomy in a patient who has already undergone a metastasectomy. There is an increasing number of tumours markers (CEA, CA 125, AFP, CA-50, etc.) but none is specific for liver metastasis.

# Bile duct tumours

In terms of clinical presentation, neoplasms of the biliary tree can be divided into three groups according to their site of origin: intrahepatic biliary tree, extrahepatic biliary tree and gallbladder. Tumours originating from the intrahepatic ducts present much like other liver lesions. Signs and symptoms are often non specific and jaundice is uncommon unless disease is widespread. On the other hand, jaundice is the hallmark of tumours of the extrahepatic biliary tree. Neoplasms of the gallbladder have a more insidious onset at presentation and are usually discovered incidentally or when disease is advanced. A more comprehensive classification of biliary tree neoplasms is outlined in Table 8.2. Most of these tumours are rare and only those encountered most frequently are discussed.

## Biliary cystadenoma cystadenocarcinoma

Tumours originating from the intrahepatic bile ducts behave clinically like other intrahepatic tumours. Although classified as a benign tumour, cystadenoma has the potential for malignant transformation and surgical excision is indicated. Furthermore, there is no way to distinguish between cystadenoma and cystadenocarcinoma on the basis of imaging criteria alone.[14] There is a strong female preponderance and 90% of these tumours arise from the intrahepatic bile ducts. When small these tumours are usually discovered serendipitously during evaluation of the upper abdomen with ultrasound or CT. When large enough to cause symptoms, these are usually non-specific and include right upper quadrant discomfort and only rarely jaundice. On both ultrasound and CT examinations these appear as multiloculated cysts with thickened septations and mural nodules.

## Adenoma of the gallbladder

Benign neoplasms of the biliary tree are rare, with the exception of adenomas of the gallbladder. These are most often an incidental finding during abdominal ultrasound and present as solitary, small polyps originating from the wall. They are not mobile and do not produce acoustic shadowing. Malignant potential is low and they

**Table 8.2** Pathologic classification of neoplasms of the bile duct and gall-bladder.

### Bile duct

*Benign neoplasms*

    papillary adenoma
    cystadenoma
    granular cell tumour
    mesenchymal tumours
    heterotopic gastric mucosa

*Malignant neoplasms*

    cholangiocarcinoma
    periampullary carcinoma
    embryonal rhabdomyosarcoma

### Gallbladder

*Benign neoplasms*

    adenoma
    granular cell tumour
    mesenchymal tumours

*Malignant neoplasms*

    primary adenocarcinoma
    mesenchymal sarcoma
    metastatic carcinoma

are usually followed sonographically. Criteria for surgical excision include a size greater than 1 cm, a solitary lesion, associated gallstones, age greater than 50 years and progression on serial ultrasound examinations.[15]

## Adenocarcinoma of the gallbladder

Adenocarcinoma of the gallbladder is more common in older female patients and is associated with gallstones in 90% of cases. Porcelain gallbladder is associated with an increased incidence of carcinoma of the gallbladder.[16] Jaundice is not as commonly seen as in cholangiocarcinoma, unless the disease is widespread. Adenocarcinoma of the gallbladder has a propensity to spread locally, invading the liver, the common hepatic and common bile ducts, and adjacent intestinal structures.

In patients with right upper quadrant pain but no jaundice the initial imaging study is undoubtedly abdominal ultrasound. The presence of a mass in the gallbladder fossa, a poorly discernible gallbladder and the presence of gallstones are compatible with the diagnosis (Fig. 8.4). In fact, gallbladder carcinoma is more commonly associated with a solitary stone, especially if it is displaced by a mass or focal wall thickening.[17] The diagnosis is not always easy to make and one must maintain a

high degree of clinical suspicion in the proper clinical context.

CT plays a complementary role and helps confirm the diagnosis and determine the extent of tumour spread. Ultrasound and CT are usually sufficient to diagnose carcinoma of the gallbladder and can guide percutaneous biopsy when necessary. Usually, the malignant nature of the disease process is not in doubt and imaging serves to confirm the diagnosis and determine surgical resectability.

## Cholangiocarcinoma

Cholangiocarcinoma is most commonly extrahepatic in location; however, 20% of cholangiocarcinomas occur intrahepatically and their clinical presentation is indistinguishable from other intrahepatic focal lesions. Intrahepatic cholangiocarcinomas can be further subdivided into peripheral and central lesions. The peripheral tumours are mass lesions occurring deep in the liver parenchyma while central lesions, also known as Klatskin's tumour, involve the bile duct bifurcation and are rarely identified as a mass lesion.[17-20] Cholangiocarcinoma involving the extrahepatic bile ducts invariably presents with jaundice. Clinically it is usually indistinguishable from other periampullary tumours which include carcinoma of the ampulla, pancreatic cancer and duodenal carcinoma.

Ultrasound is the screening test of choice to eliminate hepatic causes of cholestatic jaundice.[21] Cholangiocarcinomas are often small and not seen on imaging studies which show biliary dilatation to the point of obstruction, usually the distal common hepat-

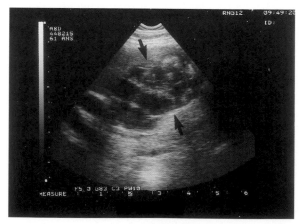

***Figure 8.4*** — Adenocarcinoma of the gallbladder. Sonographic examination of the gallbladder: The poorly defined mass (arrows) invading the liver in the gallbladder fossa represents adenocarcinoma of the gallbladder.

ic duct or the proximal common bile duct. This should suggest the diagnosis.

The site of obstruction can usually be reliably determined by a combination of ultrasound and CT. These modalities also allow elimination of extrinsic compression (e.g. liver masses, hilar adenopathy) as a cause of obstruction.

Confirmation of the site of obstruction is usually obtained by direct opacification of the bile duct either endoscopically (i.e. endoscopic retrograde cholangiography) or transhepatically (i.e. transhepatic cholangiography). Cholangiography reveals a severe segmental stenosis, an abrupt cut-off, or, more uncommonly, a filling defect. The transhepatic approach is usually favoured because of the risk of contamination with enteric organisms with a retrograde approach.[22]

Magnetic resonance cholangiography is a new technique which may represent a non-invasive alternative to depict the biliary tree.[23]

*What should be done in practice?* The purpose of imaging is to establish the diagnosis, but also to determine the extent of disease and the possibility of surgical cure. The combination of ultrasound and CT allows the assessment of hepatic metastases, local and regional lymph nodes and contiguous spread to adjacent organs. Vascular invasion can be assessed with angiography; however, new techniques with spiral CT and 3-dimensional vascular recon-

structions may preclude the use of angiography (Fig. 8.5a and b). Although there are reports of MRI in the evaluation of tumours of the biliary tree, this modality is not used routinely in the work-up of these patients.

# Pancreatic neoplasms

The pancreas functions both as an endocrine and an exocrine gland. Neoplasms can be classified according to the cell type of origin (Table 8.3). In terms of clinical presentation, however, these tumours can be divided into three groups: tumours of the head of the pancreas, tumours of the body of the pancreas and islet cell tumours. This is not a histologic classification but, from the perspective of imaging work-up, it is useful to divide pancreatic neoplasms in this way. Tumours of the head of the pancreas often present with jaundice and are indistinguishable, on purely clinical grounds, from cholangiocarcinomas and periampullary tumours. Neoplasms of the body and tail of the pancreas usually present with epigastric pain radiating to the back, anorexia and weight loss. These tumours are usually discovered later than those of the head of the pancreas and are subsequently larger at the time of diagnosis.

## Ductal adenocarcinoma

The commonest neoplasm of the pancreas is ductal adenocarcinoma.

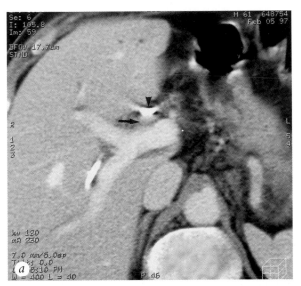
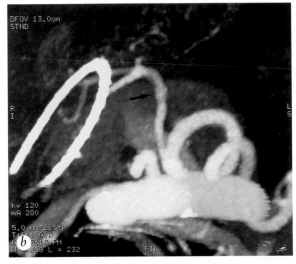

***Figure 8.5*** — Cholangiocarcinoma. *a)* CT of the liver: Small tumour (arrow) in the porta hepatis is a cholangiocarcinoma. There is a an endoprosthesis in the bile duct (arrowhead). *b)* Three-dimensional vascular reconstruction following spiral CT shows partial encasement of the hepatic artery (arrow).

**Table 8.3** Classification of pancreatic neoplasms

*Duct cell origin*
    Solid: duct cell adenocarcinoma
           solid and papillary epithelial neoplasm
           variant carcinoma
    Cystic: congenital cyst
           microcystic adenoma
           mucinous cystic adenoma

*Acinar cell origin*
        acinar cell carcinoma
        acinar cell cystadenocarcinoma

*Islet cell origin*
        insulinoma
        gastrinoma
        glucagonoma
        somatostatinoma
        VIPoma

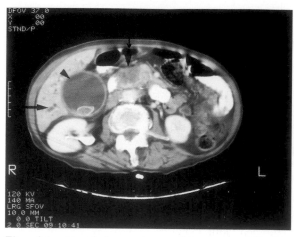

***Figure 8.6*** — Ductal adenocarcinoma of the pancreas. CT of the abdomen: Hypoattenuating mass in the head of the pancreas (short arrow) with intrahepatic bile duct dilatation (long arrow) and gallbladder distension (arrowhead).

Ultrasound is a useful initial imaging test to rule out hepatic causes of jaundice, but CT is the examination of choice for the diagnosis and staging of pancreatic cancer.[15] With proper technique, over 95% of tumours are detected. CT after intravenous contrast administration typically demonstrates lesions as hypoattenuating masses within the pancreas (Fig. 8.6). Associated pancreatic duct and biliary duct dilatation is also seen. When the tumours are large, areas of necrosis with cystic changes can be seen centrally. Less commonly, adenocarcinoma presents as diffuse involvement of the gland. When the tumour is small, only the indirect sign of pancreatic duct dilatation is seen. Imaging is important in staging disease to determine surgical resectability.

Findings that render lesions inoperable include regional lymph node metastases, distant metastases (e.g. liver), vascular encasement, contiguous spread to adjacent organs (e.g. kidney, bowel) and ascites. CT and angiography have traditionally been used to rule out vascular involvement, but spiral CT (i.e. CT-angiography) with or without 3-dimensional vascular reconstructions, as well as Doppler ultrasound, are now more widely used and may replace angiography for this particular purpose.[24,25]

At times very small tumours can only be demonstrated at endoscopic retrograde pancreatography (ERCP), which shows abrupt cut-off or short segmental stenosis with proximal dilatation. Dilatation of the pancreatic duct and the common bile duct (i.e. the double duct sign) is a classic finding.

The role of MRI was recently evaluated in a multicentre study and was found to offer no significant advantage over CT.[26]

Biopsy is not indicated if surgical cure is possible because of the risk of tumour seeding along the biopsy needle tract. Biopsy is sometimes requested to obtain histologic confirmation of the disease when the tumour is deemed inoperable.

## Cystic tumours of the pancreas

Cystic tumours of the pancreas are much less common and include microcystic adenomas (serous cystadenoma) and macrocystic adenomas (mucinous cystadenoma). Both have a higher incidence in female patients. Microcystic adenomas are found in older patients and have no malignant potential, whereas macrocystic adenomas occur in younger patients and have malignant potential.

Distinguishing features can be demonstrated both by ultrasound and CT. Microcystic adenomas contain numerous small cysts whose diameters do not exceed 1–2 cm. Septa are usually thin and there is sometimes a central scar that can calcify. These tumours can occur anywhere in the pancreas, but are more frequent in the head. Macrocystic adenomas are multiloculated with multiple cystic lesions each measuring more than 2 cm in diameter (Fig. 8.7). Septa are thick and can contain calcifications. These tumours tend to be larger than microcystic adenomas with mean diameter of 10 cm and tend to occur in the body and tail of the pancreas. Biopsy can aid in differentiating these two cystic tumours since microcystic adenomas contain glycogen with little or no mucin, while macrocystic adenomas contain mucin.[27]

## Islet cell tumours

Islet cell tumours are dealt with separately because of their different histologic origin (i.e. the endocrine gland) and their distinctive clinical presentation. These neoplasms include gastrinomas, insulinomas, glucagonomas, VIPomas and somatostatinoma. Most are hormonally active and cause symptoms associated with hypersecretion of the hormone produced. Although most of these lesions are adenomas, the biologic behaviour is better assessed by the presence of regional spread or metastatic disease.

CT and nuclear medicine are the initial imaging modalities used. The detection rate with CT varies from 75% to 85% and lesions usually appear as hyperattenuating nodules after intravenous administration of iodinated contrast. When these modalities fail to identify the tumour, more invasive procedures such as angiography, portal vein venous sampling and even intraoperative ultrasound are used.[28,29] Approximately 20% of islet cell tumours are non-functioning or produce hormone levels that are subclinical. These neoplasms are the third most common of the islet cell tumours after insulinomas and gastrinomas and pre-

sent quite late and are usually large and widespread at diagnosis. Clinically, they present much like other neoplasms of the body and tail of the pancreas. An imaging feature that distinguishes these lesions from the more common adenocarcinoma of ductal origin is the presence of calcification which is seen in up to 20% of tumours. Although once thought to be uncommon, necrosis or cystic degeneration and vascular invasion can be seen with large tumours.[30]

## References

1. Okuda K, Korio M, Okuda H. Neoplasms of the liver. In: Schiff L, Schiff ER (eds) *Diseases of the Liver*. Philadelphia: WB Saunders,1993, pp. 1236–1296.

2. Ros PR, Li KC. *Radiology of Malignant and Benign Liver Tumors: Part11: Benign Liver Tumors*. St Louis: Year Book Medical Publishers,1989 (Current Problems in Diagnostic Radiology, vol 18).

3. Vogl S, Koperna T, Satzinger U, Schulz F. Nonparasitic liver cysts. Overview of therapy with long-term results. *Langenbecks Arch Chir* 1995; **380**: 340–344.

4. Valls C, Rene M, Gil M, Sanchez A, Narvaez JA, Hidalgo F. Giant cavernous hemangioma of the liver: atypical CT and MR findings. *Eur Radiol* 1996; **6**: 448–450.

5. Lin ZY, Chang WY, Wang LY et al. Duplex pulsed Doppler sonography in the differential diagnosis of hepatocellular carcinoma and other common hepatic tumours. *Br J Radiol* 1992; **65**: 202–206.

6. Freeny PC, Marks WM. Patterns of contrast enhancement of benign and malignant hepatic neoplasms during bolus dynamic and delayed CT. *Radiology* 1986; **160**: 613–618.

7. Mungovan JA, Cronan JJ, Vacarro J. Hepatic cavernous hemangiomas: lack of enlargement over time. *Radiology* 1994; **191**: 111–113.

8. Wanless IR, Mawdsley C, Adams R. On the pathogenesis of focal nodular hyperplasia of the liver. *Hepatology* 1985; **5**: 1194–1200.

9. Mathieu D, Rahmouni A, Anglade MC et al. Focal nodular hyperplasia of the liver: assessment with contrast-enhanced turboflash MR imaging. *Radiology* 1991; **180**: 25–30.

10. Arrive L, Flejou JF, Vilgrain V et al. Hepatic adenoma: MR findings in 51 pathologically proved lesions. *Radiology* 1994; **193**: 507–512.

11. Kadoya M, Matsui O, Takashima T, Nonmura A. Hepatocellular carcinoma: correlation of MR images and histopathologic findings. *Radiology* 1992; **183**: 819–825.

12. Khakoo SI, Grellier LF, Soni PN, Bhattacharya S, Dusheiko GM. Etiology, screening, and treatment of hepatocellular carcinoma. *Med Clin North Am* 1996; **80**: 1121–1145.

13. Adson MA. Mass lesions of the liver. *Mayo Clin Proc* 1986; **61**: 362–368.

14. Pitt HA, Dooley WC, Yeo CJ, Cameron JL. Malignancies of the biliary tree. *Curr Prob Surg* 1995; **32**: 1–90.

15. Freeny P, Traverso. L, Ryan J. Diagnosis and staging of pancreatic adenocarcinoma with dynamic computed tomography. *Am J Surg* 1993; **165**: 600–606.

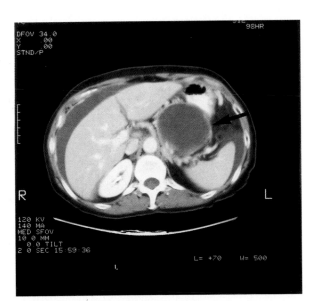

**Figure 8.7** — CT of the abdomen: Mucinous cystadenoma of the pancreas. The cystic mass (arrow) originates from the body and tail of the pancreas.

16. Fromm D. Carcinoma of the gallbladder In: David C, Sabiston Jr (eds) *Textbook of Surgery: The Biological Basis of Modern Surgical Practice*, 15th edn. Philadelphia, WB Saunders, 1997. 16. pp. 1148–1151

17. Wibbenmeyer LA, Sharafuddin MJA, Wolverson MK, Heiberg EV, Wade TP Shields JB. Sonographic diagnosis of unsuspected gallbladder cancer: Imaging findings in comparison with benign gallbladder conditions. *AJR* 1995; **165**: 1169–1174.

18. Soyer P, Bluemke DA, Reichle R *et al*. Imaging of intrahepatic cholangiocarcinoma: 2. Hilar cholangiocarcinoma. *AJR* 1995; **165**: 1433–1436.

19. Soyer P, Bluemke DA, Reichle R et al. Imaging of intrahepatic cholangiocarcinoma: 1. Peripheral cholangiocarcinoma. *AJR* 1995; **165**: 1427–1431.

20. Neumaier CE, Bertolotto M, Perrone R, Martinoli C, Loria F, Silvestri E. Staging of hilar cholangiocarcinoma with ultrasound. ??? 1995; **23**: 173–178.

21. Robledo R, Muro A, Prieto ML. Extrahepatic bile duct carcinoma: US characteristics and accuracy in demonstration of tumors. *Radiology* 1996; **198**: 869–873.

22. Vauthey JN, Blumgart LH. Recent advances in the management of cholangiocarcinomas. *Sem Liver Di* 1994; **14**: 109–114.

23. Reinhold C, Bret P. Current status of MR cholangiopancreatography. *AJR* 1996; **166**: 1285–1285.

24. Angeli E, Venturini M, Vanzulli A *et al*. Color Doppler imaging in the assessment of vascular involvement of pancreatic carcinoma. *AJR* 1997; **168**: 193–197.

25. Cameron JL, Hruban RH, Pitt HA, Siegelman SS, Soyer P, Fishman EK. Potentially resectable pancreatic adenocarcinoma: spiral CT assessment with surgical and pathologic correlation. *Radiology* 1995; **197**: 381–385.

26. Megibow A, Zhou X, Rotterdam H *et al*. Pancreatic adenocarcinoma: CT versus MR imaging in the evaluation of resectability – report of the diagnostic oncology group. *Radiology* 1995; **195**: 327–332.

27. Lewandrowski K, Lee J, Southern J, Centeno B, Warshaw A. Cyst fluid analysis in the differential diagnosis of pancreatic cysts: a new approach to the preoperative assessment of pancreatic cystic lesions. *AJR* 1995; **164**: 815–819.

28. Van Hoe L, Gryspeerdt S, Marcha l, Baert AL, Mertens L. CT for the preoperative localization of islet cell tumors of the pancreas: value of arterial and parenchymal phase images. *AJR* 1995; **165**: 1437–1439.

29. Yamamoto K, Ishii Y, Furudate M *et al*. Phase 3 multicenter clinical study of 111In-DTPA-D-octreotide (MP-1727) in patients with gastrointestinal hormone producing tumors. *Jpn J Nuclear Med* 1995; **32**: 1269–1280.

30. Buetow PC, Parrino TV, Buck JL *et al*. Islet cell tumors of the pancreas: pathologic-imaging correlation among size, necrosis and cysts, calcification, malignant behavior, and fuctional status. *AJR* 1995; **164**: 1175–1179.

# 9

# THE KIDNEY, BLADDER, PROSTATE AND TESTES

Walter Curati and Gordon Williams

Renal tumours
Bladder tumours
Prostate tumours
Testicular tumours

Over the last 10 years medical imaging has considerably improved the diagnosis and staging of renal, bladder, prostate and testicular tumours. For the kidney alone, the incidental discovery of a solid space-occupying lesion during an abdominal ultrasound investigation amounts to approximately one-third of all renal cell carcinomas.[1,2]

The 'classic' presentation of haematuria, pain and mass is rare and only occurs in large tumours.[3] In up to 50% of cases two symptoms are present. Haematuria alone is present in 33% of cases and means that the neoplastic lesion extends into the pelvicalyceal system.

In a patient found to have a renal mass, ultrasound will differentiate a cyst from a solid tumour much more reliably than CT. The smaller the cyst, the more difficult the assessment is by CT. If ultrasound rules out a simple cyst, Doppler studies, in particular power Doppler, and more recently ultrasound contrast agents, can assess its vascularity as consistently as a contrast-enhanced CT. CT has a role in staging as statistically 85% of all solid renal tumours are renal cell carcinomas and almost all tumours of the pelvicalyceal system are malignant.

This chapter focuses on imaging techniques for the renal tract and establishes algorithms for a logical investigative process.

# Renal tumours

Renal tumours represent approximately 3% of all malignancies in the adult population. Males between the ages of 50 and 70 are most likely to develop such a tumour. Renal cell carcinoma (adenocarcinoma, hypernephroma) is responsible for approximately 90% of all primary renal tumours and the transitional renal cell carcinoma of the pelvicalyceal system for approximately 10%.

## Renal cell carcinoma

Renal cell carcinoma has an incidence of 3.5 per 100 000 population per year. It is a tumour found in adults with a M:F sex ratio of approximately 2:1. It is a solitary tumour in 80% of cases. Multiple primaries are commonly linked with the von Hipple-Lindau hereditary syndrome. The renal cell carcinoma presents genetically with a DNA alteration (a deletion) on chromosome 3. This is also found in patients with von Hipple-Lindau syndrome. In about half of these cases an additional deletion occurs on chromosome 5.

Renal cell carcinoma most commonly develops within the renal cortex. The more peripheral it is, the more the outline of the organ is distorted. The vascularity of the tumour involves enlarged feeding arteries and draining veins. These characteristics are obviously valuable diagnostic features for Doppler ultrasound (power Doppler, in particular, with contrast-enhancing agents), contrast-enhanced CT and angiography. Part of the course of these tumours is frequent necroses and haemorrhages leading to cystic spaces. Some tumours, however, are initially cystic[4] with thick, irregular walls comprising one or more mural nodules.

There are three other types of renal cell carcinoma:

- Chromophobe cell carcinoma (renal 'C' adenocarcinoma)

- Tubulo-papillary carcinoma (renal 'TP' adenocarcinoma)

- Collecting tubule carcinoma (renal 'B' adenocarcinoma)

which together represent approximately 15% of all renal cell carcinomas.

The TNM classification for staging renal cell carcinoma is:

T0:  No evidence of tumour
T1:  Less than 2.5 cm, intrarenal
T2:  More than 2.5 cm, still intrarenal
T3a: Tumour invades the adrenal or the fat within Gerota's fascia
T3b: Tumour invades the inferior vena cava still under the diaphragm
T3c: Tumour invades the inferior vena cava above the diaphragm
T4:  Tumour extends beyond Gerota's fascia

Carcinosarcomas, as the name suggests, are poorly differentiated and invasive and have a poor prognosis.

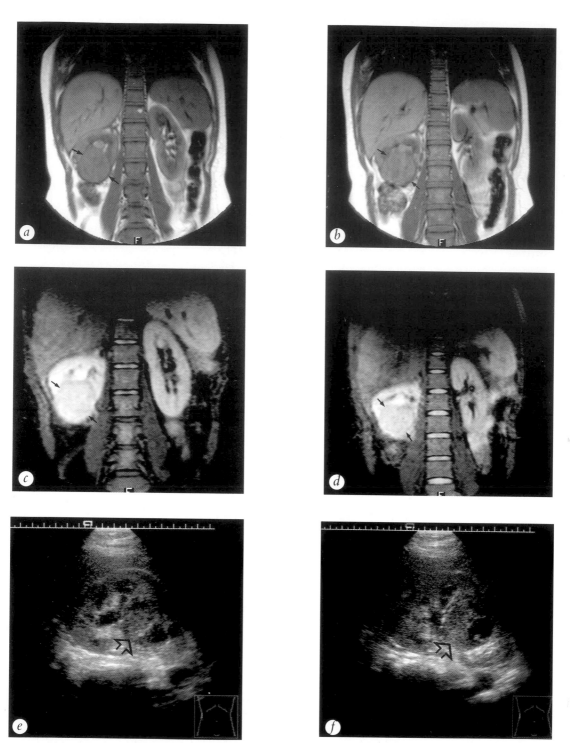

***Figure 9.1*** — Right renal cell carcinoma diagnosed and resected during pregnancy in a 24-year-old patient. a) and b) MRI contiguous T1-weighted SE coronal sections demonstrating a 5 cm intermediate signal mass at the right lower pole. c) and d) MRI contiguous STIR coronal sections: same lesion with lower signal return than the rest of the kidney. e) and f) US mixed echoic pattern within a 5 cm mass of the lower pole of the right kidney (arrows delineate the mass).

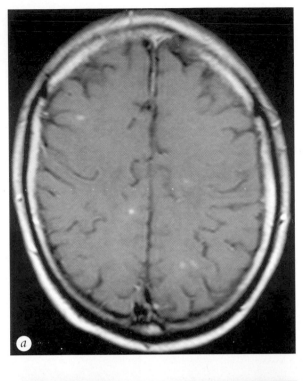

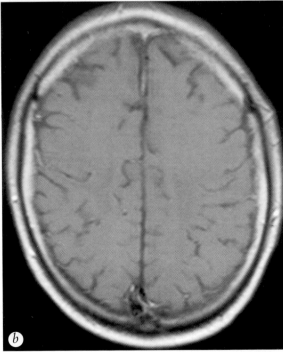

*Figure 9.2* — MRI scans of the brain. a) Post contrast enhanced T1-weighted SE axial image above the lateral ventricles: multiple small high signal lesions are identified. b) 2 months later the disappearance of the metastases is demonstrated.

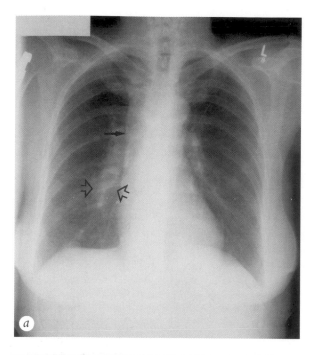

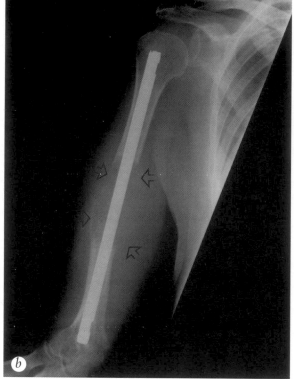

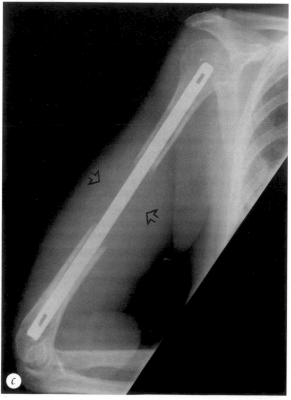

*Figure 9.3* — Metastatic renal cell carcinoma in a 64-year-old female patient. a) Postero-anterior (PA) chest radiograph: widening of the right upper mediastinum (arrow) and right hilum (open arrows) and metastatic lymph nodes are seen. b) Frontal and c) oblique views of the right humerus. Internal fixation to prevent pathological fracture secondary to a large osteolytic metastasis of the mid-diaphysis with periosteal reaction and soft tissue involvement (arrows).

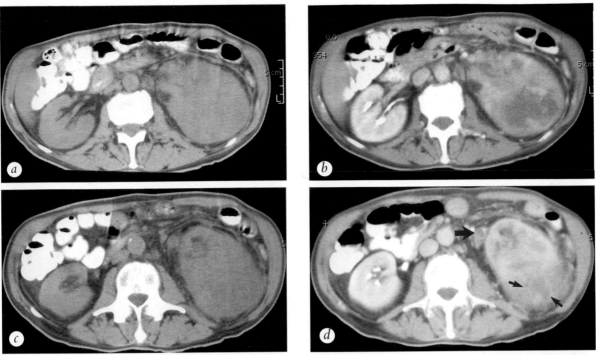

***Figure 9.4*** — Renal cell carcinoma in a 60-year-old male patient. CT a) pre- and b) post-contrast images at the level of the hilum of the left kidney. CT c) pre- and d) post-contrast images at the lower pole. An enhancing mass with a large area of necrosis (small arrows) extends beyond the capsule and accesses the Gerota's fascia. The left renal vein is invaded by tumour (large arrow).

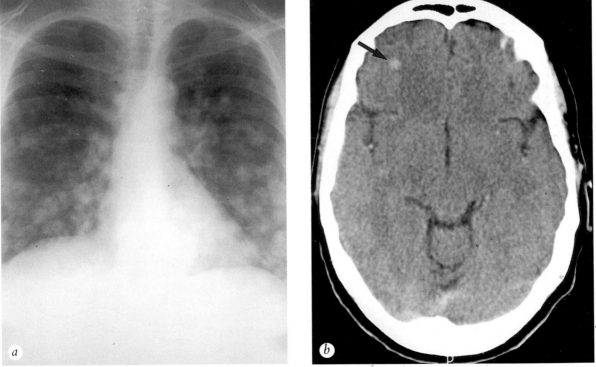

***Figure 9.5*** — Metastatic renal cell carcinoma in a 51-year-old female patient. a) Chest X-ray showing multiple large pulmonary and hilar metastases. b) Contrast-enhanced CT of the brain showing small right frontal metastasis (arrow).

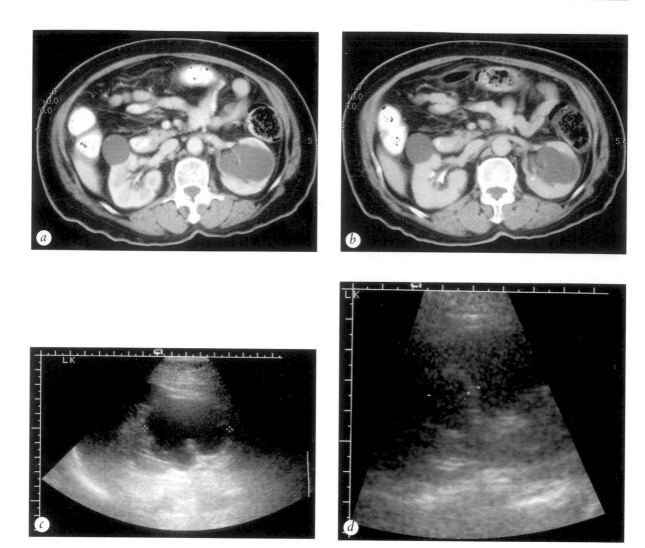

***Figure 9.6*** — A 63-year-old male patient with a complicated cyst in the left kidney and simple cysts in the right kidney. a) and b) Contrast-enhanced CT at 1 cm intervals. Contiguous section at the interpolar region of the left kidney showing irregular system and soft tissue posteriorly. c) and d) Ultrasound coronal section with magnified area detailing a thick septum. On colour Doppler the vascular signal is returned.

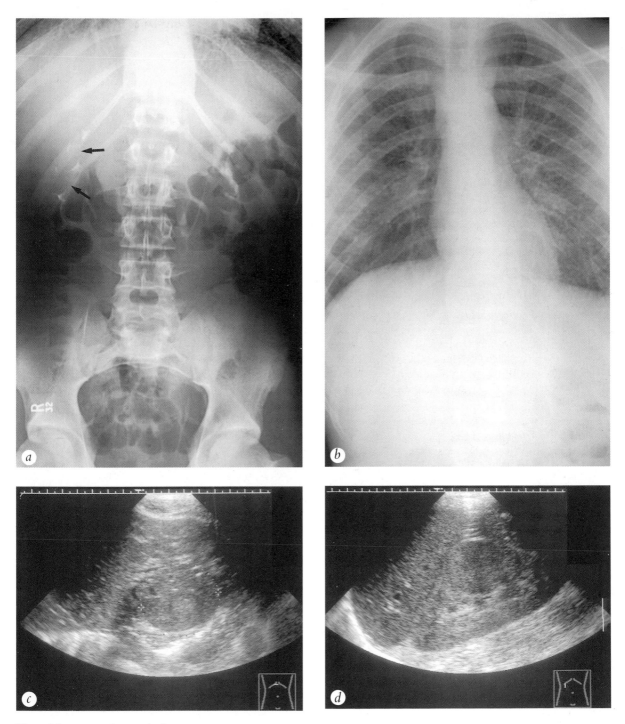

***Figure 9.7*** — see caption overleaf

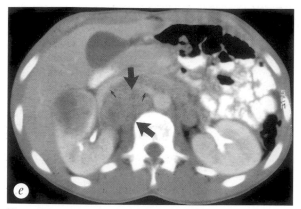
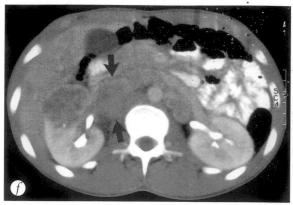

*Figure 9.7* — Metastatic renal cell carcinoma in a 20-year-old male patient. a) Intravenous urogram showing deformity of the right pelvicalyceal system with mass effect (arrows). b) Chest X-ray showing nodoreticular pattern which is consistent with lymphangitis. (c) & (d) US: 5 cm mixed echoic mass in axial and coronal planes. (e) & (f) Contrast enhanced CT: Contiguous scans. Mixed attenuation 5 cm mass at the level of right hilum – large retroperitoneal nodes (large arrows) displacing renal veins and right renal artery (small arrows).

Less malignant renal tumours are:

1. *Oncocytomas* are characterized by masses containing exclusively cells with eosinophilic cytoplasm. They are usually unique but can be found in kidneys presenting with renal cell carcinoma.[5] Oncocytomas are well circumscribed, partly encapsulated tumours and can grow up to 10 cm in diameter. They rarely recur or metastasize.[6]

2. *Renal adenomas* are, as far as imaging is concerned, a very artificial subdivision of renal cell carcinomas as they are small but can metastasize. However, it is true that genetically they present a trisomy 7 or 17 and the alteration of chromosome 3 is absent. They are very commonly small (< 1 cm) and well circumscribed.

3. *Angiomyolipomas* occur in 80% of patients presenting with tuberous sclerosis. They are single in 80% of the cases. Middle-aged females are more frequently affected with a F:M sex ratio of 2:1. In total they represent only 1% of all operated renal tumours. Angiomyolipomas are lobulated and by definition contain blood vessels, muscular bundles and fat tissue in variable proportions. They are benign but of high morbidity if more than 4 cm in diameter[8,9] as they bleed repeatedly.

## Transitional cell carcinoma

These urothelial tumours are histologically identical to urothelial bladder tumours. They represent 7% of all malignant tumours of the kidney. Macroscopically and radiologically they grow within the pelvicalyceal system and ultimately tend to occupy it entirely. They can also infiltrate the renal parenchyma.

They can be classified as follows:

- Grade 1: well differentiated cells
- Grade 2: moderately differentiated cells
- Grade 3: poorly differentiated cells.

The majority of the transitional cell carcinomas are Grade 2.[10]

In one-third of patients, the tumours are multiple. The multiplicity rate is highest for Grade 3. As demonstrated in cases of simple nephrectomy, further tumours can develop down the ureter in approximately 50% of cases. Transitional cell carcinomas are bilateral in 10% of patients. Metastases to bone, lung and liver (one-third each) occur in less than 20% of patients and usually relate to Grade 3 tumours.

There are several interesting epidemiological aspects of transitional cell carcinomas. Its incidence is 100 times higher in patients with Balkan nephropathy (along the Danube River, south of Belgrade).[11] Risk factors include tobacco (a 6-fold increase in male smokers and 8-fold in females[12]), chemicals (aniline, benzidine, solvents) and phenacetin (above a cumulative dose of 1 kg). The chromosomal abnormality is directly related to carcinogen exposure: urothelial abnormalities are more sensitive to carcinogens.[13]

The TNM staging for transitional cell carcinoma is:

T0: No evidence of tumour
Ta: Non-invasive papillary carcinoma
Tb: Carcinoma *in situ*
T1: Tumour infiltrating the submucosa

T2: Tumour infiltrating the muscular wall

T3: Tumour infiltrating the renal pelvic fat or the kidney

T4: Tumour extending through the kidney into the perirenal fat or adjacent organs

## Squamous cell carcinoma, cholesteatoma and mucinous adenocarcinoma

Squamous cell carcinoma of the renal pelvis is a rare tumour of the kidney. It is very infiltrative and commonly presents with metastases. Chronic infections and calculi are predisposing factors with calculi present in more than 50% of cases.

Cholesteatoma (or squamous metaplasia) is related to infected stones and presents as irregular filling defects of the collecting system.

Mucinous adenocarcinoma is a variant of adenocarcinoma and is rarely encountered.

## Metastases

According to large autopsy series, renal metastases are three times more common than primary tumours. Bilateral involvement is demonstrated in 50% of cases. The percentage of primary tumours presenting with renal metastases is shown in Table 9.1.

At autopsy the kidneys are involved in 60% of cases of non-Hodgkin's lymphomas, 15% of Hodgkin's lymphomas and 20–60% of various leukaemias (according to type).

# Bladder tumours

Bladder carcinoma is the most frequent malignant neoplasm of the urinary tract. Carcinoma of the bladder is most prevalent in the 50–70 year age group and is more

**Table 9.1** Percentage of primary tumours presenting with renal metastases.

| Primary tumour | Renal deposits (% of cases) |
| --- | --- |
| Bronchus | 20 |
| Breast | 15 |
| Pancreas | 12 |
| Colon | 12 |
| Ovaries | 8 |
| Rectum | 6 |
| Prostate | 4 |
| Melanoma | 2 |

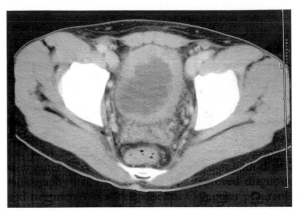

*Figure 9.8* — Large transitional cell carcinoma of the bladder in a 49-year-old patient. Contrast-enhanced CT section at the mid-pelvic level. Note the marked irregular thickening of the bladder walls. The tumour remains confined to the pelvic fat with strands of soft tissues surrounding the bladder.

common in men than in women with a M:F sex ratio of 3:1.[14] Transitional cell carcinomas represent approximately 90% of all bladder tumours and develop as papillary or sessile growth. Amongst the other tumours (10% in total), adenocarcinomas, leiomyomas, fibromas (non-malignant) and leiomyosarcomas and fibrosarcomas (malignant) are classical. Metastases from other organs are rare. It should be remembered that the pheochromocytomas (endocrine), endometriosis (endocrine-sensitive) and haemangiomas of the benign type are very symptomatic and are therefore worth mentioning here.

The TNM classification for staging bladder cancer:

Ta: Confined to mucosa

T1: Invades the submucosa (lamina propria)

T2: Invades superficial muscle

T3a: Invades deep muscle

T3b: Invades perivesical fat

T4: Invades pelvic organs.

# Prostate tumours

*Benign prostatic hypertrophy* is mentioned here as it should be included in the differential diagnosis for carcinoma of the prostate. Benign prostatic hypertrophy with intravesical enlargement causes elevation of the trigone resulting in a 'J' or fish-hook deformity of the ureters. Bladder outlet obstruction produces trabeculations of the bladder with in some cases diverticular formation.

## Carcinoma of the prostate

Carcinoma of the prostate is the commonest cancer identified at autopsy from the age of 50 (30%) to 90 (90%) with a linear progression. More than 95% of all tumours are adenocarcinomas. The clinical presentation varies from frequent micturition (most commonly without haematuria) to symptoms of bone or low back pain secondary to bone metastases and less commonly to renal failure due to ureteric obstruction by tumour infiltration or haemorrhages due to the release of prostatic fibrinolysin in the systemic circulation. The diagnosis is established by histological confirmation following biopsy.

The zonal model describes three main zones within the prostate:

- peripheral zone (70% of all cancers)
- central zone (10%)
- transitional zone (20%).

Staging is particularly important for prostate cancer as in recent years nerve sparing radical prostatectomy techniques have been developed and can cure the patient. The Jewitt & Whitmore classification[15] for prostate cancer staging is shown in Table 9.2,

Prostatic specific antigen (PSA) assays and increased awareness of symptoms and signs lead to earlier diagnosis of prostatic cancer and improved long-term outcome.

Transrectal ultrasound (TRUS) has the advantage of allowing precise assessment of the capsular integrity or penetration (the most relevant parameter as mentioned above). Ultrasound-guided biopsies of sites of possible extension also allow assessment of degree of tissue differentiation (stages T1a or A1) and are key to accurate staging.

CT scanning is used for the staging of prostate cancer but not for the primary localization of the tumour as direct visualization is not possible (which also means that stages T1 and T2 (TNM) or A and B (Jewitt & Witmore) are not seen on CT examination). CT is used for the evaluation of suspected direct periprostatic extension: pelvic soft tissues (fat planes) or organs such as seminal vesicles, bladder and rectum, and local or distant adenopathies. The further problem when using CT for staging is the lack of definition of internal architecture in normal sized nodes (<1 cm) potentially containing small areas of metastates and in enlarged nodes with fibrotic changes only and thought to be metastatic. CT, however, allows precise targeting of enlarged nodes for biopsies.

**Table 9.2**  Jewitt & Witmore classification15 for prostate cancer staging.

| TNM | Stage | Definition |
|---|---|---|
| | A | Non-palpable cancer |
| T1a | A1 | <5% of tissue (well differentiated tissue) |
| T1b | A2 | >5% of tissue (or poorly differentiated tissue) |
| T1c | | |
| | B | Palpable nodule confined within the prostatic capsule |
| T2a | B1 | Palpable nodule <1.5 cm in diameter |
| T2b | B2 | Palpable nodule >1.5 cm in diameter |
| T3–T4 | C | Extension beyond the prostatic capsule without distant metastases |
| | D | Metastases |
| N | D1 | Metastases to regional lymph nodes |
| M | D2 | Metastases to bone or viscera |

MRI is the imaging modality of choice for the anatomical assessment of the lobes of the prostate and the seminal vesicles: the outline of the tumour is a clear interface between its low signal (on T2-weighted images) and the high signal of the normal gland, the periprostatic venous plexus and the seminal vesicles. The invasion of the adjacent organs and the metastatic lymph node involvement is also seen more clearly with MRI than CT due to the multiplanar capability of MRI: primary acquisitions in

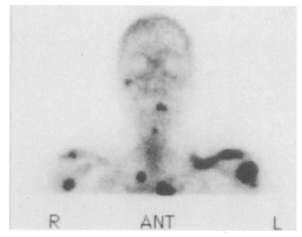

***Figure 9.9*** — Metastatic adenocarcinoma of the prostate in an 82-year-old patient. The nuclear medicine bone scan shows multiple areas of focal increased uptake which is consistent with metastases.

coronal and sagittal planes improve the assessment of integrity of neighbouring structures. These considerations apply both to body coil and endorectal coil MRI. The conventional body coil technique provides a broad field of view for the pelvis whereas the endorectal coil technique provides high resolution imaging for the accurate preoperative staging of localized prostate cancer.[16]

# Testicular tumours

Testicular tumours normally present with a painless lump in the testicle. The practice of testicular self-examination with increased awareness of testicular neoplasm has led to patients presenting at an earlier stage of the disease. This positive trend is somewhat offset by the increased incidence of testicular cancer in the second half of this century.[17]

Of all testicular tumours, 90% arise from germ cells and are malignant. They can be divided into two groups: seminomas and non-seminomatous tumours. The former are the most frequent and they present around the age of 40 and are highly radiosensitive. The non-seminomatous group presents during the teenage years. The staging for testicular cancer is shown in Table 9.3.

The non-seminomatous tumours include:

| Type | Incidence | Age | Prognosis |
|---|---|---|---|
| Embryonal carcinoma | 20% | 30yrs | Poor (metastases +) |
| Teratomas | 10% | 10–30yrs | Good |
| Choriocarcinoma | rare | 20–30yrs | Poor (metastases + +) |
| Yolk sac carcinoma | rare | <10yrs | Poor (metastases + +) |
| Mixed pattern teratocarcinoma | 30% | Variable | Variable |

Spread occurs via the regional lymphatics (except for choriocarcinoma and yolk sac carcinoma) along the spermatic vein to sentinel nodes lateral to the paralumbar nodes on the left in the renal perihilar region at the level of L1/L2 and on the right in the paracaval region below the renal artery and vein (L1–L3). From the retroperitoneal level the lymphatic spread extends via the thoracic duct into the mediastinum and lungs. (Choriocarcinoma and yolk sac carcinoma present with hematogenous spread).

**Table 9.3**  Staging for testicular cancer

| AJC TNM (American Joint Committee) | UICC TNM (Union Internationale Centre le Cancer) | | |
|---|---|---|---|
| Stage I | T1 | : | Tumour occupying less than half of testis surrounded by palpably normal gland |
| | T2 | : | Tumour occupying half or more of testis with no enlargement or deformity |
| | T3 | : | Tumour confined to testis, causing enlargement or deformity |
| | T4a | : | Tumour extending to epididymis |
| Stage II | T4b | : | Tumour invading other local structures |
| | N0 | : | No deformity of regional lymph nodes on lymphangiography |
| | N1 | : | Regional lymph nodes deformed on lymphangiography |
| | N2 | : | Fixed, palpable lymph nodes |
| Stage III | N1 | : | Metastases to nodes outside the abdomen or to viscera |
| Stage IV | | | Metastases to lung and liver |

Lymphangiography, CT and MRI can all assess the retroperitoneum. Lymphangiography, the earliest technique, demonstrates involvement even in non-enlarged lymph nodes but is invasive and time consuming (up to fours hours for the initial phase of the investigation). Its success rate is similar to that of CT. CT has advantages over lymphangiography in that it is non-invasive (except for intravenous administration of contrast ), can assess the viscera and the non-opacified lymph nodes and in particular screens the liver and the lungs. CT is also the routine modality for follow-ups. MRI is as sensitive as CT in imaging the pelvis, retroperitoneum and liver but is of little value in the chest. CT should still therefore be performed for the lungs.

# References

1.  Nakano E, Iwasaki A and Seguchi T. Incidentally diagnosed renal cell carcinoma, Eur Urol 1992; **21**: 294–298.

2. Özen H, Colowick A and Freiha FS. Incidentally discovered solid renal masses: what are they? *Br J Urol* 1993; **72**: 274–276.

3. Chisolm GD. Nephrogenic ridge tumours and their syndromes. *Ann NY Acad Sci* 1974; **230**: 402–423.

4. Davidson AJ, Hartman DS and Choyke PL. Radiographic assessment of renal masses: Implications for patient care. *Radiology* 1997; **207**: 297–305.

5. Lense E, Siegel R and Hewan-Lowe K. *In situ* oncocytic change is association with multiple renal cell adenocarcinomas. *Arch Pathol Lab Med* 1991; **115**: 1067–1069.

6. Licht MR, Novick AC and Tubbs RR. Renal oncocytoma: Clinical and biological correlates. *J Urol* 1993; **150**: 1380–1383.

7. Kovacs G. Application of molecular cytogenetic techniques to the evaluation of renal parenchymal tumours. *J Cancer Res Clin Oncol* 1990; **116**: 318–323.

8. Blute ML. Angiomyolipoma: Clinical metamorphosis and concepts for management. *J Urol* 1988; **139**: 20–24.

9. Wills JS. Management of small renal neoplasm and angiomyolipoma: a growing problem. *Radiology* 1995; **197**: 583–586.

10. Guinan P, Vogelzang NJ and Randazzo R. Renal pelvic cancer: a review of 611 patients in Illinois 1975–1985. *Urology* 1992; **40**: 393–399.

11. Cukuranovic R, Ignjatovic M and Stefanovic V. Urinary tract tumours and Balkan nephropathy in the south Moravia River basin. *Kidney Int* 1991; 40: 580–584.

12. McLaughlin JK, Silverman DT and Hsing AW. Cigarette smoking and cancers of the renal pelvis and ureter. *Cancer Res* 1992; **52**: 254–257.

13. Greenland JE, Weston PM and Wallace DM. Familial transitional cell carcinoma and the Lynch syndrome II. *Br J Urol* 1993; **72**: 177–180.

14. Heiken JP, Forman HP and Brown JJ. Neoplasms of the prostate, bladder and testis. *Radiol Clin N Am* 1994; **32**: 81–98.

15. Whitmore WF Jr. Natural history staging of prostate cancer. *Urol Clin North Am* 1984; **11**: 205–220.

16. Cavanagh PM. Staging of prostate cancer: the role of MRI. *Clin MRI* 1997; 7: 4–10.

17. Richie JP. Neoplasms of the testis. In: Walsh PC, Retik AB, Stamey TA, and Vaughan ED (eds) *Campbell's Urology, 6th* Edition. Philadelphia 1992, WB Saunders, vol.2, pp 1222–1263.

# 10

# THE ENDOCRINE SYSTEM

Daniel A Darko and Karim Meeran

**Pituitary gland**
**Thyroid gland**
**Adrenals**
**Gut hormone tumours**
**Testicular tumours**
**Ovarian tumours**
**Bone**

Endocrine cells produce and secrete specific substances which act as messengers to cells at different sites. In addition, many produce receptors for other hormones, such as somatostatin. Techniques that visualize these unique features make endocrine malignancy amenable to imaging. In addition, the fact that some endocrine malignancies secrete large amount of hormones enables angiography to be combined with selective venous sampling and assay of the samples for particular hormones. However, before considering the more specialist imaging methods, it is important to remember that plain radiology is extremely important in many endocrine diagnoses.

As well as the classical endocrine system, which includes the pituitary, thyroid, adrenal glands, ovaries, testes, parathyroid and pancreas, the gut and bone are also recognized as important endocrine organs. Many of the neoplasms in endocrine disease are benign histologically but can be life threatening because of the hormones they produce. In addition, there are some inheritable neoplasias and these have been classified with eponymous names, e.g. multiple endocrine neoplasia (MEN) type 1 (Sipple syndrome), MEN 2 and Von Hippel Lindau syndrome. In MEN 1, there is an autosomal dominant risk of individuals developing parathyroid adenomata or hyperplasia (causing hypercalcaemia), pituitary adenomata (causing prolactinomas, acromegaly or Cushing's disease) or pancreatic neoplasia. The gene for MEN 1 is coded for on chromosome 11. It has recently been cloned[1,2] and the gene product has been labelled 'MENIN' but, remarkably, the function of this protein is unknown. In von Hippel Lindau syndrome, patients have an autosomal dominant risk of phaeochromocytomas, cerebellar and spinal haemangioblastomas, retinal haemangiomas and renal cell carcinoma. The gene for this condition is coded for on chromosome 3 and the protein product is a tumour suppressor gene. Patients known to have any of the inherited endocrine neoplasias are regularly screened for the development of the relevant tumours, usually by imaging the appropriate area.

# Pituitary gland

The pituitary gland sits in the pituitary fossa of the sphenoid bone of the skull. A plain lateral X-ray can show destruction of either of the clinoid processes or an enlarged fossa in pituitary adenomas. In addition, specific pituitary tumours can produce particular changes in the lateral skull X-ray. Acromegaly, for example, causes thickening of the skull vault and enlargement of

the sinuses as well as a large pituitary fossa. Other pituitary adenomas tend to be small and hence do not produce changes in a lateral skull X-ray. More than 90% of prolactinomas and almost all corticotrophinomas (Cushing's disease) are microadenomas (i.e. <1 cm in diameter) and those as small as 1 mm in diameter can be visualized using both CT and MRI scanning. It is also important to look for deviation of the stalk as this may be the only evidence of a microadenoma.

Occasionally, pituitary tumours outgrow their blood supply and hence autoinfarct. At the time of infarction, patients may present with headache, visual disturbance and diplopia, a condition known as pituitary apoplexy. This may be the first sign of any pituitary abnormality. Often, however, even the infarction goes undiagnosed and patients may have normal pituitary function. Imaging of such a patient may show no obvious pituitary tissue or an empty sella. Normal pituitary cells may be distributed at the edge of the fossa. The term 'empty sella syndrome' has been used to describe the presence of an empty sella in patients with headache who may be obese.[3]

## Suspected Cushing's disease

In patients with suspected Cushing's disease (who by definition have a pituitary tumour secreting ACTH, also known as a 'corticotrophinoma'), inferior petrosal sinus sampling (IPSS) and assay of the samples for ACTH has become routine before transsphenoidal hypophysectomy. Otherwise hypophysectomy may be erroneously carried out in patients with another cause of Cushing's syndrome, such as ectopic ACTH or adrenal adenomas. IPSS is generally performed by interventional radiologists and serves to confirm not only that the pituitary adenoma is the source of the problem, but also the side on which it lies.[4]

One catheter is inserted into each femoral vein, and threaded up under X-ray control into the inferior petrosal sinuses. As both lines traverse the inferior vena cava, where the two lines may cross over, it is important to be sure of which side each catheter is placed by injecting contrast into each line immediately before the start of the procedure.

Once each line is correctly placed, blood must be allowed to flow freely and collected drop by drop from the end of the catheter. Aspiration, if required, must be performed very slowly, as fast aspiration will draw blood from surrounding structures and may artificially lower ACTH concentrations in the samples. To ensure the catheters are correctly placed, other pituitary hormones (thyrotropin

(TSH) and prolactin) are usually measured. Two baseline samples are drawn at 5 min intervals from each inferior petrosal sinus. Peripheral samples are also drawn and are essential for final interpretation of the results and to confirm that the catheters are correctly placed. After the second baseline sample has been drawn, an intravenous bolus of corticotrophin releasing factor (CRF) is administered, and three further samples are taken at 5 min intervals. A typical set of results, confirming a left-sided pituitary adenoma, is shown in Table 10.1.[4]

Occasionally, excess ACTH comes not from the pituitary but from an ectopic source, such as a bronchial carcinoma or adenoma, or from the pancreas. Patients with ectopic ACTH usually present with profound hypokalaemia, weakness, and, if they have malignant neoplasms, classical truncal obesity may not be obvious because of weight loss. In such patients, cortisol levels usually do not suppress with either low- or high-dose dexamethasone, but occasionally suppression does occur. If IPSS is performed in these patients, the peripheral sample will have a similar (or higher) ACTH than the central ones.

## Acromegaly

These tumours are often large and can threaten nearby structures, including the optic chiasm. As stated previously, a lateral skull X-ray may show destruction of bone locally. In addition, the skull vault may be thickened and the sinuses large. A CT or MRI scan will show the size of the tumour more accurately and will indicate whether there is pressure on the optic chiasm. Hand X-rays will show spade-like hands with soft tissue enlargement and tufting of the distal phalanges (Fig. 10.1). Because these patients often have diabetes, lateral foot X-rays may show calcification of the dorsalis

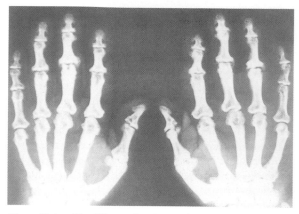

***Figure 10.1*** — Hand X-ray of patient with acromegaly.

pedis and the heel pad may be thickened. Visceral organomegaly also occurs and scanning of the abdomen may show this. Importantly, acromegalics are at risk of colonic carcinoma,[5,6] and because of their very long colon, colonoscopy may be difficult. In these instances, barium enemas need to be performed every 3–5 years. Any adenomata must be colonoscopically removed.

## Prolactinomas

Microadenomas account for 90% of prolactinomas. In women, they often present with amennorrhoea or galactorrhoea in women. In men, microadenomas go undetected because the male breast is not oestrogenized and men present either with loss of libido, or later with features of a macroadenoma, such as visual loss or seizures. The belief that men have macroadenomas while women have microadenomas may therefore be due to reporting bias, although there is some evidence that prolactinomas in males are more aggressive and less responsive to medical therapy.[7,8] CT or MRI of the pituitary may confirm the adenoma, and if very small, often the only feature is deviation of the pituitary stalk. Prolactinomas often respond to dopamine agonists such as bromocriptine or cabergoline. Prolactin levels fall and the tumour shrinks. Rescanning after a year of dopamine agonist treatment is useful to confirm this. Patients whose tumours grow despite dopamine agonists may require surgery or radiotherapy.

# Thyroid gland

The thyroid gland is unique in that normal thyroid cells as well as differentiated thyroid tumours usually take up iodine. Cold iodine has a molecular weight of 127. Two

**Table 10.1** Typical ACTH levels for a left-sided pituitary corticotrophinoma.

| Time* | ACTH level | | |
|---|---|---|---|
| | | Inferior petrosal sinus samples | |
| | Peripheral sample | Left | Right |
| –5 | 25 | 95 | 25 |
| 0 | 27 | 93 | 30 |
| +5 | 85 | 4560 | 140 |
| +10 | 125 | 2990 | 155 |

* Time from CRF bolus (min)

isotopes of iodine, [131]I and [123]I, have a relatively short half-life and can therefore be used *in vivo*, both in the diagnosis and treatment of thyroid dysfunction. In addition, thyroid C-cells (which are embryologically derived from neural crest cell that migrate into the 3rd and 4th branchial arches amongst others to form the amine precursor uptake and decarboxylation (APUD) cell series take up metaiodobenzylguanidine (MIBG) and patients with medullary thyroid carcinoma have a high uptake of this compound. Adrenal medullary chromaffin cells (classical APUD cells), which are also of neural crest origin, take up MIBG and high adrenal uptake is seen in patients with phaeochromocytomas (see below). The MEN 2 syndrome is an autosomal dominant disorder and is secondary to a mutation of the specific proto-oncogene RET, which codes for a tyrosine kinase on chromosome 10. There are three subtypes of MEN 2 (Table 10.2).[9]

## Thyrotoxicosis

This is caused by an excess of thyroid hormone in the circulation. It can occur either because of a toxic hyper-secreting thyroid nodule within a normally suppressed thyroid gland, or because of Graves' disease, where an autoantibody may stimulate the entire gland to become overactive. Radioactive iodine uptake can also be quantified and gives a measure of thyroid activity. It can be particularly useful in distinguishing viral ('De Quervain's') thyroiditis from Graves disease'. Both can cause hyperthyroidism but radioactive iodine uptake is suppressed in viral thyroiditis (Fig. 10.2) and increased in Graves' disease (Fig. 10.3). In patients with hyperthyroidism, [99m]Tc-pertechnetate is used to distinguish a toxic nodule (Fig. 10.4) from Graves' disease (Fig. 10.3). Fig. 10.5 shows a normal [99m]Tc-pertechnetate scan from the same patient as shown in Fig. 10.4 but after a therapeutic dose of radioiodine.

**Table 10.2** Characterization of three types of the multiple endocrine neoplasia (MEN) syndrome type 2.

|  | MEN 2a | MEN 2b | FMTC |
|---|---|---|---|
| Parathyroid hyperplasia | ✓ | ✗ | ✗ |
| Phaeochromocytoma | ✓ | ✓ | ✗ |
| medullary thyroid carcinoma (MTC) | ✓ | ✓ | ✓ |
| Marfanoid habitus | ✗ | ✓ | ✗ |
| Bowel ganglioneuromatosis | ✗ | ✓ | ✗ |

FMTC = familial medullary thyroid carcinoma.

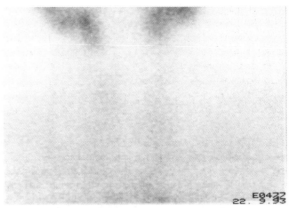

*Figure 10.2* — 99mTc-pertechnetate scan in patient with De Quervain's thyroiditis.

## Thyroid carcinoma

Plain X-rays rarely provide useful information in the management of thyroid neoplasms but on occasion may show bony or lung secondaries.

For many patients with a thyroid mass, an ultrasound scan is often the first evaluative test they have. A high-resolution ultrasound in the hands of a good operator can assess nodules as small as 5 mm in diameter. Malignant thyroid nodules are often poorly defined with irregular margins and are hyperechoic,[10] while benign thyroid cysts have a typical smooth wall with no internal echoes, although they occasionally contain some debris. Calcification within or around a cyst is associated with neoplasia and invasion of neck muscles or vasculature is highly suggestive of malignancy.[11] Finally, ultrasound can be used for the localization and biopsy of small tumours and local recurrent disease.

CT provides high-definition images of the thyroid, especially any retrosternal extension. It poorly differentiates benign from malignant masses and its main use is to define the anatomy of the neck region prior to surgery. Spiral CT is superior to conventional CT in this respect because it collates images faster and thereby eliminates movement artifact. MRI is similar to CT for imaging the thyroid but is more expensive. It has been described in combination with proton spectroscopy to distinguish follicular adenomas from carcinomas.[12]

Thyroglobulin assays are the mainstay for the detection of recurrence or metastases. However, imaging in addition to clinical examination provides useful information. Radioiodine is trapped and organified by the thyroid and aberrant thyroid tissue or metastases,

anterior

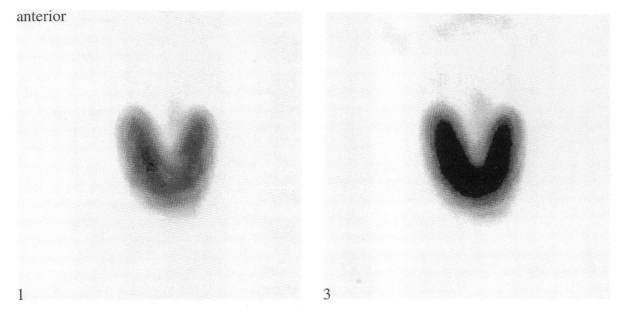

**Figure 10.3** — 99mTc-pertechnetate scan in patient with Graves' disease.

anterior anterior

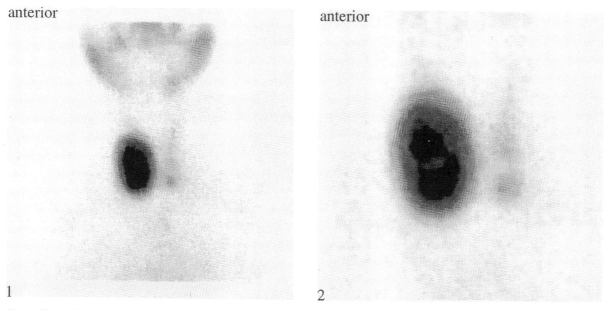

**Figure 10.4** — 99mTc-pertechnetate scan in patient with a toxic nodule.

anterior

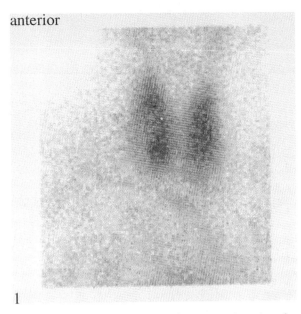

1

**Figure 10.5** — Normal 99mTc-pertechnetate scan in patient after therapeutic iodine.

making it a highly specific test. The sensitivity of radioiodine is influenced by diet, drugs (especially amiodarone) and tumour histology.

[123]I has a short half-life (13 hours) and releases short-energy γ-rays. It is the ideal isotope for thyroid imaging. [131]I has a longer half-life (8 days) and emits a high-energy γ-ray and a β particle, making it best suited for treatment, but because it is cheaper, easier to obtain and can be stored for longer before use than [123]I, it is widely used for imaging as well as treatment. Use of [131]I in imaging requires knowledge of the the physiological sites of iodine concentration and the causes of artifacts, in order to avoid potential suppression of active thyroid tissue during diagnostic scanning (thyroid stunning). Many centres limit the amount of radioiodine administered to 74–111 Mbq.[13] To maximize TSH stimulation of the remaining thyroid tissue, thyroxine therapy should be stopped 4–6 weeks before radioiodine body scanning. In patients unable to tolerate the hypothyroidism that this induces, a switch to tri-iodothyronine (T3) for 3–4 weeks after thyroxine is discontinued is advised. T3 is then stopped 8 days before scanning. As amiodarone has a half-life of 30 days and a large excess of cold iodine ([127]I), patients on amiodarone cannot be imaged with radioiodine. Patients must discontinue amiodarone for at least 6 months if radioiodine scanning is required. Alter-

natively, thallium scans may be used for the detection of local and cervical metastatic disease. These are less sensitive than [131]I in therapeutic doses but may show up metastases that are not seen with any other modality.[14]

Anaplastic carcinoma of the thyroid poorly concentrates iodine and often does not express thyroglobulin. For this reason nuclear scanning with radioiodine for diagnosis or treatment is not used. Debulking surgery or radiotherapy may be carried out to relieve tracheal or airway obstruction.

For well-differentiated thyroid carcinoma, current common practice for surveillence involves radioiodine scanning after surgery at 6–9 months and then yearly for the next 3 years and a repeat scan at 5 years.[15]

## Parathyroid disease

Primary hyperparathyroidism is a common condition affecting about 1% of the population. It is often is discovered incidentally. The diagnosis is made by the combination of a high calcium with a non-suppressed parathyroid hormone (PTH). Asymptomatic cases are often observed for a number of years, but the only successful treatment is removal of the offending parathyroid. Multiple adenomata are present in 20% of cases and imaging of the parathyroids before surgery is useful.

Simple imaging such as ultrasound can be used to demonstrate lesions. Thallium scanning shows total blood flow to the thyroid and parathyroid, and the parathyroids can thus be visualized using digital subtraction of [99]Tc (which shows the thyroid) from thallium. [99]Tc-sestamibi scanning (Fig. 10.6) is more sensitive and specific for the diagnosis of primary hyperparathyroidism than thallium-technetium subtraction scanning[16] or CT or MRI scanning.[17]

Medullary thyroid carcinoma (MTC) often presents with a neck mass or raised calcitonin or CEA levels. Ultrasound and CT are efficient at picking up tumours >1 cm in diameter. MIBG has been used in the same way as for the detection of phaeochromocytomas but has a low specificity.[18] Newer compounds being evaluated for visualization of MTC include octreotide.

# Adrenals

## Phaeochromocytomas

These are usually (90%) benign and come from adrenal chromaffin cells and are hence APUD cells and take up MIBG. Fig. 10.7 shows an MIBG scan from a patient with bilateral phaeochromocytomas. The diag-

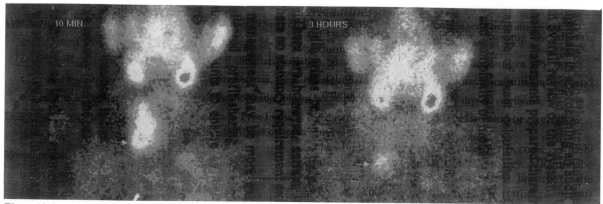

*Figure 10.6* — Sestamibi scan in patient with parathyroid adenoma (arrow).

nosis is made when there are high urinary cate-cholamines and patients often present with episodic hypertension. Adrenal phaeochromocytomas usually secrete adrenaline whereas extra-adrenal phaeochro-mocytomas may secrete more noradrenaline. Ninety per cent of phaeochromocytomas occur in the adren-als with 10% being extra-adrenal (Fig. 10.8). Phaeocromocytomas are associated with the MEN 2 syndrome, von Hippel-Lindau syndrome and neurofi-bromastosis. Approximately 10% of these tumours are malignant and metastatic lesions often deposit along the skeletal axis. The natural history of malignant phaeochromcytoma is variable and there are several case reports in the literature of >5-year survival with medical treatment.

Patients with phaeochromocytomas need imaging before surgery to localize the lesion. Plain chest X-rays are useful and provide information about metastases and any degree of heart failure. Flush aortography is an invasive technique that carries the real risk of provoking a hypertensive crisis and is now rarely used.

Ultrasound may be useful to investigate large masses within the adrenal gland. MIBG scanning combined with CT scanning of any hot areas (Fig. 10.9) is now the major method for imaging phaechromocytomas.

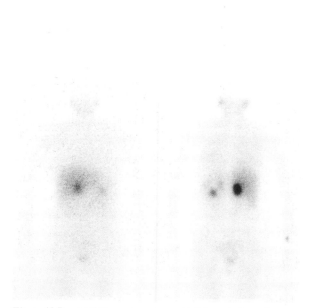

*Figure 10.7* — MIBG scan in patient with bilateral phaeochromo-cytomas.

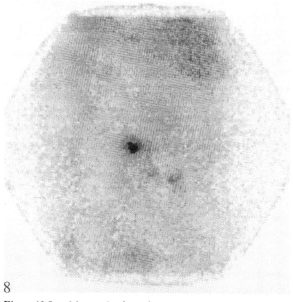

*Figure 10.8* — Metastatic phaeochromocytoma.

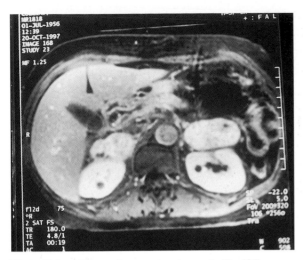

*Figure 10.9* — CT scan from same patient as in Fig. 10.7.

CT scan of the patient with bilateral phaeochromocytomas whose MIBG scan is shown in Fig. 10.7.

## Conn's syndrome

Primary hyperaldosteronism accounts for <2% of cases of hypertension. The diagnosis should be suspected in all hypertensive patients with a low serum potassium but, to confirm the diagnosis, plasma aldosterone levels must be high and renin levels sampled at the same time must be low. The temptation to scan patients with unexplained hypokalaemia but no biochemical evidence of Conn's syndrome should be avoided because up to 5% of abdominal CT scans detect incidental masses in the adrenal glands. CT can detect adrenal masses <1 cm in diameter. Adrenal hyperplasia is always bilateral and both glands are enlarged. Adrenocortical carcinoma, which is very rare (1% of cases), is commoner in tumours >3 cm. The commoner adrenocortical adenoma is often smaller.

Following intravenous administration, MIBG is actively concentrated in chromaffin cell granules and scintinography is considered to have >95% specificity for the detection of phaeochromocytomas. $^{131}$I and $^{123}$I have both been used for radiolabelling and the latter isotope allows the operator to combine MIBG scaning with single photon emission tomography (SPECT) to provide clearer definition and anatomy. Our approach to initial imaging is to scan the whole body using MIBG, followed by high-resolution (spiral) CT of areas with abnormally high uptake. Fig. 10.9 shows the

### IODOCHOLESTEROL SCINTINOGRAPHY

6-$^{131}$Iodomethyl-19-norcholesterol (iodocholestrerol) is widely employed in the imaging of Conn's syndrome. Patients are prepared by the ingestion of dexamethasone for a week prior to adminstering iodocholesterol in order to suppress cortisol production from the normal gland. They are also given saturated solution of iodine or potassium iodide (60 mg tds) to protect the thyroid from radioactive iodine in the tracer. Adrenal adenomas show up as early unilateral uptake in the affected gland (Fig. 10.10). In hyperplasia there is bilateral uptake after

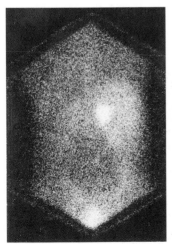
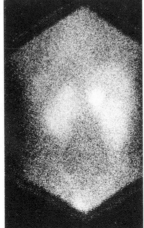

ADRENAL IMAGING

+ 7 DAYS

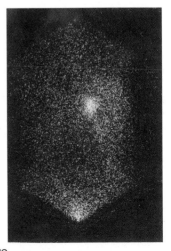

POSTERIOR VIEWS

+ 14 DAYS

*Figure 10.10* — Iodocholesterol scan in patient with Conn's syndrome.

an average 3–5 days. Adrenocortical carcinomas typically show reduced uptake on the side of the tumour.

This method is the 'gold standard' for tumour localization but is technically difficult because of frequent failure to cannulate the right adrenal vein. It is undertaken in cases where iodocholesterol and CT scanning fail to localize the tumour adequately. Throughout the procedure a continuous infusion of ACTH is maintained to stimulate a fixed cortisol production rate from both adrenals. Cortisol and aldosterone are measured from both adrenal veins, which enables correction in the case of inaccurate placement of adrenal vein cannulae.

# Gut hormone tumours

The gastrointestinal tract has an important endocrine role and many neurotransmitters are involved in signalling nutritional status: insulin (stimulates peripheral glucose utilization), gastrin (stimulates gastric acid production), vasoactive intestinal polypeptide (stimulates colonic secretions), and many other hormones. Tumours of endocrine cells of the gut are rare but can result in specific syndromes. They can form in any part of the gastrointestinal system but the commonest areas include gastrin cells of the duodenum, serotonin-secreting enterochromaffin cells commonly found in the small intestine and oxyntic cell tumours of the stomach. Commonly recognized syndromes secondary to excess secretion of hormones include Zollinger–Ellison, carcinoid and Verner–Morrison syndrome.

The carcinoid syndrome occurs with excess secretion of serotonin (5-hydroxy tryptamine) and results in increased urinary excretion of 5-hydroxy indolacetic acid (5-HIAA). Such tumours need to be localized before surgery. Ultrasound, CT and MRI, which are relatively non-invasive, are often useful. However, these modalities give no functional data and angiography with intra-arterial provocation provides functional as well as anatomical localization in some tumours.[19,20]

The liver is a common port for metastatic disease from gut endocrine tumours. Unlike other malignancies, such metastases do not herald imminent death. They are very slow growing and obtain their blood supply from the hepatic artery. The normal liver has a dual blood supply from portal triads. If the blood supply via the hepatic artery is cut off therefore, the tumour will infarct in preference to the liver hepatocytes which can survive on the portal circulation. This is the basis of hepatic emboliza-

tion as a therapeutic modality. Inert plastic microspheres are injected selectively into the hepatic arterioles supplying the metastases in order to infarct them. After embolization, tumour load is reduced and often the symptoms of flushing, diarrhoea and headache resolve.

Patients with Zollinger–Ellison syndrome present with multiple ulcers of the small bowel, which are caused by a tumour of the pancreas secreting gastrin. Gastrinomas can also be localized using intra-arterial injection of secretin[21,22] or calcium. This invasive method currently is the most sensitive technique available.

In 1958 the first case report of Verner–Morrison syndrome concerned 2 patients with hypokalaemia, a profuse watery diarrhoea and achlorhydria associated with non-β cell adenocarcinoma of the pancreas. It was not until 1973 when Bloom *et al* reported raised VIP levels in plasma from patients with this syndrome.[23] Vipomas are predominantly pancreatic, although 10% are found in extrapancreatic sites such as the adrenal medulla or autonomic nervous system. Vipomas have been localized using ultrasound. Gut endocrine tumours can express octreotide receptors and radioactive octreotide or analogues can be used to demonstrate the distribution of such tumours.

Insulinomas are usually located in the tail of the pancreas. Patients present with hypoglycaemia relieved by food and the diagnosis is confirmed when inappropriately high insulin levels occur in the face of hypoglycaemia (glucose <2.2 mM). Such patients require removal of the tumour, but the lesions are often too small to be seen by ultrasound, CT or MRI scanning. In addition, non-secreting incidentalomas of no consequence are often found on CT and MRI scanning. For this reason, the source of insulin needs to be determined. The most sensitive and specific test for localizing a functional insulinoma is intra-arterial calcium injection and portal venous sampling.[19]

Glucagonomas present with a necrolytic migratory erythema, usually to dermatologists who may recognize the condition from the skin lesions alone. Some patients have diabetes. The incidence of glucagonomas is about 1 per 10 million per annum. Diagnosis is confirmed by measuring a fasting plasma glucagon. The treatment is usually symptomatic with octreotide and zinc creams for the rash. Hepatic metastases can be treated with embolization (see above)

The first report of the use of somatostatin (SST) receptor analogues in scanning endocrine tumours was in 1989.[24] Further work lead to the development of $^{111}$In-DTPA-$_D$-Phe$^1$-octreotide (also known as $^{111}$Inpentreatide), the standard somatostatin receptor (SSTR) radioligand which binds to SSTR2 and SSTR5.

Several gut tumours show cross-reactivity to VIP and SST analogues[25] and the high level of expression by tumour cells of peptide receptors by carcinoid, neuroendocrine tumours, melanoma and lymphomas allows them to be localized by these analogues. Vasoactive intestinal peptide (VIP) receptor scintinography is a more recent development[26] and early work in small series suggests it may have a high sensitivity for vipomas. $^{111}$In-DTPA-$_D$-Phe$^1$-octreotide has a high sensitivity for the visualization of gastrinomas, carcinoid tumours (primary and secondary disease), glucagono-

mas and APUDomas.[27] It has also been applied in the imaging of MTC.[28] Fig. 10.11 shows an octreotide scan in a patient with a pancreatic gastrinoma.

# Testicular tumours

Tumours of the testes rarely present to the endocrinologist but occasionally the rare referral for gynaecomastia could have a testicular cancer since androgens may be isomerized to oestrogens. Germinal cell tumours, in particular of embryological type, which are commonest in children, may secrete gonadotrophins which are commonly used as tumour markers (e.g. human chorionic gonadotrophin). The primary approach to localization before surgical resection consists of a chest radiograph and ultrasound. Pelvic CT to stage disease

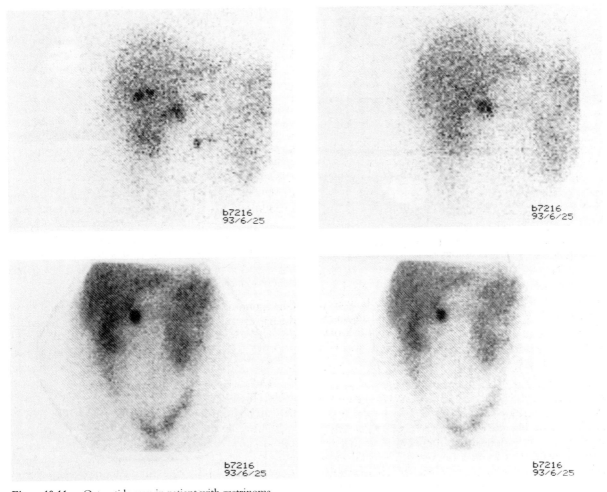

*Figure 10.11* — Octreotide scan in patient with gastrinoma.

prior to surgery is being advocated to detect early nodal metastasis.[29] Post-surgery patients typically undergo life-long follow-up with regular clinical examination, chest X-ray and tumour marker profiling.

## Ovarian tumours

Ovarian cancer remains a common cause of cancer-related death in the UK. Survival largely depends on early detection and nationally there are studies to detect the efficacy of screening in large populations. Ultrasound scanning using Doppler flow techniques are utilized to detect abnormal flow patterns (secondary to neovascularization) characteristic of malignancy. Further imaging with CT is occasionally carried out, but the common approach once the diagnosis is suspected is surgical visualization using laparoscopy. In disease greater than stage I (FIGO classification), postoperative abdomino-pelvic CT scanning is advocated[30] to guide adjuvant therapy. MRI in a few series has both been described as oversensitive[31] and superior[32] to ultrasound in its diagnostic value.

## Bone

### Paget's disease

The incidence and prevalence of Paget's disease is difficult to quantify since only 1% of patients with the condition have symptoms. The prevalence, however, is very low under the age of 40 years. It rises after this from about 3% of people over 40 years old to over 10% in people over 80 years of age. Geographical differences in its prevalance also exist; it is rare in Japan and the Nordic countries. The aetiology is as yet unknown, but its epidemiology and ultrastructural features[33] suggest an infectious origin.[34]

The bone in Paget's disease has a highly disorganized architecture. The typical X-ray findings are areas of focal bone resorption and a disordered trabecular pattern, seen as areas of lysis and sclerosis. Overall bone size appears enlarged and the cortices are thickened (Fig. 10.12). The sclerosis may be so extensive that it may be confused with metastatic disease from prostate, breast, lung, thyroid or pancreas associated with sclerotic bony metastases. Classically, Paget's disease presents with involvement from one end of the bone to the other. Although the risk of transformation to osteosarcoma is now judged to be about 1%, it is important to remember that Paget's disease and malignancy may coexist.

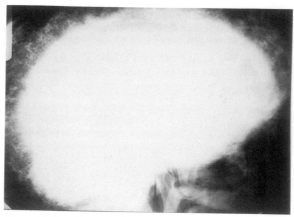

***Figure 10.12*** — Pagets skull.

## Bone in malignant disease

The bone is a common site for metastatic disease and bronchus, breast, kidney, thyroid and prostatic carcinoma in particular target bone. In addition, multiple myeolma can cause lytic lesions of the bone. Prostatic carcinoma can cause sclerotic lesions and most other malignancies cause lytic lesions.

Bone involvement in multiple myeloma classically produces extensive bone destruction with pain and susceptibility to fracture. Skeletal X-rays reveal osteoporosis, lytic lesions and fractures. Characteristic skeletal lesions are punched-out lytic areas which are sharply circumscribed. The vertebrae, skull, thoracic cage and pelvis are the commonest sites of involvement. Pathological fractures are common and should suggest the possibility of multiple myeloma. In contrast to patients with metastatic carcinoma, the vertebral pedicles are rarely involved in myeloma.

## Summary

Imaging in endocrinological malignancy has a particularly useful role because tumours often express receptors that enable them to be localized with particular ligands, they may secrete hormones that can be measured at the time of angiography and, when they spread to the liver, hepatic embolization is a useful therapeutic option. The prognosis in most endocrine tumours is far better than it is for most other solid tumours and for this reason the role of the interventional radiologist is particularly valuable.

# Acknowledgement

The authors would like to thank Dr R Jewkes who supplied most of the figures used to illustrate this chapter.

# References

1. Chandrasekharappa SC, Guru SC, Manickam P *et al*. Positional cloning of the gene for multiple endocrine neoplasia-type 1. *Science* 1997; **276**: 404–407.

2. Lemmens I, Van de Ven WJ, Kas K *et al*. Identification of the multiple endocrine neoplasia type 1 (MEN1) gene. The European Consortium on MEN1. *Hum Mol Genet* 1997; **6**: 1177–1183.

3. Catarci T, Fiacco F, Bozzao L, Pati M, Magiar AV, Cerbo R. Empty sella and headache. *Headache* 1994; 34: 583–586.

4. Oldfield EH, Doppman JL, Nieman LK *et al*. Petrosal sinus sampling with and without corticotropin-releasing hormone for the differential diagnosis of Cushing's syndrome. *N Engl J Med* 1991; **325**: 897–905.

5. Ituarte EM, Petrini J, Hershman JM. Acromegaly and colon cancer. *Ann Intern Med* 1984; **101**: 627–628.

6. Sharma S, Longo WE, Baniadam B, Vernava AM. Colorectal manifestations of endocrine disease. *Dis Colon Rectum* 1995; **38**: 318–323.

7. Daunt N, Mowat P. Computed tomographic appearances and clinical features of prolactin-secreting pituitary adenomas in young male patients. *Clin Radiol* 1985; **36**: 227–231.

8. Delgrange E, Trouillas J, Maiter D, Donckier J, Tourniaire J. Sex-related difference in the growth of prolactinomas: a clinical and proliferation marker study. *J Clin Endocrinol Metab* 1997; **82**: 2102–2107.

9. Eng C, Clayton D, Schuffenecker I *et al*. The relationship between specific RET proto-oncogene mutations and disease phenotype in multiple endocrine neoplasia type 2. International RET mutation consortium analysis. *JAMA* 1996; **276**: 1575–1579.

10. Simeone JF, Daniels GH, Mueller PR *et al*. High-resolution real-time sonography of the thyroid. *Radiology* 1982; **145**: 431–435.

11. Solbiati L, Cioffi V, Ballarati E. Ultrasonography of the neck. *Radiol Clin North Am* 1992; **30**: 941–954.

12. Mackinnon WB, Delbridge L, Russell P *et al*. Two-dimensional proton magnetic resonance spectroscopy for tissue characterization of thyroid neoplasms. Diagnosis of follicular thyroid lesions by proton magnetic resonance on fine needle biopsy. *World J Surg* 1995; **80**: 1306–1311.

13. Cavalieri RR. Nuclear imaging in the management of thyroid carcinoma. *Thyroid* 1996; **6**: 485–492.

14. Brendel AJ, Guyot M, Jeandot R, Lefort G, Manciet G. Thallium-201 imaging in the follow-up of differentiated thyroid carcinoma. *J Nucl Med* 1988; **29**: 1515–1520.

15. Singer PA, Cooper DS, Daniels GH *et al*. Treatment guidelines for patients with thyroid nodules and well-differentiated thyroid cancer. American Thyroid Association. *Arch Intern Med* 1996; **156**: 2165–2172.

16. Rauth JD, Sessions RB, Shupe SC, Ziessman HA. Comparison of Tc-99m MIBI and TI-201/Tc-99m pertechnetate for diagnosis of primary hyperparathyroidism. *Clin Nucl Med* 1996; **21**: 602–608.

17. Peeler BB, Martin WH, Sandler MP, Goldstein RE. Sestamibi parathyroid scanning and preoperative localization studies for patients with recurrent/persistent hyperparathyroidism or significant comorbid conditions: development of an optimal localization strategy. *Am Surg* 1997; **63**: 37–46.

18. Skowsky WR, Wilf LH. Iodine 131 metaiodobenzylguanidine scintigraphy of medullary carcinoma of the thyroid. *South Med J* 1991; **84**: 636–641.

19. O'Shea D, Rohrer Theurs AW, Lynn JA, Jackson JE, Bloom SR. Localization of insulinomas by selective intraarterial calcium injection. *J Clin Endocrinol Metab* 1996; **81**: 1623–1627.

20. Hammond PJ, Bloom SR. Searching for gastrinomas. *Br Med J* 1993; **307**: 4–5.

21. Doppman JL, Miller DL, Chang R *et al*. Gastrinomas: localization by means of selective intraarterial injection of secretin. *Radiology* 1990; **174**: 25–29.

22. Gibril F, Doppman JL, Chang R, Weber HC, Termanini B, Jensen RT. Metastatic gastrinomas: localization with selective arterial injection of secretin. *Radiology* 1996; **198**: 77–84.

23. Bloom SR, Polak JM, Pearse AG. Vasoactive intestinal peptide and watery-diarrhoea syndrome. *Lancet* 1973; **2**: 14–16.

24. Krenning EP, Bakker WH, Breeman WA *et al*. Localisation of endocrine-related tumours with radioiodinated analogue of somatostatin. *Lancet* 1989; **1**: 242–244.

25. Virgolini I, Yang Q, Li S *et al* Cross-competition between vasoactive intestinal peptide and somatostatin for binding to tumor cell membrane receptors. *Cancer Res* 1994; **54**: 690–700.

26. Virgolini I, Raderer M, Kurtaran A *et al*. Vasoactive intestinal peptide-receptor imaging for the localization of intestinal adenocarcinomas and endocrine tumors. *N Engl J Med* 1994; **331**: 1116–1121.

27. Hammond PJ, Arka A, Peters AM, Bloom SR, Gilbey SG. Localization of metastatic gastroenteropancreatic tumours by somatostatin receptor scintigraphy with [111In-DTPA-D-Phe1]-octreotide. *Q J Med* 1994; **87**: 83–88.

28. Lamberts SW, Reubi JC, Krenning EP. Validation of somatostatin receptor scintigraphy in the localization of neuroendocrine tumors. *Acta Oncol* 1993; **32**: 167–170.

29. White PM, Howard GC, Best JJ, Wright AR. The role of computed tomographic examination of the pelvis in the management of testicular germ cell tumours. *Clin Radiol* 1997; **52**: 124–129.

30. Dobson M, Carrington BM, Radford JA, Buckley CH, Crowther D. The role of computed tomography in the management of ovarian tumours of borderline malignancy. *Clin Radiol* 1997; **52**: 280–283.

31. Mascaretti G, Carta G, Renzi E *et al*. Transvaginal ultrasonography and nuclear magnetic resonance. Comparison of techniques in the evaluation of ovarian lesions. *Minerva Ginecol* 1994; **46**: 591–595.

32. Acar B, Posaci C, Dicle O, Topuz A, Erten O. Diagnostic value of magnetic resonance imaging in gynaecology. *Aust N Z J Obstet Gynaecol* 1992; **32**: 252–255.

33. Rebel A, Basle M, Pouplard A, Malkani K, Filmon R, Lepatezour A. Bone tissue in Paget's disease of bone. Ultrastructure and immunocytology. *Arthritis Rheum* 1980; **23**: 1104–1114.

34. Holdaway IM, Ibbertson HK, Wattie D, Scragg R, Graham P. Previous pet ownership and Paget's disease. *Bone Miner* 1990; **8**: 53–58.

# 11

# THE OVARIES, ENDOMETRIUM AND CERVIX

N M deSouza and W P Soutter

**Imaging techniques**
**The ovaries**
**The uterus**
**Cervical cancer**

# Imaging techniques

Cross-sectional imaging plays a crucial role in the detection, assessment and follow-up of gynaecological malignancy. Ultrasound, X-ray, computed tomography (CT) and magnetic resonance imaging (MRI) are all widely used and can offer complementary information depending on the clinical situation.

For transabdominal ultrasound a 3.5–5 MHz transducer is used, while for endovaginal sonography a 5.0–7.5 MHz probe is appropriate. Endovaginal ultrasound is superior for near field lesions but its field of view and penetration are limited. Transabdominal ultrasound may be used for assessment of abdominal and pelvic lymphadenopathy, renal obstruction or liver metastases. Colour flow and duplex Doppler imaging may be used with either probe: the former allows identification of vascularity and the latter can be used to characterize arterial waveform patterns and resistive indices.

With CT a meticulous scanning technique is essential to look for metastases. The complete scanned field ranges from the dome of the diaphragm to the inguinal region. Contrast opacification of the bowel is mandatory and 8–10 mm thick slices through the abdomen and 5 mm slices through the pelvis are optimal. Intravenous contrast opacification aids differentiation between iliac vessels and lymph nodes. In general, CT scanning of the pelvis is not as helpful as in the upper abdomen and ultrasound and MRI are preferred.

Similar imaging volumes to include the abdomen and pelvis are required when using MRI. With this modality multiple imaging planes for lesion visualization are a distinct advantage. In the pelvis T2-weighted images provide maximal tissue contrast. Fat-suppressed or short T1 inversion recovery (STIR) sequences in the coronal plane show pelvic lymphadenopathy to best advantage. To reduce bowel motion the patient is advised to remain nil by mouth for 6 hours prior to scanning. In addition, glucagon or buscopan may be administered intramuscularly. The use of a phased array multicoil wrapped around the lower abdomen markedly improves signal to noise ratios and hence image quality. Respiratory motion may be controlled with respiratory gating and vascular motion with the use of pre-saturation bands.

# The ovaries

## Normal anatomy and variations

The ovaries vary in appearances with their functional status. Infantile ovaries are small (except in the neonate when hypertrophy and follicular growth stimulated by maternal hormones may surprise the inexperienced) and they enlarge before puberty. They are ovoid in shape, approximately 2.5–4 cm long and can be anywhere within the true pelvis. Follicular development begins before menstruation but cycles in young women and perimenopausal women are often imperfect, so that follicles may persist and continue enlarging for several months. Normally ovulation occurs at a follicle size of 20–25 mm diameter and the echo-free follicle is replaced by a corpus luteum which can be cystic or solid. Corpora lutea produce a confusing variety of appearances, whose only consistent feature is their relative transience. In doubtful cases, repeated scans after an interval of several weeks may be needed to resolve the question.

On MRI normal ovaries are often difficult to define but they may be recognized on STIR sequences as very high signal ovoid structures.

## Ovarian carcinoma

The risk of ovarian cancer increases with age and becomes significant after the menopause. (Serov et al, 1973): 15.7 of 100 000 women aged 40–44 years and 54 of 100 000 women aged 75–79 years will develop ovarian cancer.[2] Nulliparous women are at increased risk for developing ovarian cancer.[3] Early menopause and long-term oral contraception appear to protect against ovarian cancer possibly because of the reduced frequency of ovulation.[4] Familial ovarian cancer is responsible for 3–5% of cases. Environmental factors, both dietary[1,2] and chemical such as herbicides,[5] asbestos and talc[6] have all been linked with an increased risk of ovarian cancer.

SCREENING

Ovarian cancer is diagnosed late because of a lack of symptoms and the intraperitoneal location of the ovaries. The overall 5-year survival is 30%[7] and the majority of patients have extrapelvic spread at initial presentation.[2] The goal of screening is to detect the cancer at a curable stage and to improve ovarian disease specific survival. To this end screening programmes with bimanual rectovaginal pelvic examination, CA125 testing and transabdominal as well as transvaginal sonography have all been advocated for high risk patients such as close relative with ovarian cancer.

Campbell et al[8] screened 5479 females aged 18–19 years with transabdominal sonography and found 326 to have persistently abnormal ovaries. Only 9 of these cases had tumours: 5 had Stage I ovarian cancer and 4 metastatic lesions to the ovaries. Van Nagell et al[9] screened 3220 postmenopausal women and detected 1.4% of morphologic ovarian abnormalities. Only 2 cases had Stage I ovarian cancer, 1 had more advanced disease and the other lesions were benign. Attention should therefore focus on high risk groups to improve the risk: benefit ratio.

Other early detection studies coupled conventional ultrasound techniques with colour Doppler imaging in an attempt to visualize early physiologic changes, such as angiogenesis,[10] that occur before morphologic changes in ovarian architecture can be detected. Colour Doppler imaging (CDI) is based on the principal that fast growing tumours contain many new blood vessels that have relatively little smooth muscle in their walls. The resistance to blood flow within these vessels is therefore less than the resistance to flow within vessels of benign lesions. In practice, however, clinical studies of CDI have revealed that normal physiologic changes in the premenopausal ovary at the time of ovulation have low impedance flow characteristics similar to those seen in malignancy.[11] Carter et al[12] examined 123 women with suspected pelvic masses using both conventional transvaginal sonography and CDI. A comparison of findings between the benign and malignant tumours was made by analysing different thresholds of the intratumoral pulsatility and resistance index values by means of receiver-operator characteristic curves. The area under the curve indicated the efficiency of the pulsatility and resistance index values at predicting malignancy. Malignant tumours were generally larger and had a complex or solid pattern. Absent colour flow was found equally among benign and malignant tumours. There was no difference in systolic, diastolic or mean velocities between benign and malignant tumours. No significant difference existed in performance of either the pulsatility or resistance index in predicting malignancy, although the best thresholds for predicting malignancy were obtained with a pulsatility index of 1.0 and a resistance index of 0.6. This relatively poor specificity, difficulties in reproducibility and subjectivity of results have limited the usefulness of CDI in ovarian cancer screening.

CA125 is elevated (>35 U/ml) in ~80% of patients with epithelial ovarian cancer but is also elevated in hepatic cirrhosis, endometriosis, the first trimester of pregnancy and advanced intra-abdominal malignancy.[3] Only 50% of patients with Stage I disease have elevated CA125 levels,[3] indicating that half the patients would not be detected by CA125 levels at a potentially curable stage.

The National Cancer Institute's consensus conference on ovarian cancer[14] concluded that 'there is no evidence available yet that the current screening modalities of CA125 and transvaginal sonography can be used effectively for widespread screening to reduce mortality from ovarian cancer nor that their use will result in decreased rather than increased morbidity and mortality'. Women from a family with a hereditary cancer syndrome should be referred to a specialist to discuss the appropriate use of diagnostic testing and prophylactic surgery. The optimal interval for screening interventions also remains unknown.

## CLINICAL PRESENTATION

Ovarian cancer presents with nausea, dyspepsia and abdominal discomfort: in the later stages abdominal distension and an abdominal mass may be noted by the patient.

## STAGING

Staging is based on the disease site and extent at exploratory laparotomy. (Table 11.1) Definitive staging requires abdominal hysterectomy with bilateral salpingo-oophorectomy, excision of omentum, biopsy of pelvic and abdominal nodes and cytological examination of effusions. Without rigorous staging, patients are generally understaged. Spread is by surface shedding and seeding to other organs, the subphrenic space and diaphragm. Lymphatic dissemination and obstruction produce omental implants and 'caking' and result in ascites. All peritoneal surfaces are involved including the bowel wall. Haematogenous spread to liver, lungs and bone is rare.

The dramatic difference in cure rates between patients with local disease (80–90%) and those with distant disease (15–25%), means that imaging to detect ovarian cancer early is desirable.

## IMAGING
*Primary site*

Imaging is used to assess tumour size, wall thickness, internal architecture, including septations, calcifications, cystic and solid components and papillary nodules. Thin-walled unilocular cysts with few septations and no papillary projections suggest a benign lesion.[15–17] Papillary projections are highly indicative of malignancy.[15,16,18] The findings of thick walls and septa >3 mm (Fig 11.1) are less reliable signs of malignancy.[19] In addition, pelvic, omental and mesenteric involvement may be noted. Ascites is non-specific and is found in 40% of patients without metastases.[1]

The probability of malignancy is also related to tumour size.[20,21] Goldstein et al[21] did not find any cancer among 52 postmenopausal women with thin-walled unilocular

**Table 11.1** FIGO staging for primary ovarian carcinoma

| Stage | FIGO definition |
|---|---|
| I | Growth limited to ovaries |
| Ia | Growth limited to one ovary no ascites; no tumour on external surface; capsule intact |
| Ib | Growth limited to both ovaries no ascites; no tumour on external surfaces; capsule intact |
| Ic | Tumour either Stage Ia or Ib but tumour on surface of one or both ovaries; or with capsule ruptured; or with ascites present containing malignant cells; or with positive peritoneal washings |
| II | Growth involving one or both ovaries with pelvic extension |
| IIa | Extension and/or metastases to the uterus or tubes |
| IIb | Extension to other pelvic tissues |
| IIc | Tumour either Stage IIa or IIb but tumour on surface of one or both ovaries; or with capsule ruptured; or with ascites present containing malignant cells; or with positive peritoneal washings |
| III | Growth involving one or both ovaries with peritoneal implants outside the pelvis or positive retroperitoneal or inguinal nodes. Superficial liver metastases equals Stage III |
| IIIa | Tumour grossly limited to the true pelvis with negative nodes but with histologically confirmed microscopic seeding of abdominal peritoneal surfaces |
| IIIb | Tumour with histologically confirmed implants on abdominal peritoneal surfaces none exceeding 2 cm in diameter. Nodes are negative |
| IIIc | Abdominal implants greater than 2 cm in diameter or positive retroperitoneal or inguinal nodes |
| IV | Growth involving one or both ovaries with distant metastases. If pleural effusion is present there must be positive cytology to allot a case to Stage IV. Parenchymal liver metastasis equals Stage IV |

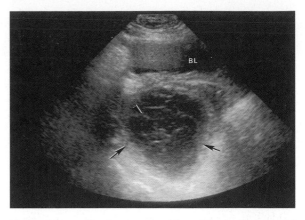

***Figure 11.1*** — Ovarian cancer: Transabdominal ultrasound image in longitudinal section showing a large cystic mass (arrows) with multiple septations within it (arrowhead) typical of a cystic ovarian neoplasm. BL = bladder.

ovarian lesions of <5 cm in diameter. Rulin & Preston[20] found that in 150 postmenopausal patients the malignancy rate was 3% for lesions <5 cm, 11% for lesions 5–10 cm in diameter and 63% for lesions >10 cm. Haemorrhage in a unilocular cyst is typical of benign lesions. On US however, a clot may look like papillary projections and fibrous strands may be misread as septa.

A scoring system has evolved which results in false positives because of confusion between unusual appearing corpora lutea and benign tumours. Benign lesions are unilocular or multilocular with thin septa and no nodules, whereas malignant lesions are often multilocular with thick septa and nodules (Fig. 11.2). Uniformly echogenic lesions are less likely to be malignant than those of mixed echogenicity. In postmenopausal women, anechoic lesions <5 cm in diameter are unlikely to be malignant but those >5 cm carry a 10% chance of malignancy.[22] However, Campbell et al[8] were unable to identify any morphological characteristics to differentiate reliably between ovarian tumour-like conditions, benign ovarian tumours and early malignant tumours. Bourne et al[23] proposed that the false positive rate may be reduced by the use of transvaginal colour flow imaging but these studies have been reported as both disappointing[24] and useful.[25] Initially, a low resistance index (<0.4) was advocated as the best discriminator but this has proved unreliable and a high peak velocity may be a better feature.

As a tumour arising from a non-essential organ that remains primarily confined to the peritoneal cavity, ovarian cancer makes an attractive target for monoclonal antibodies. In the last decade progressive improvement in tumour imaging has been observed when one compares the best examples of early studies performed with [131]I heterosera to the best of modern images obtained with [123]I, [99m]Tc or [111]In labelled monosera. However, these antibodies are limited by problems that include antibody specificity, detectability and the immunoreactivity of the patient to the antibodies used.

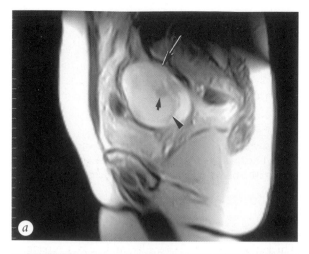

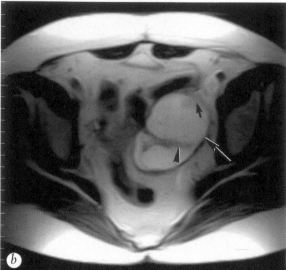

*Figure 11.2* — MR images through the pelvis using an external phased array multicoil. a) Sagittal and b) transverse T2-weighted spin-echo (2500/80 ms [TR/TE]) images show a large cystic mass (long arrow). Irregular septations (arrowhead) and papillary projections (short arrow) are seen and are indicative of malignancy.

Methods have therefore been developed to [198]Au-label a human monoclonal antibody (TC5) developed against an ovarian cell surface antigen,[26] which has a high sensitivity and specificity for detecting ovarian cancer. Antibodies coupled to drugs or biological toxins are also under investigation. Some antibodies may have direct antitumour effects through binding to biologically active receptors or through immune receptor functions. The use of antibody fragments, chimeric antibodies and genetically engineered antibodies is also under active

investigation.[27] Monoclonal antibodies have great potential for improving the diagnosis and for treatment of ovarian cancer.

The potential of positron emission tomography (PET) is being evaluated to distinguish benign from malignant tumours by comparing the results of [18]F fluoro-2-deoxyglucose ([18]F FDG) PET scans with surgical findings. The positive predictive value from one such study was 86% and, more importantly, the negative predictive value was 76%.[28] It may be possible using such techniques to identify metabolically active tumours that are not clearly seen on morphological studies.

### Pelvic and abdominal spread

CT is the most useful imaging modality to demonstrate macroscopic recurrence but may fail to show even quite large tumour masses. A variety of manifestations can be seen with CT, each of which can have a spectrum of appearances including ascites, peritoneal seeding and visceral and nodal metastases.[29] Ultrasound may also be used to detect ascites and liver metastases, although it may be difficult to differentiate benign from malignant cystic masses. MRI should be performed in women with questionable macroscopic recurrent tumour in the pelvis and negative CT examination. Although in a small study, it has been shown that MRI is at least equivalent and may be superior to CT in the evaluation of ovarian malignancy.[30] Neither CT nor MRI can exclude microscopic disease.[31]

In a correlative imaging study, Peltier *et al*[32] found that using Fab'2 fragments of [111]In labelled monoclonal antibody CA125, a positive immunoscintigram, even with a negative CT and ultrasound, was highly suggestive of recurrence in the abdomen and pelvis. [111]In CYT 103 immunoscintigraphy detected occult disease in 20 of 71 patients with surgically documented ovarian adenocarcinoma[33] and this approach may be a valuable addition to the presurgical evaluation in patients with suspected, persistent or recurrent pelvic tumour.

# The uterus

## Normal anatomy and variations

The uterus is a pear-shaped structure with an expanded fundus narrowing to a cylindrical cervix. The normal uterine cavity is triangular with the cornua and the internal cervical os as the corners.

The morphology of the normal uterus is best defined on MRI where the zonal architecture of the uterus may be recognized.[34] On T2-weighted images the endometrium is seen as a central high signal stripe which increases in thickness in the secretory phase of the menstrual cycle. The inner myometrium (junctional zone) is of lower signal intensity than the outer myometrium on T2-weighting and histologically correlates with a layer of more densely packed smooth muscle.

Fluid may be present within the cavity at menstruation. Persistent fluid or fluid in a non-menstruating woman is abnormal. In adolescence, it may be caused by vaginal atresia whilst in postmenopausal women cervical stenosis, either fibrotic or malignant, must be considered.

## Endometrial cancer

The median age of patients with endometrial cancer is 61 years, with 75–80% of women being postmenopausal and 3% being less than 40 years old. In women under 40, there is a higher incidence in those who are obese and anovulatory, e.g. in polycystic ovarian disease. The major risk factor for the development of this cancer is excessive unopposed oestrogen stimulation of the endometrium. In postmenopausal women this is caused by a circulating oestrone derived from the conversion of 4-androstenedione in fat and muscle. A marked increase in body weight thus increases circulating oestrone, promoting endometrial proliferation. Administration of exogenous unopposed oestrogens in hormone replacement therapy increases the risk of developing endometrial cancer to 7–10 times that of the general population.[35] Addition of progestagen lowers the risk to below that of the general population.

Although it reduces the death rate in women with breast cancer, tamoxifen increases the annual incidence of endometrial cancer from 0.2/1000 women to 1.6/1000 women.[36] Although the relative risk is large, the absolute risk of endometrial cancer is still very small in tamoxifen-treated women.

### SCREENING

There are no immediate prospects for mass screening. A number of tests such as endometrial biopsy, curettage, brushings, lavage, aspiration and progestagen challenge tests are available but no data support their value in reducing the morbidity and mortality of this disease.

### CLINICAL PRESENTATION

Postmenopausal bleeding is the presenting symptom in 75–80% of cases. The remainder present with discharge, pain or an abnormal cervical smear test. In pre-menopausal patients bleeding is usually irregular but can be regular and heavy.

Although curettage is mandatory in all patients with postmenopausal or irregular bleeding, imaging at this point helps establish the diagnosis and assess the extent of disease.

### STAGING

The current FIGO staging criteria are shown in Table 11.2. The overall 5-year survival is 65% and is similar to carcinoma of the cervix of an equivalent stage.

### IMAGING

*Primary site*

Thickening of the endometrium is characteristic of endometrial carcinoma and is well demonstrated on transvaginal ultrasound. However, specificity is low and Doppler has been suggested as a way to distinguish hormonal causes of thickening (weak signals) and malignancy which gives marked colour and spectral Doppler signals. Endometrial cancer is very rare if the endometrium is <4 mm thick.

In patients already proven to have endometrial cancer, the presence and depth of myometrial extension has important prognostic and therapeutic implications. Myometrial invasion may be classified as absent, superficial or deep. It may be possible to assess the depth of myometrial invasion with high resolution ultrasound probes. In a study of 20 patients, 70% of ultrasound estimations of invasion depth were within

Table 11.2  FIGO surgical staging of endometrial carcinoma.

| Stage | Description |
|---|---|
| IaG123 | Tumour limited to endometrium |
| IbG123 | Invasion <½ myometrium |
| Ic123 | Invasion >½ myometrium |
| IIaG123 | Endocervical glandular involvement only |
| IIbG123 | Cervical stromal invasion |
| IIIaG123 | Tumour invades serosa anod/or adnexae and/or positive peritoneal cytology |
| IIIbG123 | Vaginal metastases |
| IIIcG123 | Metastases to pelvic and/or para-aortic lymph nodes |
| IVa | Tumour invades bladder and/or bowel mucosa |
| IVb | Distant metastases including intra-abdominal and/or inguinal lymph nodes |

10% of the actual pathological measurement.[37] Errors in estimation occurred when the tumour was exophytic and had significant extension into the uterine cavity. False positives also occur if the uterine cavity is over distended with pus or blood when a subendometrial hypoechoic halo may be demonstrated. Ultrasound assessment of the integrity of the hypoechoic layer can be improved by the use of transvaginal or transrectal sonography.

Changes in uterine blood flow have been used to detect endometrial cancer using endometrial thickness (including tumour) and pulsatility index (PI) derived from flow velocity waveforms recorded from both uterine arteries and from within the tumour. Bourne et al[38] found an overlap in endometrial thickness between women with and without endometrial cancer but the PI was invariably lower in women with postmenopausal bleeding due to endometrial cancer than in those with other reasons for blood loss. Blood flow impedance is inversely related to the stage of cancer. PI values in healthy women increase slightly with age but decrease with oestrogen replacement therapy. Therefore, although Doppler studies may be helpful in the detection of endometrial cancer, allowance must be made for oestrogen replacement therapy.

CT may also be used to stage endometrial cancer. It depicts endometrial cancer as a hypodense lesion in the uterine parenchyma[39] or as a fluid-filled uterus due to tumour obstruction of the endocervical canal or vagina. These findings, however, are non-specific and are easily confused with leiomyomata, intrauterine fluid collections and extension of a cervical carcinoma into the uterine body. In addition, a central lucency may occur in normal postmenopausal women.

MRI appears to represent a unique method of assessing a patient with an endometrial cancer, possessing advantages over other radiological techniques in stage I and II disease, but probably equal to CT in a patient with a more advanced tumour.[40] On T2-weighted MRI, endometrial cancer has an intermediate high signal intensity, similar to that of normal endometrium, but shows some degree of variability (Fig. 11.3). The high signal makes the tumour quite distinct from the surrounding myometrium which possesses an intermediate signal intensity. In a premenopausal uterus, however, it may be difficult to differentiate tumour from adenomatous hyperplasia or indeed from the high signal of normal endometrium. Contrast-enhanced T1-weighted MRI improves the ability to assess the depth

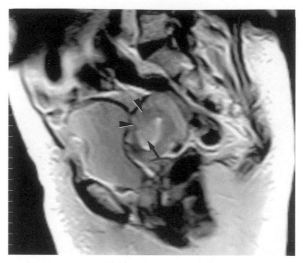

***Figure 11.3*** — Endometrial cancer: Sagittal MR image through the pelvis using an external phased array multicoil. T2-weighted spin-echo (2500/80 ms [TR/TE]) images show an intermediate signal-intensity mass (arrow) within the endometrium that is expanding the cavity. A break in the low signal stripe of the junctional zone (arrowheads) indicates myometrial invasion.

of myometrial invasion by endometrial tumour.[41] MRI has been found to have a sensitivity of 57% and a specificity of 96% for tumour confined to the endometrium, 74% and 74% for superficial invasion and 88% and 85% respectively for deep penetration.[42] However, the degree of invasion may be overestimated by exophytic polypoid tumours with significant extraluminal extension. Powell et al[40] found the low signal band of inner myometrium to be thinned or absent in those patients with deeply invasive tumours (Fig. 11.4) and this correlated well with the pathological measurement of myometrial invasion.

The sagittal plane is the most appropriate for examination of a patient with primary endometrial cancer as this provides a longitudinal view of the uterus which will include both corpus and cervix. The sagittal plane also provides the opportunity to assess anterior invasion of the tumour into the bladder and posteriorly to the rectum.

*Recurrence*

Transrectal sonography has been investigated in cases where recurrent endometrial cancer is suspected.[45] Physical examination may be difficult because of post-surgical fibrosis. Infiltration to the surrounding connective tissues and organs such as the rectum and bladder can be identified and transrectal ultrasound can

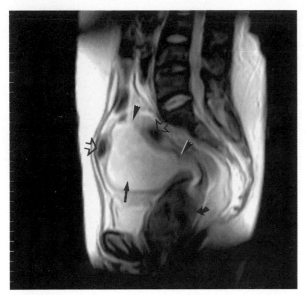

*Figure 11.4* — Advanced endometrial cancer: Sagittal MR image through the pelvis using an external phased array multicoil. T2-weighted spin-echo (2500/80 ms [TR/TE]) images show a very large intermediate signal-intensity mass (arrow) within the endometrium, expanding the uterine cavity and breaching the junctional zone in several places (arrowheads). Well-defined low signal-intensity masses within the endometrium represent incidental fibroids (open arrows). There is a large clot in the vagina (curved arrow).

be used to guide transvaginal or transperineal fine-needle biopsy. CT[46] or MRI may also be used to detect recurrent disease and metastatic carcinoma to omentum or lymph nodes.

# Cervical cancer

There is a wealth of epidemiological evidence to suggest that the risk of developing cervical neoplasia is associated with sexual behaviour. This may be due to a sexually transmitted agent, in particular human papilloma virus, as well as immunosuppressive agents present in seminal fluid which may alter the local immune response to viral infections. However, definitive evidence for these risk factors is not yet available.

### SCREENING

The use of cervical cytology to identify precancerous lesions in asymptomatic healthy women is well established. The cellular atypia detectable by cervical cytology are graded as mild (I), moderate (II) or severe (III). An international study by the IARC[47] clearly indicated

that screening every 3 years is as effective as screening every year. However, in patients with treated CIN, annual screening cytology is recommended because of a 5% risk of recurrent CIN.[48]

### CLINICAL PRESENTATION

Intermenstrual or postcoital bleeding are the most common presenting symptoms. A foul smelling vaginal discharge may occur. Pelvic and leg pain occur in the later stages of the disease due to pelvic sidewall involvement and invasion of the lumbosacral plexus. Bladder invasion causes haematuria and urinary frequency while rectal invasion causes tenesmus and bleeding.

### STAGING

This is done by bimanual examination under anaesthesia using the FIGO system (Table 11.3). Imaging does not alter the FIGO staging of the disease but its use is vital in the assessment of disease extent. MRI is the modality of choice for assessing the primary tumour and pelvic organs.

CT, transabdominal ultrasound and lymphangiography have all been used to assess nodal involvement, but none is sufficiently accurate to advocate routine use. Lymphangiography correctly identifies only 61% of women with positive nodes,[50] while CT had a false negative rate of 34%.[51]

### IMAGING
*Primary site*

Transabdominal ultrasound is of little value in the assessment of patient with cervical cancer.[52] Poor image quality and difficulty in interpretation are the major problems. Transrectal ultrasound produces clearer views of the cervix but differentiation of tumour from normal cervix is still poor. The same difficulty limits the value of CT since both the normal cervix and cervical carcinoma have similar attenuation values so that the primary tumour can only be recognized if it alters the size and contours of the normal cervix.

Several studies have now confirmed the accuracy of MRI in the staging of early cervical cancer in comparison to the surgical stage.[53,54] Patients are best assessed using T2-weighted MRI of the primary tumour which is superior to CT in tumour detection (sensitivity 75% vs. 51%, p <0.005) and in overall tumour staging (accuracy 75–77% vs. 32–69%, p<0.025).[55,56]

The resolution of MRI of the primary tumour (Fig.11.3) may be further improved by using intracavi-

**Table 11.3**  FIGO staging classification for cervical cancer.[49]

| Stage | Description |
|---|---|
| 0 | Preinvasive carcinoma (carcinoma *in situ*, CIN) |
| I | Carcinoma confined to the cervix (corpus extension should be disregarded) |
| Ia | Invasive cancer identified only microscopically. All gross lesions, even with superficial invasion, are stage Ib cancers. Depth of measured stromal invasion should not be >5 mm and no wider than 7 mm★ |
| Ia1 | Measured invasion no >3 mm in depth and no wider than 7 mm |
| Ia2 | Measured depth of invasion >3 mm and no >5 mm and no wider than 7 mm |
| Ib | Clinical lesions confined to the cervix or preclinical lesions greater than Ia |
| Ib1 | Clinical lesions no >4 cm in size |
| Ib2 | Clinical lesions >4 cm in size |
| II | Carcinoma extending beyond the cervix and involving the vagina (but not the lower third) and/or infiltrating the parametrium (but not reaching the pelvic side wall) |
| IIa | Carcinoma involving the vagina |
| IIb | Carcinoma has infiltrated the parametrium |
| III | Carcinoma involving the lower third of the vagina and/or extending to the pelvic side wall (there is no free space between the tumour and the pelvic side wall) |
| IIIa | Carcinoma involving the lower third of the vagina |
| IIIb | Carcinoma extending to the pelvic wall and/or hydronephrosis or non-functioning kidney due to ureterostenosis caused by tumour |
| IVa | Carcinoma involving the mucosa of the bladder or rectum and/or extending beyond the true pelvis |
| IVb | Spread to distant organs |

★ The depth of invasion should not be >5 mm from the base of the epithelium, either surface or glandular, from which it originates. Vascular space involvement, either venous or lymphatic, should not alter the staging.

tary receiver coils. Endorectal coils give high resolution images of the posterior cervix but the anterior margin of the tumour and its relation to the bladder base is often difficult to define because of drop-off in signal. Endovaginal coils give very high resolution images of the cervix and adjacent parametrium.[57] The distortion of the low signal ring of inner stroma may be apparent and any breaks in the ring representing tumour extension may be identified (Fig. 11.5).

With MRI, the invasion of cervical cancer may be assessed in three planes: the coronal and axial planes may be used to determine parametrial invasion, the axial plane for extension into the bladder and rectum and the sagittal plane for extension into the uterine body, bladder and rectum.[58] The use of 3D volume imaging also provides the necessary information to calculate tumour volumes, which is of prognostic significance. Volumes obtained with MRI correlate well with those obtained by histomorphometric methods but only weakly with clinical stage.[59] The volumetry of the tumour also permits more accurate judgement of the histological findings of parametrial invasion, vascular involvement and lymph node involvement.[60]

*Parametrium*

Transrectal ultrasound, CT and MRI have all been used to assess parametrial spread. In a series of 180

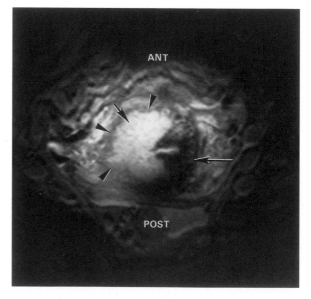

***Figure 11.5*** — Cervical carcinoma: Transverse T2-weighted MR image (2500/80 ms [TR/TE]) image of the cervix using an endovaginal receiver coil. A high signal intensity mass (short arrow) is seen expanding the cervix on the right with a rim of normal low signal stroma around it (arrowheads). This indicates that the tumour is confined to the cervix at this level. Normal looking low signal-intensity cervical stroma is present on the left (long arrow).

patients, good correlation was found between ultrasound and surgical findings, but significant problems arose in distinguishing between inflammatory or fibrotic change and tumour invasion.[61] Similarly, false positive diagnosis may arise from misinterpreting normal inflammatory parametrial soft tissue strands as tumour invasion on both CT and MRI. A comparison of the assessment by these modalities with histological findings after radical hysterectomy showed an accuracy rate for parametrial involvement of 87–90% for MRI, 55–80% for CT and 82.5% for examination under anaesthesia.[54,56] Extracervical extension on MRI is best defined using contrast enhancement and varied pulse sequences. MRI therefore yields valuable information for treatment planning[62] and should be used routinely in conjunction with clinical staging to determine the appropriate therapy in patients with cervical carcinoma. An intravenous urogram (IVU) may sometimes be useful in estimating the pelvic extent of cervical carcinoma by demonstrating partial or complete ureteric obstruction and/or displacement and distortion of the bladder outline. The IVU is abnormal in 2.1% of stage I cases, in 5.1% of stage II, in 26.8% of stage III and in 48.9% of stage IV.[63] The presence of a hydronephrosis or nonfunctioning kidney due to stenosis from tumour invasion of the ureter puts the patient into stage III even if, according to the other findings, the case should be allotted to an earlier stage.

Barium enema abnormalities are rare in cervical cancer and proctoscopy is also positive if an abnormality is observed on the enema.

### Nodal involvement

The role of lymphangiography in the staging of cervical cancer is controversial with up to 71% false positives and 16% false negatives. Percutaneous fine-needle aspiration biopsy of nodes may improve the results obtained with pelvic lymphangiography. CT has proved to be a reliable method for staging and following lymph node disease in patients with lymphoma but the major drawback for epithelial tumours is that the nodes must be enlarged to be detected. Thus metastases <2 cm will not be identified.

MRI is superior to CT in pelvic lymph node evaluation (accuracy 88% vs. 83%, p <0.01).[55] However, like CT it relies on changes in the size of the lymph nodes since the tumour deposits themselves are not highlighted (Fig. 11.6). Although an *in vitro* study has shown that lymph nodes containing metastases have a significantly longer T2 than normal or hyperplastic nodes, *in vivo* tissue characterization based on relaxation times or signal intensities does not support this data.

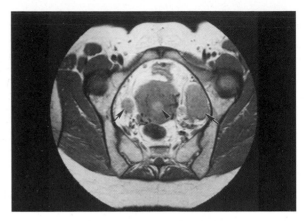

***Figure 11.6*** — Advanced cervical carcinoma: Transverse proton density-weighted MR image (2500/20 ms [TR/TE]) image of the cervix using a whole body receiver coil. The cervix is expanded with a centrally situated tumour (arrowhead). Large intermediate signal-intensity lymph node masses are seen bilaterally at the pelvic side-walls (arrows).

A small patient study suggested that [123]I-labelled epidermal growth factor may be used to recognize cervical cancer lymph node metastases because these tumours express high levels of the receptor.[65]

### Distant spread

Even in advanced pelvic spread, involvement of distant sites is the exception rather than the rule. In only 1 of 160 patients was bone scan positive and this patient had stage 4 disease with liver metastases.[66] Patients with stage I and stage II cervical cancer do not need to have bone scans.

A chest X-ray is a routine pretreatment investigation but the yield of lung metastases at first presentation is likely to be no more than 2%.

### Response and recurrence

In conjunction with clinical examination, MRI may provide a more objective comparison of surgery and radiotherapy. Serial MRI may be used before and after primary radiation therapy to assess tumour response.[67] Primary tumours with a volume of >50 cm³ are likely to have no response or a delayed response.[67] An early (2–3 months) and significant decrease in the signal intensity and volume of tumour indicates a favourable response.

With the increased use of new cytotoxic regimes for primary tumours and increased use of surgery, accurate imaging techniques become more important. Early detection of recurrent cervical cancer in order to institute cytotoxic therapy may be of value. CT and ultrasound have limited ability to differentiate between fibrosis and tumour recurrence. Although isolated reports promote MRI in distinguishing post-treatment fibrosis and recurrent pelvic neoplasm by measuring signal intensities from the different tissues on T2-weighted pulse sequences,[68] in individual cases fibrosis is often impossible to differentiate from recurrence.

# Conclusion

Until recently, management of gynaecological malignancy relied heavily on clinical findings. Newer imaging methods, particularly MRI has pushed imaging to the forefront in the assessment of gynaecological tumours. Such detailed images of the pelvis provide important information to the gynaecological oncologist in planning treatment.

# References

1. Serov SF, Scully RE, Sobin LH. *International Classification of Tumours no. 9. Histological Typing of Ovarian Tumours*. Geneva: World Health Organization, 1973.

2. Young RC, Perez CA, Hoskins WJ. Cancer of the ovary. In: De Vita VT, Hellman S, Rosenberg SA (eds). *Cancer. Principles and Practices of Oncology*. Philadelphia: JB Lippincott Company, 1993, vol. 1, pp. 1226–1263.

3. Smith LH, Oi RH. Detection of malignant ovarian neoplasm. A review of literature. 1. Detection of patient at risk: Clinical, radiological and cytological detection. *Obstet Gynecol Surv* 1984; **39**: 313–328.

4. Cramer DW, Hutchinson GE, Welch WR, Scully RE, Knapp RC. Factors affecting the association of oral contraceptives and ovarian cancer. *N Engl J Med* 1982; **307**: 1047–1051.

5. Donna A, Crosignani B, Robutti F *et al*. Triazine herbicides and ovarian epithelial neoplasm. *Scand J Work Environ Health* 1989; **15**: 47–53.

6. Longo DL, Young RC. Cosmetic talc and ovarian carcinoma. *Lancet* 1979; **2**: 349–351.

7. Webb MJ. Screening for ovarian cancer. *Br Med J* 1993; **306**: 1015–1016.

8. Campbell S, Bhan V, Royston P, Whitehead MI, Collins WP. Transabdominal ultrasound screening for early ovarian cancer. *Br Med J* 1989; **299**: 1363–1366.

9. Van Nagell JR Jr, DePriest PD, Puls LE *et al*. Ovarian cancer screening in asymptomatic postmenopausal women by transvaginal sonography. *Cancer* 1991; **68**: 458–462.

10. Folkman J, Watson K, Ingber D, Hanahan D. Induction of angiogenesis during the transition from hyperplasia to neoplasia. *Nature* 1989; **339**: 58–61.

11. Karlan BY, Platt LD The current status of ultrasound and color Doppler imaging in screening for ovarian cancer. *Gynecol Oncol* 1994; **55**: S28–33.

12. Carter J, Saltzman A, Hartenbach E, Fowler J, Carson L, Twiggs LB. Flow characteristics in benign and malignant gynecologic tumors using transvaginal color flow Doppler. *Obstet Gynecol* 1994; **83**: 125–130.

13. Johnson RJ. Radiology in the management of ovarian cancer. *Clin Rad* 1993; **48**: 75–82.

14. Trimble EL. The NIH Consensus Conference on Ovarian Cancer: screening, treatment, and follow-up. *Gynecol Oncol* 1994; **55**: S1–3.

15. Outwater EK, Mitchell DG. Magnetic resonance imaging techniques in the pelvis. *MRI Clin N Am* 1994; **2**: 161–188.

16. Outwater EK, Dunton CJ. Imaging of the ovary and adnexa: Clinical issues and applications of MR imaging. *Radiology* 1995; **194**: 1–18.

17. Buy JN, Ghossain MA, Sciot C *et al*. Epithelial tumors of the ovary: CT findings and correlation with US. *Radiology* 1991; **178**: 811–818.

18. Granberg S, Wikland M, Jansson I. Macroscopic characterization of ovarian tumors and the relation to the histological diagnosis. Criteria to be used for ultrasound evaluation. *Gynecol Oncol* 1989; **33**: 139–144.

19. Stevens SK, Hricak H, Stern JL. Ovarian lesions. Detection and characterization with gadolinium-enhanced MR imaging at 1.5T. *Radiology* 1991; **181**: 481–488.

20. Rulin MC, Preston AL. Adnexal masses in postmenopausal women. *Obstet Gynecol* 1987; **70**: 578–581.

21. Goldstein SR, Subramanyan B, Synder JR, Beller U, Raghavendra BN, Beckman EM. The postmenopausal cystic adnexal mass: the potential role of ultrasound in conservative management. *Obstet Gynecol* 1989; **73**: 8–10.

22. Andolf E, Jorgensen C. Cystic lesions in elderly women, diagnosed by ultrasound. *Br J Obstet Gynaecol* 1989; **96**: 1076–1079.

23. Bourne T, Campbell S, Steer C, Whitehead MI, Collins WP. Transvaginal colour flow imaging: a possible new screening technique for ovarian cancer. *Br Med J* 1989; **299**: 1367–1370.

24. Hata K, Hata T, Manabe A, Sugimura K, Kitao M. A critical evaluation of transvaginal Doppler studies, transvaginal sonography, magnetic resonance imaging and CA 125 in detecting ovarian cancer. *Obstet Gynecol* 1992; **80**: 922–926.

25. Kawai M, Kano T, Kikkawa F, Maeda O, Ogichi H, Tomoda Y. Transvaginal Doppler ultrasound with colour flow imaging in the diagnosis of ovarian cancer. *Obstet Gynecol* 1992; **79**: 163–167.

26. Chaudhuri TR, Zinn KR, Morris JS, McDonald GA, Llorens AS, Chaudhuri TK. Detection of ovarian cancer by [198]Au-labelled human monoclonal antibody. *Cancer* 1994; **73**: 878–883.

27. Rubin SC. Monoclonal antibodies in the management of ovarian cancer. A clinical perspective. *Cancer* 1993; **71**: 1602–1612.

28. Hubner KF, McDonald TW, Niethammer JG, Smith GT, Gould HE, Buonocore E. Assessment of primary and metastatic ovarian cancer by positron emission tomography (PET) using 2-[18F] deoxyglucose (2-[18F]FDG). *Gynecol Oncol* 1993; **51**: 197–204.

29. Lee MJ, Munk PL, Poon PY, Hassell P. Ovarian cancer: computed tomography findings. *Can Assoc Radiol J* 1994; **45**: 185–192.

30. Smelka RC, Lawrence PH, Shoenut JP, Heywood M, Kroeker MA, Lotocki R. Primary ovarian cancer: prospective comparison

of contrast enhanced CT and pre and post contrast, fat suppressed MR imaging, with histological correlation. *J Mag Res Imag* 1993; **3**: 99–106

31. Prayer L, Kainz C, Kramer J et al. CT and MR accuracy in the detection of tumour recurrence in patients treatment for ovarian cancer. *J Comput Assist Tomogr* 1993; **17**: 626–632.

32. Peltier P, Wiharto K, Dutin JP et al. Correlative imaging study in the diagnosis of ovarian cancer recurrences. *Eur J Nucl Med* 1992; **19**: 1006–1110.

33. Surwit EA, Childers JM, Krag DN et al. Clinical assessment of [111]In-CYT-103 immunoscintigraphy in ovarian cancer. *Gynecol Oncol* 1993; **48**: 283–284.

34. Hricak H, Alpers C, Crooks LE, Sheldon PE. Magnetic resonance imaging of the female pelvis: initial experience. *AJR* 1983; **141**: 1119–1128.

35. Mack T M, Pike M C, Henderson B et al. Estrogens and endometrial cancer in a retirement community. *N Eng J of Med.* 1976; **294**: 1262–1267.

36. Fisher B, Costantino JP, Redmond CK, Fisher ER, Wickerham DL, Cronin WM. Endometrial cancer in tamoxifen treated breast cancer patients: findings from the National Surgical Adjuvant Breast and Bowel Project (NSABP) B-14. *J Natl Cancer Inst* 1994; **86**: 527–537.

37. Fleisher AC, Dudley SB, Entman SS, Baxter JW, Kalemeris GE, Everette JA. Myometrial invasion by endometrial carcinoma: sonographic assessment. *Radiology* 1987; **162**: 307–310.

38. Bourne TH, Campbell S, Steer CV, Royston P, Whitehead MI, Collins WP. Detection of endometrial cancer by transvaginal ultrasonography with colour flow imaging and blood flow analysis: a preliminary report. *Gynecol Oncol* 1991; **40**: 253–259.

39. Suzuki M. Role of x-ray, CT and magnetic resonance imaging in the diagnosis of gynecological malignant tumour. *Nippon Sanka Fujinka Gakkai Zasshi* 1989; **41**: 942–952.

40. Powell MC, Womack C, Buckley JH, Worthington BS, Symonds EM. Pre-operative magnetic resonance imaging of stage 1 endometrial adenocarcinoma. *Br J Obstet Gynaecol* 1986; **93**: 353–350.

41. Sironi S, Colombo E, Villa G et al. Myometrial invasion by endometrial carcinoma: assessment with plain and gadolinium-enhanced MR imaging. *Radiology* 1992; **185**: 207–212.

42. Sironi S, Taccagni G, Garancini P, Belloni C, DelMaschio A. Myometrial invasion by endometrial carcinoma: assessment by MR imaging. *AJR* 1992; **158**: 565–569.

43. Lien HH, Blomlie V, Trope C, Kaern J, Abeler VM. Cancer of the endometrium: value of MR imaging in determining depth of invasion into the myometrium. *AJR* 1991; **157**: 1221–1223.

44. Gordon AN, Fleischer AC, Dudley BS et al. Preoperative assessment of myometrial invasion of endometrial adenocarcinoma by sonography (US) and magnetic resonance imaging (MRI). *Gynecol Oncol* 1989; **34**: 175–179.

45. Squillaci E, Salzani MC, Grandinetti M et al. Recurrence of ovarian and uterine neoplasms: diagnosis with transrectal US. *Radiology* 1988; **169**: 355–358.

46. Balfe DM, Heiken JP, McClennan BL. Oncologic imaging of carcinoma of the cervix, ovary and endometrium. In: Bragg DG, Rubin P, Youker JE (eds) *Oncologic Imaging.* Oxford: Pergamon Press, 1986, pp. 437–477.

47. IARC Working Group on Evaluation of Cervical Cancer Screening Programmes. Screening for cervical squamous cancer: duration of low risk after negative results of cervical cytology and its implication for screening policies. *Br Med J* 1986; **293**: 659–664.

48. Soutter WP, Wisdom S, Brough JK, Monaghan JM. Should patients with a mild atypia in a cervical smear be referred for colposcopy? *Br J Obstet Gynaecol* 1986; **93**: 70–74.

49. Shepherd JH. Staging announcement – FIGO staging of gynaecological cancers; cervical and vulval. *Int J Gynecol Cancer* 1995; **5**: 319.

50. Lagasse LD, Ballon SC, Berman ML, Watring WG. Pretreatment lymphangiography and operative evaluation in carcinoma of the cervix. *Trans Pac Coast Obstet Gynecol Soc* 1979; **46**: 123–128.

51. Pectasides D, Kayianni H, Facou A et al. Correlation of abdominal computed tomography scanning and second-look operation findings in ovarian cancer patients. *Am J Clin Oncol* 1991; **14**: 457–462.

52. Levenback C, Dershaw DD, Rubin SC. Endoluminal ultrasound staging of cervical cancer. *Gynecol Oncol* 1992; **46**: 186–190.

53. Powell MC, Buckley JH, Wasti M, Worthington BS, Sokal M, Symonds WM. The application of magnetic resonance imaging to cervical carcinoma. *Br J Obstet Gynaecol* 1986; **93**: 1276–1285.

54. Togashi K, Nishimura K, Itoh K. Uterine cervical cancer: assessment with high field MR imaging. *Radiology* 1987; **160**: 431–435.

55. Kim SH, Choi BI, Han JK et al. Preoperative staging of uterine cervical carcinoma: comparison of CT and MRI in 99 patients. *J Comput Assist Tomogr* 1993; **17**: 633–640.

56. Ho CM, Chien TY, Jeng CM, Tsang YM, Shih BY, Chang SC. Staging of cervical cancer: comparison between magnetic resonance imaging, computed tomography and pelvic examination under anaesthesia. *J Formas Med Assoc* 1992; **91**: 982–990.

57. deSouza NM, Scoones DJ, Krausz T, Gilderdale DJ, Soutter WP. High-resolution MR imaging of stage I cervical neoplasia, using a dedicated endovaginal coil: MR features and correlation of imaging and pathologic findings *AJR* 1996; **166**: 553–559.

58. Goto M, Okamura S, Ueki M, Sugimoto O. Evaluation of magnetic resonance imaging in the diagnosis of extension in uterine cervical cancer cases with special attention to imaging planes. *Nippon Sanka Fujinka Gakki Zasshi* 1990; **42**: 1627–1633.

59. Burghardt E, Hofmann HM, Ebner F, Haas J, Tamussino K, Justich E. Magnetic resonance imaging in cervical cancer: a basis for objective classification. *Gynecol Oncol* 1989; **33**: 61–67.

60. Burghardt E, Baltzer J, Tulusan AH, Haas J. Results of surgical treatment on 1028 cervical cancers studied with volumetry. *Cancer* 1992; **70**: 648–655.

61. Yuhara A, Akamatsu N, Sekiba K. Use of transrectal radial scan ultrasonography in evaluating the extent of uterine cervical cancer. *J Clin Ultrasound* 1987; **15**: 507–517.

62. Sironi S, Belloni C, Taccagni GL, DelMaschio A. Carcinoma of the cervix: value of MR imaging in detecting parametrial involvement. *AJR* 1991; **156**: 753–756.

63. Griffin JW, Parker RG, Taylor WJ. An evaluation of procedures used in staging carcinoma of the cervix. *AJR* 1976; **127**: 825–827.

64. Weiner JL, Chako AC, Merton CW, Gross S, Coffey EL, Stein HL. Breast and axillary tissue MR imaging correlation of signal intensities and relaxation times with pathologic findings. *Radiology* 1986; **160**: 229–305.

65. Scotian C, Pateisky N, Vavra N et al. Lymphoscintigraphy with [123]I-marked epidermal growth factor in cervix cancer. *Gynakol Geburtshilfliche Rundsch* 1992; **32**: 17–21.

66. Hirule P, Mattman KP, Schmidt B, Pfiefter KH. Indications for radioisotope bone scanning in staging of cervical cancer. *Arch Gynaecol Obstet* 1990; **248**: 21–23.

67. Flueckiger F, Ebner F, Poschauko H, Tamussino K, Einspieler R, Ranner G. Cervical cancer: serial MR imaging before and after primary radiation therapy – a two year follow up study. *Radiology* 1992; **184**: 89–93.

68. Ebner F, Kressel HY, Mintz MC et al. Tumour recurrence versus fibrosis in the female pelvis: differentiation with MR imaging at 1.5T. *Radiology* 1988; **166**: 333–340.

# 12

# THE LYMPHATIC SYSTEM

Walter Curati

**Pathology and classification**
**Imaging strategies**

In the study of tumours, the lymphatic system has a dual role: *per se* it presents with its own diseases (Hodgkin's disease (HD) and non-Hodgkin's lymphoma (NHL)) and it is also involved in the metastatic spread of tumours. This 'dual role' constitutes the mainframe of pathology and classification.

The lymphatic system has two functions:

- provision of immunity-related cells (lymphocytes and macrophages) and sera to fight antigens of various sorts;

- clearance of circulating micro-organisms and cells identified as undesirable.

This combination of functions explains either the successful clearance of small clones of mutant cells or the passive acceptance and proliferation of exogenous micro-organisms carrying infections or endogenous mutants in the initial stages of tumour develpment.

The following are required to implement these functions:

- factories to produce cells and sera (thymus, spleen, liver and bone marrow);

- distribution network (lymphatic channels).

The same lymphatic channels plus interconnected nodes also act as collectors and filters for interstitial fluids and cells.

# Pathology and classification

Lymphomas account for 5–6% of adult tumours in the UK.[1] The incidence of HD peaks in the third and sixth decades, whereas that of NHL increases from the fifth decade onwards.[2] Men are affected more than women (1.4: 1 for HD and 1.1: 1 for NHL).[3]

At the time of its clinical manifestation a *lymphoma* is commonly implanted in two or more sites. In such cases, staging plays a key part in the diagnostic process as it determines treatment strategy. The Rye classification for HD is shown in Table 12.1.[4]

HD spreads along contiguous groups of nodes: cervical, thoracic, abdominal and the involvement by vicinity extension motivates the diagnostic and treatment strategies. NHL covers a broader spectrum of cell types (lymphocytes, histioytes or mixed) and of nodal and extranodal involvement and spread. Over the last 15 years, AIDS-related NHL has been described and approximately 10% of AIDS patients develop this complication and ultimately die from it.

Post-transplant lymphomaproliferative disorders are usually NHL and have a polymorphous histological appearance. They can remain limited to the allograft.

# Imaging strategies

## Diagnosis

Lymphoma can be suspected from a combination of clinical symptoms: long-standing weakness, malaise and/or fever and signs: lymphadenopathy and weight loss, or as an incidental finding of an enlarged mediastinum and/or hilar on a plain chest X-ray. How is imaging used in confirming diagnosis? Filly *et al*[5] studied 300 untreated HD and NHL and found $\frac{2}{3}$ HD and $\frac{1}{3}$–$\frac{1}{2}$ NHL patients to have thoracic nodes. The most useful imaging technique is then the one that allows local-

Table 12.1 Rye classification of Hodgkin's disease.[4]

| Histology | Distinctive features | Relative frequency in adults (%) |
|-----------|---------------------|----------------------------------|
| Lymphocytic | Abundant stroma of mature lymphocytes and/or histiocytes; no necrosis. Reed-Sternberg cells may be sparse | 10–15 |
| Nodular stenosis | Nodules of lymphoid tissue separated by bands of doubly refractile collagen: atypical 'lacunar' Hodgkin's cells in clear spaces within the lymphoid nodules | 20–50 |
| Mixed cellularity | Usually numerous Reed-Sternberg cells and mononuclear Hodgkin's cells in a pleomorphic stroma of eosinophils, plasma cells, fibroblasts and necrotic fat | 20–40 |
| Lymphocytic | Reed-Sternberg cells usually, although not always, abundant; marked paucity of lymphocytes; diffuse, non-refractile fibrosis and necrosis may be present | 5–15 |

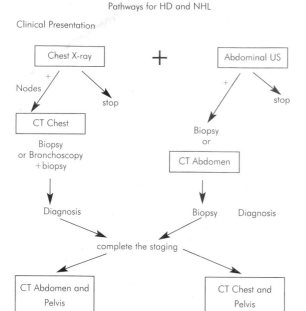

Pathways for HD and NHL

**Figure 12.1** — Pathways for diagnosis of Hodgkin's disease and non-Hodgkin's lymphoma.

ization of a lymph node for needle biopsy and histological assessment. In most cases, CT can localize the node and guide the biopsy. Alternatively, for the abdomen and pelvis, ultrasound can be used.

## Staging

Sensitivity (detection of disease without false negatives), specificity (confirmation of absence of disease without false positives) and accuracy (total sum of sensitivity and specificity) are the best criteria by which to assess the performance of staging techniques. Tolerance and compliance are additional parameters.

**Table 12.2** Staging and monitoring techniques

|  | Staging | Monitoring |
|---|---|---|
| *Whole body techniques* | | |
| CT | +++ | +++ |
| MRI | ++ | ++ |
| PET | (+++) | +++ |
| *Organ techniques* | | |
| Ultrasound | ++ | ++ |
| Lymphography | +++ | +++ |
| Plain X-rays | + | ++ |

## Modalities

*CT* is the best technique for assessing the thorax, abdomen and pelvis. It:

- delineates the anatomy: assesses infiltration and extension;
- visualizes the lymph nodes: isolated or in groups.

Once high resolution fast imaging becomes widely available in terms of costs and technology, *MRI* may be even better than CT. At present it is limited to the pelvis and abdomen (principally the retroperitoneum) in view of the limited motion artefacts, the coronal plane acquisition and the fat tissue background which is easy to suppress by means of various sequences (STIR etc.) and locally, to the brain, spinal cord, etc. by using highly sensitive sequences to suppress the CNF signal and raising the T2-weighting (FLAIR etc.).

*Positron emission tomography* (PET) localizes functional abnormalities with reasonable spatial resolution. Local metabolic hyperactivity is identified and quantified by excessive consumption of metabolites, which permits both accurate staging and monitoring but requires multidisciplinary expertise.

*Ultrasound* is restricted to areas where the presence of air or gas does not restrict anatomical view, i.e. the upper adomen (often without retroperitoneum), lower pelvis and thoracic wall. Locally it can be used to assess renal (ureteric) obstruction.

*Lymphography* was the first accurate (and universally used in oncologic centres) imaging technique for lymphomas and in particular HD. It achieves superb and long-lasting opacification of lymph nodes and allows identification of disease spread and response to treatment. The technique has two drawbacks: 1) visualization is limited to the para-aortic and iliac groups of nodes (in the case of bipedal injection) and 2) it is necessary to dissect and cannulate the superficial lymphatics with very fine needles which requires considerable expertise. Lymphography has been widely superceded by CT.

*Chest X-ray* reveal lymph nodes only in the hilar and mediastinum providing they alter the outline of these regions at a soft tissue-air interface or stand out in an area normally occupied by fat only and not obscured by bone. It is effective and simple as a method of monitoring the reduction or increase in size of groups of nodes in the hilar or mediastinal outline. *Plain abdominal X-rays* can monitor the size of the liver and spleen objectively and at a fraction of the cost of CT. *Skeletal surveys*

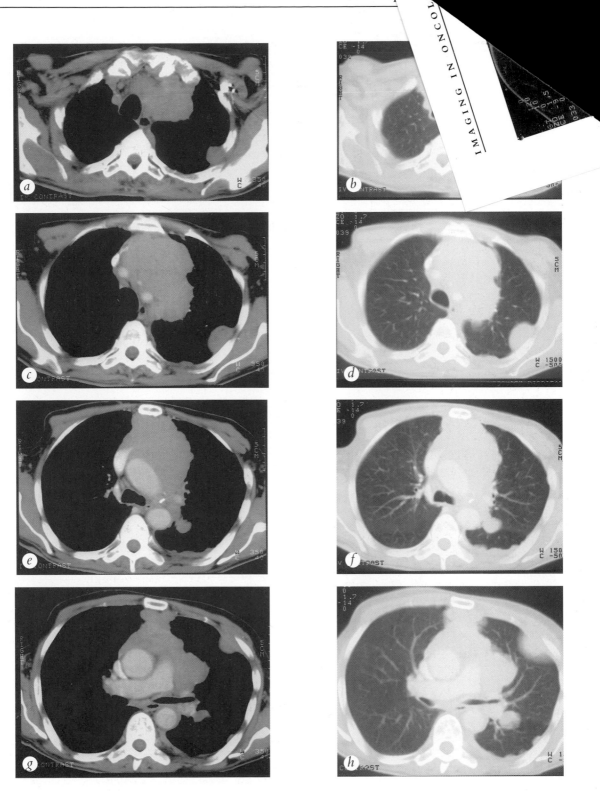

***Figure 12.2*** — Non-Hodgkin's lymphoma type T in a 72-year-old male patient. Contrast-enhanced CT of the chest at different levels with soft tissue and lung windows showing anterior and middle mediastinums.

171

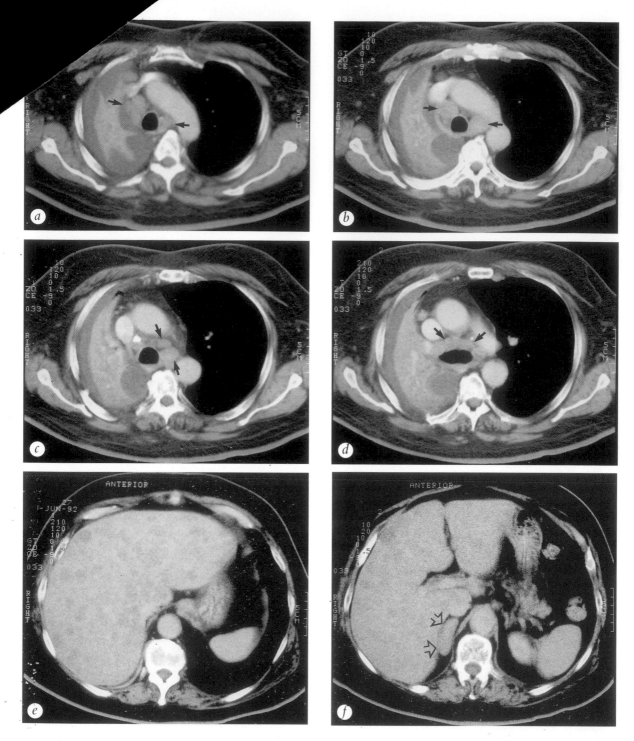

***Figure 12.3*** — Large mediastinal nodes, adrenal glands and liver in a 66-year-old male patient with metastatic right upper lobe bronchial carcinoma. Contrast-enhanced CT of the chest and upper abdomen at different levels. a)–d) Right upper lobe atelec- tasis, pleural effusion and mediastinal nodes (arrows). e) and f) Metastatic liver disease and enlarged right adrenal glands (open arrows).

are not required as bone involvement at presentation is rare (HD 4% and NHL 1%).+6

Metastatic involvement of the lymphatic system is only mentioned here as it is described in the organ-specific chapters of this book. The following rule of thumb for nodal size in relation to metastatic spread is useful in all situations:

- well-defined lymph nodes < 1 cm: normal

- well-defined lymph nodes 1–1.5 cm: questionably malignant

- any lymph node > 1.5 cm: abnormal.

## Conclusion

The single most important contribution of imaging for HD and NHL is the localization of a node for biospy. CT is the most accurate and effective imaging technique for staging and monitoring of HD and NHL.

## References

1. Bunch C, Gatter KC. The lymphomas. In: Weatherall DJ, Leadingham JC and Warrell DA (eds). *Oxford Textbook of Medicine, 3rd* Edition. Oxford: Oxford University Press, 1996, Section 22.5.3, pp.3568–3587.

2. Bragg DG. Radiology of the lymphomas. *Curr Prob Diag Radiol* 1987; **16**: 183–206.

3. Sandrasegaran K, Robinson PJ, Selby P. Staging of lymphoma in adults. *Clin Radiol* 1994; **49**: 149–161.

4. Lukes RJ, Butler JJ. The pathology and nomenclature of Hodgkin's disease. *Cancer Res* 1966; **26**: 1063–1081.

5. Filly R, Blank N, Castellino RA. Radiographic distribution of intrathoracic disease in previously untreated patients with Hodgkin's disease and non-Hodgkin's lymphoma. *Radiology* 1976; **120**: 277–281.

6. Vanrenterghem Y. Lymphoproliferative disorders in organ transplant recipients. *Eur. Radiol.* 1997; **7**: 665–667.

7. Bonnadonna G, Santoro A. Clinical evaluation and treatment of Hodgkins' disease. In: Wiernick PH, Canellos GP, Kyle RA, Schiffer CA (eds) *Neoplastic Diseases of the Blood*. New York: Churchill Livingstone,1985, vol II, pp.789–790 and 794–795.

# 13

# THE BONE AND SOFT TISSUE

Asif Saifuddin

**Primary bone tumours**
**Skeletal metastases and myeloma**
**Primary soft-tissue tumours**

Neoplasms of bone and soft tissues may be divided into primary (benign and malignant) and secondary (metastatic). Primary bone and soft-tissue tumours are rare but the skeleton is one of the commonest sites of metastatic disease. This chapter covers primary and metastatic disease of bones and soft tissues as separate entities, highlighting important clinical features and aspects of treatment but emphasizing the role played by imaging in the management of patients presenting with such diseases.

# Primary bone tumours

## Classification and incidence

Table 13.1 gives a classification of bone tumours and an indication of their relative frequencies based on referrals to the Mayo Clinic.[1] Primary bone neoplasms are rare. It has been estimated that 1500 new malignant bone tumours are recorded in the United States per year, compared to 93 000 new cases of lung carcinoma and 88 000 new cases of breast carcinoma.[1] There is no reason to believe that this ratio is different in the United Kingdom. However, sarcomas of bone account for a significant proportion of cancers occurring in childhood and adolescence. In the 0–14 year age group, they have a recorded incidence of 6.1 per million caucasian children. After the age of 14 years, they are the fifth commonest childhood malignancy, after leukaemia, CNS tumours, lymphoma and soft-tissue sarcomas.[2]

Osteosarcoma and Ewing's sarcoma are the commonest malignant bone tumours in children and adolescents. In adults, apart from multiple myeloma, chondrosarcoma is the commonest primary bone malignancy.[1]

Benign bone tumours account for just under one-quarter of all primary bone neoplasms.[1] This does not include benign tumour-like conditions, such as fibrous dysplasia, simple bone cyst (SBC) and aneurysmal bone cyst (ABC). The commonest benign neoplasms are osteochondroma, giant-cell tumour (GCT), enchondroma and osteoid osteoma.[1]

**Table 13.1** Classification and relative frequency of primary bone tumours (excluding myeloma) (Adapted from Mayo Clinic data (total 7338 cases)[1]

| Benign | Malignant |
| --- | --- |
| *Cartilaginous* | |
| Osteochondroma 872 (11.9%) | Chondrosarcoma★ 1049 (14.3%) |
| Enchondroma 335 (4.6%) | |
| Chondroblastoma 119 (1.6%) | |
| Chondromyxoid fibroma 45 (0.6%) | |
| *Osseous* | |
| Osteoid osteoma 331 (4.5%) | Osteosarcoma★★ 1718 (23.4%) |
| Osteoblastoma 87 (1.2%) | |
| *Round cell* | |
| | Ewing's sarcoma 512 (7.0%) |
| | Lymphoma 694 (9.5%) |
| *Fibrous* | |
| Benign fibrous | Malignant fibrous |
| histiocytoma 9 (0.12%) | histiocytoma 338 (4.6%) |
| Desmoplastic fibroma 12 (0.16%) | |
| *Vascular* | |
| Haemangioma 108 (1.5%) | Haemangioendothelioma 80 (1.1%) |
| | Haemangiopericytoma 13 (0.18%) |
| *Others* | |
| Giant-cell tumour 568 (7.7%) | |
| | Chordoma 356 (4.9%) |
| Lipoma 1 (0.1%) | Liposarcoma 1 (0.01%) |

★ Includes secondary, dedifferentiated and mesenchymal cs
★★ Includes central (conventional and low-grade), surface (parosteal, periosteal and high-grade), Paget's and post-irradiation os

## Clinical features

Primary bone neoplasms most commonly present with bone pain and/or a palpable mass. Alternatively, they may produce pathological fracture or may be incidental findings on radiographs obtained for other reasons.[3] Tumours of the spine not uncommonly present with neurological symptoms and signs due to neural compression.[4,5] Sciatica is also a common presentation of malignant tumours arising from the iliac bone and sacrum, while painful scoliosis is a classical presentation of spinal osteoid osteoma or osteoblastoma.[6]

Constitutional symptoms such as fever and weight loss are often seen with Ewing's sarcoma which is classically associated with a very large mass. A raised ESR is also a feature.

## Age, sex and race

Ewing's sarcoma and osteosarcoma have highest incidence in the first two decades of life, with Ewing's sarcoma having an earlier peak incidence. Osteosarcoma in older age groups occurs following Paget's disease or radiotherapy. Chondrosarcoma has its greatest incidence in the fourth to seventh decades, as do primary bone lymphoma, chordoma and malignant fibrous histiocytoma (MFH).[1] As regards benign bone tumours, the majority have their highest incidence in the second to fourth decades of life.

Some tumours, such as osteoid osteoma and osteosarcoma, show an increased incidence in males, but this is not a striking feature. Ewing's sarcoma has an extremely low incidence in children of Afro-Caribbean and Chinese origin.[2]

## Site

Most primary bone tumours arise in the distal femur, proximal tibia and proximal humerus.[7] This is particularly the case for osteosarcoma. However, there are many exceptions, such as chondrosarcoma, which is most commonly located in the pelvis or proximal femur, and Ewing's sarcoma, which has a propensity for the diaphyses of long bones and the pelvis.[1] GCT characteristically occurs in a subarticular site, whereas chondroblastoma is typically located within an epiphysis.

Primary tumours of the small bones of the hands and feet are extremely rare and are usually enchondromas. Similarly, primary tumours rarely affect the skull, mandible or sinuses.[1]

Primary malignant neoplasms are rare in the spine and tend to involve the vertebral body. Chordomas arise centrally, usually within the sacrum or clivus.[1] Conversely, benign spinal tumours, particularly osteoid osteoma and osteoblastoma, tend to involve the neural arch.[6]

## Mortality

The introduction of chemotherapy in the management of patients with conventional osteosarcoma has resulted in a dramatic increase in 5-year survival rates in tumour centres from approximately 15% to 60%.[8] Chemotherapy also facilitates tumour resection, allowing the majority of patients with extremity osteosarcoma to benefit from limb-salvage surgery. Reported 5-year survival rates for Ewing's sarcoma are in the range of 50–70%.[9]

Approximately 20% of patients will have detectable pulmonary metastases at presentation. This, and the presence of bony metastases, are poor prognostic signs. Although pulmonary metastatectomy increases disease-free survival, it rarely results in increased long-term survival.[10]

The prognosis for patients with low-grade malignant tumours such as chondrosarcoma and chordoma is much better. These tumours are rarely associated with metastatic disease and chemotherapy is not used in their management. Death is usually due to local recurrence.

## Imaging

The aims of imaging in the initial assessment of primary bone lesions are to try and answer the following questions:

- What is the most likely diagnosis?
- What is the local extent of disease (local staging)?
- If the lesion is malignant, has it metastasized (distant staging)?

DIAGNOSIS

The first investigation for a patient presenting with a suspected primary bone tumour is the plain radiograph.[7,11] Despite the introduction of bone scintigraphy, computed tomography (CT) and more recently magnetic resonance imaging (MRI), the plain radiograph remains the most valuable investigation in formulating an initial differential diagnosis. With the combination of radiographic appearance, site of the lesion and age of the patient, a correct diagnosis can be achieved in the majority of cases.

The plain radiographic features that need to be assessed include the following:

*Site of lesion*

Many tumours have a predilection for various parts of the skeleton. It is therefore important to ascertain the precise site of the lesion, not only within the skeleton but also within the individual bone. In a long bone, the lesion may be epiphyseal, metaphyseal, metadiaphyseal or diaphyseal. It may also arise within the medullary canal, the cortex or from the surface of the bone. In the spine, it may arise solely within the vertebral body or the neural arch or may involve both of these structures. In the long bones, the site of the lesion can usually be accurately determined by the combination of good quality anteroposterior (AP) and lateral radiographs. In the spine or pelvis, CT is of additional value for precise localization.

*Margin of lesion and pattern of bone destruction*

Assessment of these two factors results in an accurate assessment of the rate of growth (and therefore aggressiveness) of a solitary bone lesion. Radiographic patterns of bone destruction have been graded by Lodwick *et al*[12] as being either *geographic* (Grade IA, B or C), *moth-eaten (Grade* II) *or permeative* (Grade III). A Grade IA lesion represents the appearance produced by the most benign (or non-aggressive) of bone lesions (Fig. 13.1), whereas a Grade III lesion indicates a rapid rate of growth seen with the most malignant (or aggressive) of bone lesions (Fig. 13.2).

The type of *periosteal reaction* produced by the lesion also gives clues as to its activity. A thick, well-formed periosteal reaction indicates a slow rate of growth, whereas a rapidly growing tumour may produce no identifiable periosteal reaction at all, since the periosteum only becomes visible radiographically once it has had time to produce bone on its inner surface. Aggressive bone neoplasms may also break through the cortex of the bone, producing an extraosseous mass. This feature is generally indicative of a malignant lesion.

*Matrix of the lesion*

The matrix of a tumour refers to the extracellular tissue produced by the tumour and within which the tumour cells lie. Tumours of cartilaginous or osseous origin may produce characteristic patterns of matrix mineralization which can be recognized radiographically (Figs 13.1 and 13.2).

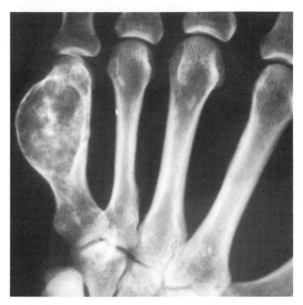

**Figure 13.1** — Anteroposterior radiograph of a patient with an enchondroma of the little finger metacarpal, appearing as a well-defined expanding lesion with a sclerotic margin and matrix calcification typical of a cartilaginous tumour.

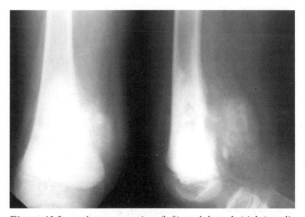

**Figure 13.2** — Anteroposterior (left) and lateral (right) radiographs of the distal femur of an 11-year-old boy with osteosarcoma, appearing as a destructive bone-forming lesion in the metaphysis.

Bone scintigraphy, CT and MRI play little role in the diagnosis of primary bone lesions. Although these techniques are more sensitive than plain radiography in the identification of medullary pathology, they lack specificity. Exceptions include the ability of CT and MRI to demonstrate lesions containing fat, such as lipomas, and scintigraphy and CT to detect and characterize osteoid osteoma and osteoblastoma, particularly in the spine (Fig. 13.3). CT and MRI can also demonstrate fluid–fluid levels, most commonly seen in aneurysmal bone cysts (Fig. 13.4). MRI may suggest a lesion to be much more aggressive than it actually is, due to the demonstration of reactive peritumoural oedema.[13]

Following the initial imaging assessment, several situations may arise. First, the radiological or imaging appearances may be pathognomonic of a non-progressive benign tumour or tumour-like lesion which needs no active treatment. Examples include non-ossifying fibroma, asymptomatic osteochondroma or enchondroma, fibrous dysplasia and some traumatic conditions, such as myositis ossificans and stress fracture.[7] A confident diagnosis of these latter two conditions is particularly important since biopsy of such lesions may result in a misdiagnosis of osteosarcoma by an inexperienced pathologist, with tragic consequences for the patient.

Secondly, the imaging features may be pathognomonic for a benign lesion following which definitive treatment can be instituted. A typical example of this is osteoid osteoma. It is now common practice to excise such lesions percutaneously using CT guidance.[14]

Thirdly, the imaging features may be characteristic of a locally aggressive benign lesion, such as a giant-cell tumour, or a malignant lesion, such as an osteosarcoma or Ewing's sarcoma. Such lesions need further imaging for local staging and, in the case of malignant tumours,

for distant staging. Following these staging procedures, biopsy is undertaken in order to obtain histological confirmation of the diagnosis.

Finally, the imaging features may not be characteristic of any lesion. In this situation, biopsy is required to make a histological diagnosis, following which the appropriate treatment can be planned.

LOCAL STAGING

Clear identification of the local extent of a focal bone lesion is vital so that complete excision can be achieved at the first attempt. For tumours arising within the appendicular skeleton, the surgeon needs to know:

- the extent of tumour within the medullary cavity (the intraosseous extent);

- whether the tumour has extended through the cortex to form an extraosseous mass, as is usually the case with osteosarcoma;

- the relationship of extraosseous tumour to adjacent structures (the extraosseous extent), in particular the neurovascular bundle and adjacent joint.

If the neurovascular bundle is encased by tumour, then amputation will usually be necessary. The primary amputation rate for osteosarcoma is approximately 8%. If there is no involvement of the neurovascular bundle, limb salvage surgery becomes possible. Involvement of the adjacent joint (usually the knee) will alter management, such that an extra-articular resection must be performed followed by arthrodesis. This results in a poorer functioning limb.

With regard to the spine, the extension of tumour into the paravertebral and extradural space and the relationship of tumour to the thecal sac must be identified.

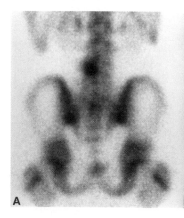 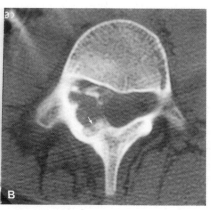

*Figure 13.3* — A 14-year-old boy with osteoblastoma of L4. A) The bone scan shows a focal region of increased activity related to the pedicle of L4. B) CT shows an expanded lytic lesion with matrix mineralization (arrow).

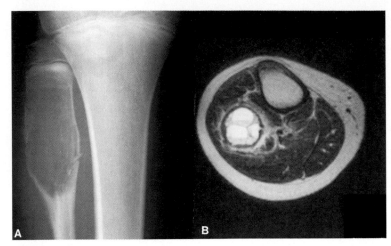

*Figure 13.4* — A 12-year-old girl with an aneurysmal bone cyst of the proximal fibula. A) Anteroposterior radiograph demonstrates an expansile lytic lesion. B) Axial MRI shows characteristic fluid – fluid levels within the lesion.

MRI is ideally suited to local staging of an aggressive benign or primary malignant bone neoplasm for several reasons. MRI can be performed in any desired plane, typically sagittal, coronal and axial. MRI is the most sensitive technique for imaging the marrow cavity and soft tissues, with the exception of tendons where ultrasound is extremely valuable. However, the latter situation is not of particular relevance to tumour imaging. The large variety of MRI sequences allows clear differentiation between intraosseous tumour and normal marrow tissue, and between extraosseous tumour, muscle and the neurovascular bundle (Fig. 13.5).[7,11] MRI can also identify 'skip' metastases (metastases to the same bone), which are a rare occurrence in appendicular osteosarcoma. Also, MRI is not associated with potentially harmful ionizing radiation, which is of importance in the young patient population that presents with primary malignant bone tumours.

MRI has some disadvantages. Infants and young children need general anaesthesia, as movement will degrade image quality. Contraindications to MRI include patients with cardiac pacemakers, aneurysm clips and cochlear implants. A small proportion of patients suffer claustrophobia, but this can usually be overcome with sedation.

The local extent of the tumour will determine whether limb-salvage surgery is possible. The MR images together with measurement films (plain radiographs of the whole limb) are then used to design an endoprosthesis.

MRI is also of established value in assessing malignant tumours of the spine, clearly demonstrating the extent of tumour within the body and neural arch, as well as extension into the epidural space. Infiltration of the dura, however, is difficult to identify. MRI will also demonstrate normality of the adjacent vertebral bodies, which is important if they are to be the site of spinal fixation following tumour excision. Benign tumours of the spine are still better imaged with CT, which allows

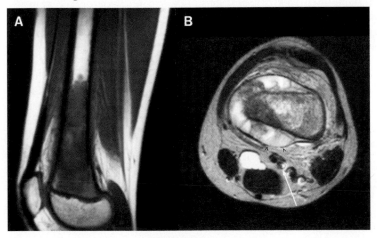

*Figure 13.5* — An 11-year-old girl with osteosarcoma of the distal femur. A) Sagittal MRI sequence identifies the intraosseous extension of tumour. B) Axial MRI sequence demonstrates the relationship of tumour (arrowheads) to the neurovascular bundle (long arrow).

a clearer definition of tumour margins, particularly for lesions arising in the neural arch (Fig. 13.3B). As regards tumours of the bony pelvis, important points in the intraosseous staging of the lesion are the relationship to the sacroiliac joint and acetabulum.

Scintigraphy no longer plays any role in the local staging of bone neoplasms. Arteriography may still be of occasional value when it is not clear from MRI if local vessels are involved. Arteriography and preoperative embolization is occasionally performed for vascular tumours around the pelvis [11].

### DISTANT STAGING

Primary bone tumours most commonly metastasize to the lungs and skeleton.[15] Spread to regional lymph nodes is rare but occasionally seen with osteosarcoma. Metastases to the liver occur with Ewing's sarcoma once tumour has spread to the lungs. All patients presenting with primary malignant bone tumours therefore require a chest radiograph and CT of the lungs and mediastinum.[15] Chest CT is far more sensitive than plain radiography for the identification of pulmonary metastases. Metastases from bone sarcomas have a predilection for the subpleural region of the lungs, where they may produce spontaneous pneumothorax.

The major role for bone scintigraphy is the identification of metastatic disease to the skeleton.[15] Bone scintigraphy is a sensitive technique for identification of skeletal pathology,[16,17] but is relatively non-specific and cannot clearly distinguish infection or trauma from neoplastic disease. Furthermore, the differentiation of benign and malignant neoplasms is unreliable. Therefore, scintigraphy has a limited role in assessment of the primary tumour other than osteoid osteoma and osteoblastoma (Fig. 13.3A). More skeletal metastases can be identified by MRI than by bone scintigraphy. However, it is not practical to image the whole skeleton with MRI in order to identify metastatic disease.[18] MRI is used as an adjunct to scintigraphy, when the appearances of the bone scan are not typical or if there is persistent focal bone pain in the presence of normal plain radiography and scintigraphy.

The identification of metastatic bone disease in patients with osteosarcoma is of particular importance since this virtually excludes the possibility of cure. This is not the case with Ewing's sarcoma.

## Biopsy

Biopsy is the next step in the investigation of primary bone neoplasms once all staging examinations have been performed. Biopsy is performed by either the surgeon or the radiologist, and may be either *open* (through a small surgical incision) or *closed* (by a percutaneous needle technique).[19] It is of overriding importance that the biopsy takes place in the institution where definitive surgical treatment is to be performed. An inappropriate biopsy site may preclude limb-salvage surgery.[20]

The practice of the London Bone Tumour Service is to utilize percutaneous needle biopsy, usually by a radiologist in the X-ray department. There are several advantages to this method. With the aid of the plain radiographs and MR images, the radiologist will be able to target the biopsy to the part of the tumour that is most likely to give a positive diagnosis. The biopsy may be guided either by fluoroscopy, ultrasound or CT. A short general anaesthetic is used for children, whereas the vast majority of adults tolerate the procedure as outpatients under local anaesthesia.

When examined by an experienced bone tumour pathologist, needle biopsy has a diagnostic accuracy of over 95%.[21] Histological examination of the biopsy specimen not only enables a definitive diagnosis, but also establishes the grade of malignancy, which is one of the criteria for surgical staging of the tumour.

## Surgical staging

The combination of local extent, metastatic spread and histological grade allows the tumour to be graded according to one of the several surgical staging systems available.[22] Correct surgical staging is important for predicting prognosis and for planning treatment.

## Treatment

With the establishment of a definitive diagnosis, local and distant staging of the lesion, an appropriate treatment plan can be formulated. This will include a variety of surgical procedures for benign neoplasms and some malignant tumours, such as low-grade chondrosarcoma or parosteal osteosarcoma. High-grade malignant tumours of the long bones, including osteosarcoma and Ewing's sarcoma, will be treated initially by neoadjuvant chemotherapy followed by endoprosthetic replacement where appropriate (Fig. 13.6). Radiotherapy may also be used for patients presenting with pathological fracture.

During the period of chemotherapy, the radiologist's role is to assess the response of the tumour to chemotherapy. This is usually attempted by serial MRI,[23,24] but Doppler ultrasound may be of value by demonstrating reduced vascularity within the tumour.[25]

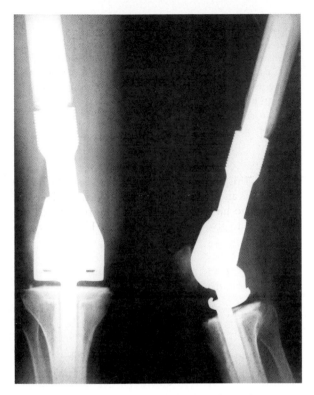

*Figure 13.6* — A 38-year-old man with distal femoral Ewing sarcoma. Anteroposterior and lateral radiographs showing appearances of an endoprosthetic replacement.

While the patient is undergoing chemotherapy, the endoprosthesis is designed and manufactured. This takes 4–6 weeks.

Following surgery for high-grade malignant neoplasms, pathological examination of the excised specimen allows an assessment of the degree of tumour necrosis. Based on this, decisions are made as to the choice of post-operative (adjuvant) chemotherapy.

## Radiological follow-up

The purpose of postoperative radiological follow-up of primary bone tumours is essentially two-fold; first, to assess the effects of surgery and, secondly, to identify tumour recurrence.

Many benign neoplasms are treated by local excision with or without filling of the surgical defect by bone graft or cement. Serial radiography will demonstrate adequate healing of surgical defects and satisfactory incorporation of bone grafts. Recurrence of tumours treated by curettage and methyl methacrylate cement

installation (cementoma) can be identified radiologically several months prior to recurrence of symptoms.[26]

Potential complications of endoprosthetic replacement include mechanical loosening and infection. Both of these can be identified by plain radiography. Swelling at the site of an endoprosthesis can be due to either chronic infection or tumour recurrence. The presence of a metallic implant makes assessment with CT and MRI difficult, although not impossible (Fig. 13.7). Ultrasound, which is not subject to metal artefact, can be very useful in this situation. Identification of any mass lesion adjacent to a prosthesis can be followed by ultrasound-guided needle biopsy.

Where endoprosthetic replacements have not been used, possible tumour recurrence is best investigated by MRI. MRI is effective at distinguishing between recurrent tumour, postoperative fibrosis and radiotherapy changes. If recurrent tumour is suspected, needle biopsy is usually performed for histological confirmation prior to further treatment.

Follow-up of patients with osteosarcoma and Ewing's sarcoma also requires serial chest radiography and CT to assess the response of pulmonary metastatic disease to chemotherapy or to identify new metastatic disease.

The development of any new bone pain should be investigated with plain radiography and whole-body bone scintigraphy. MRI may be performed if these two investigations are normal. It should be remembered that bone pain does not necessarily indicate skeletal metastatic disease but may be a consequence of treatment. Osteonecrosis is a well recognized complication of radiotherapy and can be differentiated from metastasis by MRI.

# Skeletal metastases and myeloma

Skeletal metastases and myeloma are considered together since they occur in the same age group and are the two major differential diagnoses in patients presenting with multifocal destructive bone lesions.

Metastases are the commonest tumours to occur in the skeleton and the skeleton is one of the commonest sites of metastatic disease. The reported incidence of skeletal metastases from postmortem studies in patients dying of cancer is 12–70%.[27] Skeletal metastases are estimated to be 25 times more common than primary bone tumours and approximately 9% are solitary.[28] Therefore, in a patient over the age of 40, a solitary metastasis is more common-

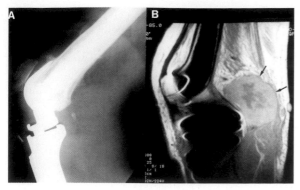

*Figure 13.7* — A 52-year-old man with recurrent pain and swelling after endoprosthetic replacement for proximal tibial chondrosarcoma. A) Lateral radiograph shows satisfactory appearances of the endoprosthesis. B) Sagittal MRI sequence demonstrates the recurrent tumour (arrows).

ly encountered than a primary bone tumour. The commonest cancers to metastasize to bone are prostate, breast, lung, renal and thyroid. Occasionally, patients present with metastatic disease to bone of unknown origin.[15]

Skeletal metastases may occur in any bone but the spine, pelvis, proximal femur, ribs and skull are the commonest sites.[27] Over 80% of metastatic deposits occur in the axial skeleton.[16]

*Multiple myeloma* is the commonest primary bone malignancy.[1] The condition is commoner in males and the peak incidence is in the sixth to seventh decades of life. The sites of occurrence in the skeleton mirror those of metastatic disease. Patients may also present with a solitary lesion, termed *plasmacytoma,* which usually progresses to multiple myeloma.

## Clinical features

Pain is the commonest symptom in patients with either skeletal metastases or myeloma. However, 30–50% of patients with skeletal metastases have no pain.[29]

Pathological fracture is also a common presentation. When this involves a vertebral body, it is frequently associated with spinal cord compression. Asymptomatic skeletal metastases may also be identified by bone scintigraphy as part of the staging process of patients with known cancer.[16,17]

## Imaging

### INITIAL ASSESSMENT

The initial imaging investigation in any patient presenting with a possible metastatic lesion or myeloma is the plain radiograph, which may show a variety of appearances (lytic, sclerotic or mixed).

In a patient over 40 years of age presenting with focal bone pain and a destructive lesion on plain radiography, the working diagnosis is metastasis or myeloma. The next step in the diagnostic pathway is the demonstration of multiple lesions, which is best achieved by whole body bone scintigraphy (Fig. 13.8). Metastases typically appear as multiple asymmetric areas of increased activity located predominantly in the axial skeleton. Occasionally, lesions appear as focal areas of reduced activity, usually seen with renal carcinoma metastases. Another well recognized pattern is the 'superscan'. This occurs when there is widespread osteoblastic metastatic disease involving the skeleton and is most often seen in prostatic and breast cancer.[16]

In patients presenting with metastatic disease of unknown origin, the lung and kidney are the most likely primary sites.[15] The bone scan should be followed by chest radiography and ultrasound or CT of the abdomen. If a primary site is not identified, needle biopsy of the presenting lesion is indicated.

The further imaging of a skeletal metastasis depends upon the effects it is producing. Surgical intervention is indicated in several circumstances. First, in patients presenting with vertebral lesions causing spinal cord

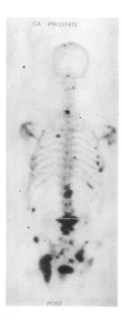

*Figure 13.8* — Bone scan in a patient with metastatic prostate cancer. Metastases typically appear as multiple areas of increased activity in the axial skeleton.

compression, either due to pathological collapse or extradural extension, MRI is indicated to determine the exact local extent of tumour so that surgical resection can be planned (Fig. 13.9). MRI is also of value in the differentiation of osteoporotic and malignant collapse.[18] Secondly, in a patient presenting with a solitary extremity metastasis, treatment may be by wide excision and endoprosthetic replacement. Local staging with MRI is then required, as for a primary malignant bone neoplasm. Thirdly, surgery may be required either prophylactically or for an established pathological fracture. This risk of pathological fracture is proportional to the extent of cortical destruction.[29]

In contrast to skeletal metastases, the bone scan is less sensitive than plain radiography in the detection of myeloma deposits.[16,17] The diagnosis is usually established by a combination of laboratory tests and bone marrow aspirate. Needle biopsy is indicated for plasmacytoma, in which case the typical serum protein abnormalities may not be present.[1] As with metastatic disease, further imaging with MRI is indicated for local staging prior to spinal cord decompression or excision of solitary lesions. Plain radiographs of painful lesions should be obtained to assess the likelihood of pathological fracture.

FOLLOWING TREATMENT

The treatment of skeletal metastases is primarily palliative, the aims being to relieve pain, prevent pathological fracture, improve mobility and function and, if possible,

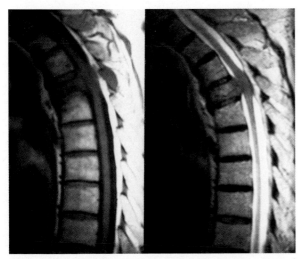

*Figure 13.9* — A 70-year-old man with prostatic cancer. Sagittal MRI sequences showing metastasis to the thoracic spine with spinal cord compression.

prolong survival. Treatment options, apart from pain relief, include endocrine therapy, chemotherapy, targeted radiotherapy, biphosphonates and external beam radiotherapy,[30] in addition to surgery, as described above.

Treatment response can be assessed, although not very accurately, by serial radiography or scintigraphy. As yet, MRI is not a sensitive technique for identifying response since abnormal appearances may remain despite successful medical treatment.[18]

# Primary soft-tissue tumours

Primary soft-tissue tumours are a highly heterogeneous group of tumours that may arise from muscle, fat, fibrous tissue, vessels and nerves. They may be benign or malignant (in which case they are termed *sarcomas*). It is estimated that benign tumours are 100 times commoner than malignant tumours.[31] Soft-tissue sarcomas account for approximately 1% of cancers in the United States and 2% of cancer deaths. The lower limbs are the commonest site of occurrence (40%), followed by the upper limbs (20%), head and neck (10%) and trunk or retroperitoneum (30%).[32]

The commonest soft-tissue sarcomas are malignant fibrous histiocytoma (MFH), liposarcoma and synovial sarcoma. The commonest benign soft-tissue tumours are intramuscular lipoma, fibromatosis, haemangioma and nerve-sheath tumours.[15] However, it should also be remembered that metastatic disease and lymphoma, as well as non-neoplastic lesions, such as ganglion cyst, abscess and post-traumatic ossification or aneurysm, can present as soft-tissue masses.

## Clinical features

Soft-tissue tumours most commonly present as painless masses. Features that suggest malignancy include pain and rapid enlargement.[33] Also, extremity masses arising deep to the fascia and that are larger than 5 cm in diameter, are more likely to be malignant. However, almost one-third of sarcomas are subcutaneous and smaller than 5 cm.[15]

## Imaging

INITIAL ASSESSMENT

The aims of initial imaging of soft-tissue masses are diagnosis and staging. The initial assessment is with plain radiography which, however, is not as valuable a diagnostic aid for soft-tissue tumours as it is for bone lesions. Most soft-tissue tumours are isodense to muscle. A mass with fat density indicates a diagnosis of lipoma or liposarcoma. Phleboliths (small rounded calcifications) are characteristic of soft-tissue haemangioma. The plain radiograph may also show extrinsic pressure erosion of bone or periosteal reaction.[15]

Ultrasound is of value in differentiating solid and cystic masses and can give some indication of tumour size. If the mass is completely cystic (especially if related to a joint), superficial and less than 5 cm in diameter, it is probably benign. Larger solid masses are more likely to be sarcomas, in which case it is advisable to refer the patient to a specialist centre.[15]

MRI has a greater diagnostic capability for soft-tissue masses than for bone lesions. Benign soft-tissue tumours that can be diagnosed include lipoma, haemangioma, fibromatosis, myxoma and nerve sheath tumours (based on their relationship to major nerves). Non-neoplastic masses identifiable by MRI include ganglion cyst, enlarged bursa and haematoma.[34]

MRI is of less value in allowing a pre-biopsy diagnosis for soft-tissue sarcoma. Characteristic features are seen with well-differentiated liposarcoma (Fig. 13.10), myxoid sarcomas and malignant peripheral nerve sheath tumours. However, the majority of soft-tissue sarcomas show an indeterminate pattern (Fig. 13.11).[35] The differentiation between benign and malignant lesions on MRI is not clear-cut, although masses showing marked heterogeneity and internal septation appear more likely to be malignant.[36]

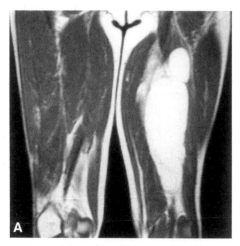

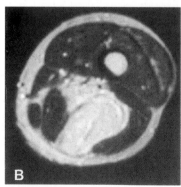

*Figure 13.10* — A 50-year-old man with low-grade liposarcoma of the left thigh. A) Coronal and B) axial MRI sequences show a large mass in the medial aspect of the thigh with the signal characteristics of fat.

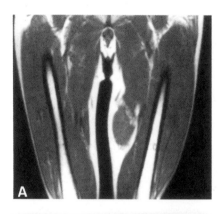

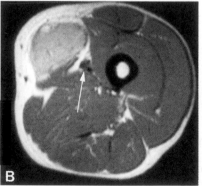

*Figure 13.11* — A 68-year-old man with a high-grade liposarcoma of the left thigh. A) Coronal and B) axial MRI sequences show a mass in the medial aspect of the thigh. The lesion has no characteristic features but the relationship to the neurovascular bundle (arrow) is clearly shown.

MRI is the technique of choice for local staging of soft-tissue sarcomas,[15,32] allowing the clearest identification of tumour margins and the relationship to the neurovascular bundle and adjacent bone (Fig. 13.11). Patients with soft-tissue sarcomas also require distant staging as for malignant bone tumours.[15]

Following staging, biopsy is indicated for those masses which are indeterminate in nature based on clinical and imaging findings. Percutaneous needle biopsy with ultrasound-guidance is usually a successful technique. Biopsy of deep lesions that are not identified by ultrasound can be guided with CT.

### ASSESSMENT OF RECURRENCE

Surgery is the mainstay of treatment for primary soft-tissue sarcoma. Wide local excision may be combined with radiotherapy. The role of neoadjuvant chemotherapy for soft-tissue sarcomas is unclear,[37] although it is beneficial for rhabdomyosarcoma and synovial sarcoma. The evaluation of potential tumour recurrence (estimated to occur in 10–20% of cases) is therefore hampered by changes resulting from the surgical procedure and radiotherapy. Local recurrence will usually occur within 2 years of therapy and since it can be effectively treated with further surgical excision or radiotherapy, early detection with MRI is important. MRI can also characterize benign masses at the resection site such as seromas, abscesses and chronic haematomas.[37]

Radiotherapy produces characteristic changes limited to the radiation portal within subcutaneous tissues and muscle. Recurrent tumour typically appears as a relatively well-defined nodule or mass which can be differentiated from postoperative fibrosis by dynamic enhanced MRI techniques.[38] Where any doubt persists, further needle biopsy is indicated.

# Conclusion

The successful treatment of a patient with a suspected primary bone or soft-tissue neoplasm requires close cooperation between surgeons, radiologists and pathologists, as well as radiotherapists, oncologists and paramedical staff. Because of their relative rarity, such tumours are best treated in specialist centres. Therefore, as soon as the diagnosis of a potential primary bone tumour or soft-tissue sarcoma has been made by clinical and initial radiographic findings, and ideally prior to biopsy, the patient should be referred to a tumour unit for further management.

# Acknowledgements

The author would like to thank Mr Stephen Cannon, FRCS and Dr Jane Edge for their helpful comments, Ms Veronika Aurens for typing the manuscript and Mr Dirk de Camp, Department of Medical Photography, Institute of Orthopaedics, UCL, for the illustrations.

# References

1. Unni KK. *Dahlin's Bone Tumors. General Aspects and Data on 11,087 Cases*, 5th edn. Philadelphia: Lippincott-Raven, 1996.

2. Souhami R. Incidence and aetiology of malignant primary bone tumours. *Clin Oncol* 1987; **1**: 1–20.

3. Letson GD, Greenfield GB, Heinrich SD. Evaluation of the child with a bone or soft-tissue neoplasm. *Orthop Clin N Am* 1996; **27**: 431–451

4. Weinstein JN, McLain D, McLain RF. Primary tumors of the spine. *Spine* 1987; **12**: 843–851.

5. Dreghorn CR, Newman RJ, Hardy GJ et al. Primary tumours of the axial skeleton. Experience of the Leeds Regional Bone Tumour Registry. *Spine* 1990; **156**: 137–140.

6. Pettine KA, Klassen RA. Osteoid osteoma and osteoblastoma of the spine. *J Bone Joint Surg (Am)* 1986; **68-A**: 354–361.

7. Stoker DJ. The place of radiology in diagnosis and management. *Clin Oncol* 1987; **1**: 65–96.

8. Bramwell VH, Burgers M, Sneath R et al. A comparison of two short intensive chemotherapy regimens in operable osteosarcoma of limbs in children and young adults: the first study of the European Osteosarcoma Intergroup. *J Clin Oncol* 1992; **10**: 1579–1591.

9. Jurgens H, Exner U, Gadner H et al. Multidisciplinary treatment of primary Ewing's sarcoma of bone: a 6-year experience of a European cooperative trial. *Cancer* 1988; **61**: 23–32.

10. Bloem JL, Kroon HM. Osseous lesions. *Radiol Clin N Am* 1993; **31**: 261–278.

11. Stoker DJ. Management of bone tumours – the radiologist's role. *Clin Radiol* 1989; **40**: 233–239.

12. Lodwick GS, Wilson AJ, Farrell C et al. Determining growth rates of focal lesions of bone from radiographs. *Radiology* 1980; **134**: 577–583.

13. Seeger LL, Durgan DH, Eckardt JJ, Bassett LW, Gold RH. Nonspecific findings on MR imaging. The importance of correlative studies and clinical information. *Clin Orthop* 1991; **270**: 306–312.

14. Bemard R, Berlin M-F, Wiolard M, Grenier P. Osteoid osteoma: CT-guided percutaneous excision confirmed with immediate follow-up scintigraphy in 16 outpatients. *Radiology* 1996; **201**: 239–242.

15. Simon MA, Finn HA. Diagnostic strategy for bone and soft-tissue tumours. *J Bone Joint Surg (Am)* 1993; **75-A**: 622–631.

16. Brown ML. Bone scintigraphy in benign and malignant tumours. *Radiol Clin N Am* 1993; **31**: 731–738.

17. Brown ML, Collier D, Fogleman 1. Bone scintigraphy: part 1. Oncology and infection. *J Nucl Med* 1993; **34**: 2236–2240.

18. Traill Z, Richards MA, Moore NR. Magnetic resonance imaging of metastatic bone disease. *Clin Orthop* 1995; **312**: 76–88.

19. Simon MA, Biermann JS. Biopsy of bone and soft-tissue lesions. *J Bone Joint Surg (Am)* 1993; **75-A**: 616–621.

20. Springfield DS, Rosenberg A. Biopsy: complicated and risky (editorial). *J Bone Joint Surg (Am)* 1996; **78-A**: 639–643.

21. Stoker DJ, Cobb JP, Pringle JAS. Needle biopsy of musculoskeletal lesions. A review of 208 procedures. *J Bone Joint Surg (Br)* 1991; **73-B**: 498–500.

22. Finn HA, Simon MA. Staging systems for musculoskeletal neoplasms. *Orthopedics* 1989; **12**: 1365–1371.

23. Fletcher BD. Response of osteosarcoma and Ewing's sarcoma to chemotherapy: imaging evaluation. *Am J Roentgenol* 1991; **157**: 825–833.

24. Erlemann R, Sciuk J, Bosse A *et al*. Response of osteosarcoma and Ewing's sarcoma to preoperative chemotherapy: assessment with dynamic and static MR imaging. *Radiology* 1990; **175**: 791–796.

25. Van der Woude H-J, Bloem JL, Schipper J *et al*. Changes in tumor perfusion induced by chemotherapy in bone sarcomas: color Doppler flow imaging compared with contrast-enhanced MR imaging and three-phase bone scintigraphy. *Radiology* 1994; **191**: 421–431.

26. Remedios D, Saifuddin A, Pringle JAS, Giant-cell tumour of bone: radiological versus clinical recurrence following cementation. *J Bone Joint Surg (Br)* 1997 79-B: 26–30.

27. Brage ME, Simon MA. Metastatic bone disease. Evaluation, prognosis and medical treatment considerations of metastatic bone tumours. *Orthopedics* 1992; **15**: 589–596.

28. Stoker DJ. Bone tumours: malignant lesions. In: Grainger R, Allison DJ (eds) *Diagnostic Radiology – An Anglo American Textbook of Imaging,* 2nd edn. Edinburgh: Churchill Livingstone. 1992: 1527–1554.

29. Galasko CSB. Diagnosis of skeletal metastases and assessment of response to treatment. *Clin Orthop* 1995; **312**: 64–75.

30. Houston SJ. The systemic treatment of bone metastases. *Clin Orthop* 1995; **312**: 95–104.

31. Enzinger FM, Weiss SW. *Soft-Tissue Tumors*, 3rd edn. St. Louis: Mosby Year Book. 1995.

32. Moreau G, Bush CH, Scarborough MT, Enneking WF. Surgical considerations in the diagnostic imaging evaluation of musculoskeletal masses. *MRI Clin N Am* 1995; **3**: 577–590.

33. Frassica FJ, Thompson RC. Evaluation, diagnosis and classification of benign soft-tissue tumours. *J Bone Joint Surg (Am)* 1996; **78-A**: 126–140.

34. Sundaram M, Sharafuddin MJA. MR imaging of benign soft-tissue masses. *MRI Clin N Am* 1995; **3**: 609–628.

35. Hanna SL, Fletcher BD. MR imaging of malignant soft-tissue tumours. *MRI Clin N Am* 1995; **3**: 629–650.

36. Weatherall PT. Benign and malignant masses: MR imaging differentiation. *MRI Clin N Am* 1995; **3**: 669–694.

37. Varma DGK, Jackson EF, Bullock RE, Benjamin RS. Soft-tissue sarcoma of the extremities. MR appearances of post-treatment changes and local recurrence. *MRI Clin N Am* 1995; **3**: 695–712.

38. Vanel D, Shapeero L, De Baere T *et al*. MR imaging in the follow-up of malignant and aggressive soft-tissue tumors: results of 511 examinations. *Radiology* 1994; **190**: 263–268.

# 14

# THE CARDIOVASCULAR SYSTEM

Craig A Hackworth and Martin J Lipton

Nature and incidence of cardiac neoplasia
Mechanisms of tumour extension
Clinical manifestations of neoplastic heart disease
Primary tumours of the heart
Malignancy and the great vessels
Differential diagnosis of cardiac tumours
Future impact of digital imaging on tumour diagnosis

# Nature and incidence of cardiac neoplasia

Primary tumours of the heart are rare, with an incidence of 1 in 2000 autopsies.[1] Approximately 75% of these primary cardiac neoplasms are benign. Cardiac metastases on the other hand, are 20–40 times more frequent. However, any benign or malignant cardiac lesion may produce a range of symptoms and mimic a wide spectrum of heart disease. Early diagnosis of primary cardiac tumours permits the opportunity for a complete cure by surgical resection. The success of surgery depends on diagnostic imaging studies, which define the site and nature of a tumour as well as its relationship to cardiac, pericardial and other adjacent structures. Therefore, early diagnosis is critical as it may avoid serious complications and even prevent sudden death.

Since the diagnostic approach is similar for any suspected cardiac neoplasm, a solid understanding of the wide spectrum of pathology encountered is essential. The heart is involved in approximately 10% of all patients with malignancies, and of these, tumour is present in the pericardium in 85%. Pericardial infiltration accounts for both cardiac dysfunction and symptoms which are found in nearly all patients. The physiological effect is usually secondary to pericardial thickening with or without effusion. Frequently a malignant effusion is haemorrhagic, as compared to the serous type seen commonly with other forms of heart disease. Pericardial effusion associated with malignancy may be secondary to hypoalbuminaemia, chemotherapy response and radiation therapy. Almost any tumour, except neurogenic neoplasms can metastasize to the heart.[2] However, the most common sources of cardiac metastases are lung carcinoma in men and breast cancer in women. Approximately 10% of these patients will develop metastases to the heart. Melanoma is a much less common tumour, but has the highest incidence of metastases to the myocardium, followed by leukaemia and lymphoma.

# Mechanisms of tumour extension

The route of tumour spread is dependent on the site of the primary malignancy. Carcinoma of lung, breast and oesophagus usually reach the heart by direct extension. However, approximately 50% of patients with lung and breast carcinoma develop cardiac metastases without evidence of direct extension. These isolated cardiac metastases exhibit retrograde tumour spread via lymphatics with microscopic nodules deposited throughout the myocardium.

Another well known route of spread is by venous extension. Renal cell carcinoma and hepatoma are notorious for metastasizing in this fashion. Tumour thrombus exits a major draining vein and classically grows along the inferior vena cava (IVC). These tumour thrombi may extend into the right atrium.

Finally, haematogenous spread is the main route of dissemination in the case of sarcoma, lymphoma, leukemia and melanoma. Chapter 4 deals with tumours involving the lungs and mediastinum.

McAllister and Fenoglio[1] reviewed 533 cases of primary tumours and cysts of the heart and pericardium at the Armed Forces Institute of Pathology in Washington, DC. The incidence of various cardiac tumours found in their series is given in Table 14.1.

**Table 14.1** Tumours and cysts of the heart and pericardium[1] (reproduced with permission).

| Type | Number | Percentage |
|---|---|---|
| **Benign** | | |
| Myxoma | 130 | 24.2 |
| Lipoma | 45 | 8.4 |
| Papillary fibroelastoma | 42 | 7.9 |
| Rhabdomyoma | 36 | 6.8 |
| Fibroma | 17 | 3.2 |
| Hemangioma | 15 | 2.8 |
| Teratoma | 14 | 2.6 |
| Mesothelioma of the AV node | 12 | 2.3 |
| Granular cell tumour | 3 | |
| Neurofibroma | 3 | |
| Lymphangioma | 2 | |
| Subtotal | 319 | 59.8 |
| Pericardial cyst | 82 | 15.4 |
| Bronchogenic cyst | 7 | 1.3 |
| Subtotal | 89 | 16.7 |
| **Malignant** | | |
| Angiosarcoma | 39 | 7.3 |
| Rhabdomyosarcoma | 26 | 4.9 |
| Mesothelioma | 19 | 3.6 |
| Fibrosarcoma | 14 | 2.6 |
| Malignant lymphoma | 7 | 1.3 |
| Extraskeletal osteosarcoma | 5 | |
| Neurogenic sarcoma | 4 | |
| Malignant teratoma | 4 | |
| Thymoma | 1 | |
| Leiomyosarcoma | 1 | |
| Liposarcoma | 1 | |
| Synovial sarcoma | 1 | |
| Subtotal | 125 | 23.5 |
| TOTAL | 533 | 100.0 |

# Clinical manifestations of neoplastic heart disease

It is important to recognize that any space occupying lesion in the heart carries a risk of functional cardiac impairment, embolism or sudden death. Neoplastic disease of the heart, whether primary or secondary, can only present with a limited number of signs and symptoms (Table 14.2). Modern surgical techniques may allow complete resection of a tumour and offer the potential for a cure. Therefore, the physician is obligated to make the diagnosis early and to define as precisely as possible the extent and nature of the tumour. Recent radiological techniques, as discussed below, provide improved diagnosis and tissue characterization as well as 3D imaging and display.

# Primary tumours of the heart

## Cardiac myxomas

Cardiac myxomas represent one-half of all primary myocardial neoplasms. These lesions are intracardiac and are normally attached by a pedicle. Myxomas usually, but not exclusively, lie near the foramen ovale. Over 75% arise in the left atrium, 20% occur in the right atrium and the remainder in either ventricle.[3] Myxomas have a gelatinous consistency and range in size from 1 to 15 cm (average 5 cm). Tumours may contain haemorrhage, thrombus or calcification.

Patients may be asymptomatic, or exhibit a triad of embolic, obstructive and constitutional symptoms. Indeed, systemic illness occurred in 90% of patients in some series.[4,5] The typical patient is between 30 and 60 years old. The clinical presentation may mimic that of mitral valve disease. However, atypical symptoms including syncope, weight loss, fatigue, fever, anemia, elevated sedimentation rate and abnormal serum proteins may occur. Haemolytic anaemia is typically associated with calcified myxomas, especially in a right atrial location. Atrioventricular valve obstruction secondary to prolapse of the tumour may produce stenosis of the atrioventricular valve and/or regurgitation resulting in the 'wrecking ball' phenomenon. A syndrome myxoma is also described. This is characterized by skin pigmentation and the presence of endocrine neoplasms in addition to the myxoma.[6,7] Tumour embolism occurs in approximately 50% of myxomas. Surgical embolectomy is usually necessary, since these emboli are resistant to percutaneous interventional

techniques. Histopathologic evaluation of the embolus often provides the first evidence of a cardiac myxoma.

The clinicopathological features of 107 atrial myxomas were reviewed at the Armed Forces Institute of Pathology.[8] Table 14.3 illustrates the wide spectrum of symptoms. It is noteworthy that local recurrence may occur after myxoma excision. Even more remarkable is that neurological symptoms may progress and even appear after resection. Numerous reports emphasize that late diagnosis is common, especially when symptoms are remote from the heart.[8,9] Therefore, it is essential to have a high index of suspicion and be vigilant in considering this diagnosis, since appropriate diagnostic studies will otherwise not be requested. The diagnostic procedures now available to identify cardiac tumours are listed in Table 14.4.

Most patients with a suspected myxoma are referred to a cardiologist, who usually performs a 2D echocardiogram that reveals the tumour. Doppler assessment of mitral valve flow provides haemodynamic evaluation. The plain chest radiograph is usually normal, but may reveal left atrial enlargement, elevated pulmonary venous pressure and pulmonary arterial hypertension. CT and MRI are newer, equally non-invasive techniques that frequently offer more information. MRI is an excellent technique for displaying, not only the cardiac chamber cavities, but also the myocardial wall (Fig. 14.1a and b). Both these relatively new imaging tech-

**Table 14.2** General manifestations of neoplastic heart disease[1] (reproduced with permission).

Pericardial involvement
    Pericarditis, pain
    Pericardial effusion
    Radiographic enlargement
    Arrhythmia, predominantly atrial
    Tamponade
    Constriction
Myocardial involvement
    Arrhythmias, ventricular and atrial
    Electrocardiographic changes
    Radiographic enlargement: generalized, localized
    Conduction disturbances and heart block
    Congestive heart failure
    Coronary involvement: angina, infarction
Intracavitary tumour
    Cavity obliteration
    Valve obstruction and valve damage
    Embolic phenomena: systemic, neurologic, coronary
    Constitutional manifestations

**Table 14.3**  Presenting symptoms in 107 patients with cardiac myxoma[8] (reproduced with permission).

|  | All sites | Left atrium | Right atrium | Other sites |
|---|---|---|---|---|
| Embolic symptoms★ | 22 | 21 | 0 | 1 |
| Asymptomatic | 19 | 12 | 5 | 2 |
| Constitutional | 19 | 14 | 2 | 3 |
| Dyspnoea | 18 | 16 | 1 | 1 |
| Syncope | 8 | 3 | 5 | 0 |
| Palpitations | 7 | 6 | 1 | 0 |
| Chest pain | 4 | 3 | 1 | 0 |
| Haemoptysis | 3 | 1 | 0 | 2 |
| Sudden death | 3 | 3 | 0 | 0 |
| Ankle oedema | 2 | 0 | 2 | 0 |
| Mean duration of symptoms (mo) | 16.6 (n=30) | 17.7 (23) | 13.6 (5) | 12.5 (n=2) |

Values are no. of cases.

★ Cerebrovascular accident, 10; cerebrovascular accident with other peripheral emboli. 4; haemaniopsia. 2; leg weakness, pulselessness or gangrene, 4; Lariche's syndrome, 1; flank pain and haematuria (renal artery embolism), 1.

In 19 cases the presenting symptoms included malaise, sudden vertigo, fever of unknown origin (2 related to bacterial endocarditis), weight loss, and combination of non-specific constitutional symptoms.

Precise length of symptoms was known in 30 cases only.

niques are continually being refined and applied more widely. Myxomas can also be diagnosed by ECG-gated radionuclide scan using technitium-99m labelled red blood cells.

DIFFERENTIAL DIAGNOSIS

The location, appearance and mobility of myxomas is characteristically diagnostic. However, large vegetations on the mitral or tricuspid valve, thrombus and other tumours must be excluded (Fig. 14.2). Neither echocardiography nor MRI are tissue specific.

However, MRI may be advantageous when the 2D echocardiogram cannot delineate the extent of cardiac chamber wall involvement. Spin echo and gradient echo MRI imaging techniques can survey the whole heart in unrestricted multiple planes. Both MRI and electron beam or conventional CT scanning made the correct diagnosis and were more precise in lesion characterization in 30 of 107 myxomas evaluated by Burke & Virmani.[8]

Myxoma may also be diagnosed by angiography. Coronary arteriography may demonstrate a tumour

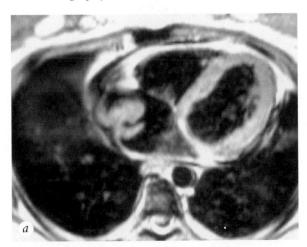

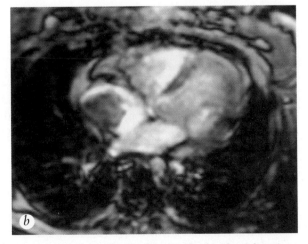

*Figure 14.1* — a) Axial T1-weighted MRI. A round mass as identified in the right atrium immediately opposite to the tricuspic valve. This represents a surgically proven right atrial myxoma. b) Axial gradient echo MRI. The round mass in the right atrium appears as a low signal defect. Flowing blood in the right atrium, right ventricle and left atrium appears as high signal in these flow sensitive images. (Courtesy of Murray Baron, MD.)

**Table 14.4**  Diagnostic cardiac imaging methods

Clinical examination
Electrocardiogram
Chest radiograph
Echocardiography and Doppler ultrasound
Computer tomography
Magnetic resonance imaging and angiography
Nuclear medicine studies
Invasive angiocardiography

blush. Ventriculography invariably can demonstrate the mass and its motion, including atrio-ventricular prolapse. However, invasive catheterization carries the risk of tumour embolism[10] and should now be replaced by safer non-invasive studies.

A thrombus within a cardiac chamber can usually be distinguished by its shape and location. Most thrombi are not mobile. CT may be helpful in differentiating a thrombus from other tissues on the basis of density (Hounsfield Units).[11] CT can identify clot in the atrial appendage of patients with mitral stenosis with excellent reliability. MRI interpretation can be more difficult. Slow blood flow around a thrombus, most often related to a hypokinetic myocardial segment near the ventricular septum or free wall, may produce indeterminate MRI signal, which makes interpretation difficult. However, gradient echo and other MRI pulse sequences may resolve this question.

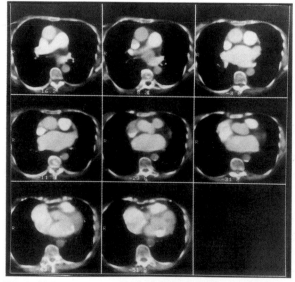

***Figure 14. 2*** — Contrast-enhanced CT. A heavily calcified mass is identified within the left atrium immediately adjacent to the atrioventricular junction. A large calcified mitral valve vegetation was recovered at surgery.

## Other benign cardiac tumours

Lipomas occur throughout the heart and pericardium. Lesions reside in the myocardial free wall or the septae. They are frequently round in appearance and vary in size from 2 to 8 cm. Lipomas are easily recognized with MRI because they have such high signal intensity, due to their short $T_1$ relaxation time and a long $T_2$ consistent with fat.[12] Recent studies have shown that transoesophageal echocardiography can provide more diagnostic information than transthoracic echocardiography when evaluating lipomas.[13] Patients with cardiac lipomas may present with pericardial effusion, supraventricular tachycardia and sudden death. Other lesions, such as pericardial and parasitic cysts, must be differentiated from lipomas. However, the clinical presentation is often helpful in distinguishing these other entities.

Rhabdomyoma is the most common cardiac tumour in infants and children. It is considered to be a hamartoma rather than a true neoplasm.[14-18] Multiple lesions are usually present. These masses tend to be pedunculated and are most frequently found in the left ventricle. Conduction problems or obstruction produce the symptoms which bring most patients to their physicians. Hypoxic episodes, similar to those associated with tetralogy of Fallot, have also been reported. Rhabdomyomas may be diagnosed during the evaluation of children with tuberous sclerosis, 30% of whom will manifest lesions. The diagnosis is frequently made by cross-sectional imaging. Intrauterine echocardiography has also been successful in identifying rhabdomyomas. Currently, surgery is performed for multiple tumours only.

## Paragangliomas and other infrequent neoplasms

Phaeochromocytoma, or chemodectomas, arise in the thorax from neuroectodermal elements. These tumours are exceedingly uncommon and only 2% of all phaeochromocytomas occur in the chest. Lesions may or may not be visible by plain radiograph. Recently [131]I-MIBG (iodine-131 metaiodobenzylguanidine) radionuclide scanning followed by CT and MRI has shown promise in the diagnosis of cardiac paragangliomas.[19,20] This dual modality approach may greatly benefit diagnosis and exact tumour localization which will aid patient care and surgical planning.

A number of other rare benign tumours occur in the heart. Case reports of fibroma, mesothelioma of the atrioventricular node and haemangiomas are described.[1,2]

## Malignant primary tumours of the heart

Sarcomas account for nearly all primary malignant cardiac neoplasms. These tumours exhibit a strong male prevalence. The right atrium or pericardium are the predominant sites of origin (Fig. 14.3).[21] One-quarter of these neoplasms are intracavitary. Patients may present with obstructive symptoms, heart failure and/or a haemorrhagic pericardial effusion. Diagnosis is usually made by echocardiography. Coronary arteriography can demonstrate angiomotous vasculature. CT and MRI both provide more global anatomic information of these rare tumours. The clinical course is rapid, often with widespread metastases.

True rhabdomyosarcoma is the second most frequent primary malignant cardiac tumour. This tumour also exhibits a male preponderance. No single chamber is affected more frequently. The prognosis for cardiac rhabdomyosarcoma is also dismal.

Extremely rare primary cardiac involvement by fibrosarcoma, liposarcoma, haemangiopericytoma and primary lymphoma have been reported (Fig. 14.4a and b). Fibrous histiocytoma has been identified in the left atrium also. This specific tumour has an association with Dacron vascular grafts which raises the question of a carcinogenic link to this material.[22]

## Pericardial tumours

The commonest pericardial mass lesions are cysts. These benign lesions are often discovered incidentally on a chest radiograph in patients aged 40–60 years, with no particular sex predilection. The right costophrenic angle and upper mediastinum are their most frequent locations. Communication into the pericardial cavity is rare. Occasionally, these cysts may become symptomatic, producing chest pain, cough and dyspnoea. Surgical excision, if required, is usually curative.

## Teratoma

Teratomas occur most frequently in infants and children. Females are affected more often than males. Most tumours are intrapericardial, but extracardiac. Teratomas are rarely intracardiac. These tumours can be very large, occasionally reaching 15 cm in diameter. They routinely derive their blood supply either from the root of the aorta or the pulmonary arteries. Recurrent pericardial effusions in children should suggest the diagnosis.[23,24] Surgery is usually curative since cardiac teratomas are rarely malignant. The classical chest radiograph finding of radiopaque cartilage or a tooth remnant is uncommon. Cross-sectional imaging is extremely useful in tumour localization for surgical resection.

## Mesothelioma

Mesothelioma is the third most common primary malignant tumour involving the heart and pericardium. Most patients are males in their fourth to sixth decade.[25] This locally aggressive tumour may produce constrictive physiology or limit venous return secondary to IVC obstruction. Radiographic findings of associated asbestosis exposure should be sought in the chest. However, mesotheliomas often occur in the absence of this history. Treatment is usually palliative and the prognosis is poor.

## Metastatic disease to the heart

Secondary malignant tumours of the heart are usually carcinomas rather than sarcomas. Cardiac metastases eventually occur in 2–21% of all cancer patients.[26–28] Improved patient treatment with increased survival appears to account for an increasing incidence of cardiac metastases. Numerous cell lines including those from primary carcinomas, sarcomas, leukaemia and lymphoma may metastasize to the heart. However, only melanoma has a predilection for the myocardium. Cardiac metastases have been reported in up to 50% of patients with melanoma.[29]

Finally, direct cardiac invasion can occur. Mediastinal tumours are frequently responsible. This direct extension is thought to be related to the proximity of the cardiac lymphatic channels. Carcinoma of the lung and

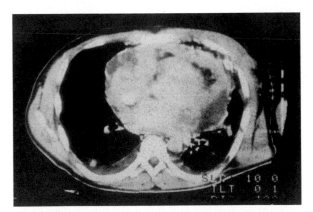

*Figure 14.3* — Contrast-enhanced CT. Diffuse pericardial thickening with effusion is noted. Encasement and deformation of the superior vena cava is also present. This process extended caudad to involve the right ventricle. Open biopsy revealed aggressive spindle cell sarcoma of ventricular origin.

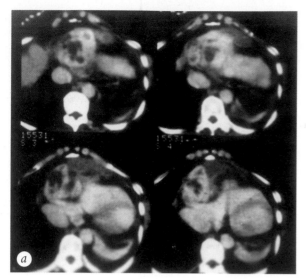

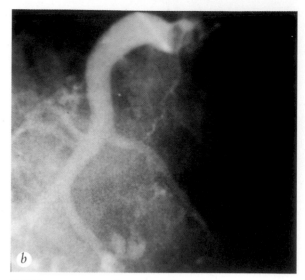

*Figure 14.4* — a) Contrast-enhanced CT. A mixed large attenuation mass involves the right atrium. Single level region of interest (ROI) evaluation of the mass by time density curves showed pronounced vascularity. This prompted coronary arteriography.

b) Right coronary arteriogram reveals a massive coronary artery supply to the mass with neovascularity and abnormal 'pooling' of contrast medium. Surgery revealed a haemangiosarcoma of the pericardim.

breast are most notorious for cardiac invasion. Involvement of the great vessels by local tumours may also occur.[30]

Isolated metastases to the pericardium are infrequent. Patients may present with pericardial effusion, constriction and tamponade. Diagnosis is normally made by cross-sectional imaging with echocardiography, CT and MRI.

## Transplantation

Patients who have undergone heart transplantation are at risk from infection, rejection and malignant tumours. Cyclosporin-induced tumours were discussed in a series reported by Penn.[31,32] Malignant tumours developed in 33 (5%) of 721 recipients after organ transplantation. Eight of 10 malignant tumours occurring in cyclosporin-treated recipients were malignant lymphomas. The mechanism of neoplasia in these circumstances has been well described. Cyclosporin, a fungal metabolite, inhibits suppressor T-cells, which control overproduction of B cells. Although this helps suppress the rejection of transplanted organs, it also depresses the defense system and allows unrestricted proliferation of B cells infected by the Epstein-Barr virus. The malignant tumours occurring in transplant recipients treated with cyclosporin are characterized by their relatively early appearance after transplantation (in Penn's two series the latent period in untreated cases averaged

54 months, while in treated cases it was only 4 months), by their widespread involvement at the time of diagnosis and by their regression or complete resolution after the reduction of immunosuppression — specifically by lowering the dose of cyclosporin. The occurrence of tumours is often, but not always, related to cyclosporin treatment. Lesions are usually clearly seen with ultrasound and CT (Fig. 14.5a and b). These neoplasms may differ from those occurring in non-transplant patients in that they are more homogeneous, solid, and can lack the low density appearance of lymphomas in the latter.[33]

## Carcinoid heart disease

Carcinoid primary tumours do not arise in the heart, although rarely they metastasize to the myocardium.[34-36] Tumours producing the carcinoid syndrome usually originate in the gastrointestinal tract. Carcinoid tumours in the bronchus, testes and ovary have also been implicated. The morphology and chemical staining differ, depending on the location of the primary, but the carcinoid syndrome itself results from the secretion and release of humoral substances (5-HT) into the systemic circulation. These circulating vasoactive amines produce flushing of the skin, hyperactivity of the gut, bronchial and rarely, coronary artery spasm and unusual lesions in the heart.[37-39] The right side of the heart is predominantly affected.[40] Pulmonary and tricuspid valve stenosis results from the endocardial

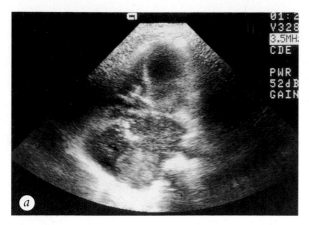

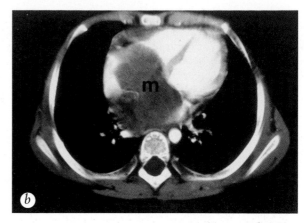

*Figure 14.5* — Oblique long axis echocardiogram of right atrium and ventricle in an 8-year-old liver transplant recipient. A lobulated mixed reflectivity mass is demonstrated in the right atrium (arrows). Contrast-enhanced CT of the same child performed to assess for additional adenopathy reveals that the mass (m) also involves the atrial septum and left atrium. Open biopsy of a mediastinal component of this mass yielded B-cell lymphoma.

deposition of a shiny yellow fibrous material. This process may also result in mitral valve regurgitation.

The treatment of carcinoid syndrome primarily involves systemic chemotherapy. Symptomatic control with α-adrenergic blockers, 5-HT antagonists and somatostatin analogues is routinely employed. However, response is variable.[41,42] Catheter-directed chemoembolic therapy may be considered in symptomatic patients with substantial hepatic tumour burden. Surgery with pulmonary and tricuspid valve excision is performed infrequently. Recurrent deposition of carcinoid plaque may occur on a valve prosthesis within a year. More recently, balloon valvuloplasty has been employed for treatment of carcinoid heart lesions.[43]

# Malignancy and the great vessels

## Superior vena cava syndrome

Superior vena cava syndrome (SVCS) occurs in approximately 5% of patients with malignancy and is a significant clinical problem. Patients most frequently present with dyspnoea, often exacerbated by supine posture. Oedema of the upper extremity and face as well as cyanosis occur. Bronchogenic carcinoma produces approximately 80% of all cases of SVCS. Lymphoma is the next most common cause. Metastatic lesions to the superior mediastinal lymph nodes and locally aggressive tumours of breast, thyroid, thymus and germ cell origin account for the remaining 9% of patients.[44]

Clinicians rely heavily on imaging, not only to provide a precise diagnosis, but also to guide and expedite ther-

apy in these clinically tenuous patients. Routine chest radiographs are frequently available and approximately 60% reveal a superior mediastinal mass.[45] Ultrasound, scintigraphy and direct venography can all be used to confirm the presence of SVC obstruction, but cross-sectional imaging such as CT and MRI have greater importance early in therapy.[46–48] These cross-sectional imaging modalities can determine the exact position of the offending obstruction. The same modalities are then used to guide the biopsy approach optimally which can decrease patient morbidity and mortality.[49]

The majority of patients with SVCS are treated with radiation therapy, with or without chemotherapy, and this usually relieves their symptoms. However, approximately one-third of this group either will not respond to the treatment or develop recurrent SVCS. Percutaneous techniques using thrombolytic infusions, angioplasty and stents have been reported. The early experience is promising and technical success in stent deployment is possible in greater than 80% of these patients. These techniques produce faster relief of symptoms and do not appear hampered by the effects of radiation therapy. The greatest problem with these percutaneous methods is recurrence of SVCS in up to 45% of patients. Tumour progression or stent thrombosis represent the two major problems. However, these can be addressed effectively with repeat stent placement, thrombolytics and long-term oral anticoagulation.[50–52]

## Vascular invasion and resectability

Imaging plays an important role in the evaluation of vascular invasion by tumour. This is especially true in the treatment of tumours affecting the IVC and aorta.

Direct vascular invasion of the IVC is most frequently due to malignancy arising from the kidneys. Five to 15% of renal tumours exhibit direct caval extension, which may involve the right atrium. Although less common, direct tumour spread from the liver, adrenal glands, pelvic organs, retroperitoneal masses and lymph nodes can also involve the IVC (Fig. 14.6a and b).[53–55] Detection of IVC involvement has been greatly advanced over the past two decades by the routine use of cross-sectional imaging (ultrasound, CT and MRI) in the evaluation of the abdomen and pelvis. Surgeons are now capitalizing on these improvements in imaging, which allow them to perform their operations more precisely and with far greater confidence. Individuals previously deemed unresectable are now surgical candidates, with acceptable morbidity and mortality from exceedingly complex procedures.[56, 57] Imaging has, therefore, made a significant contribution to patient care in this aspect of oncology.

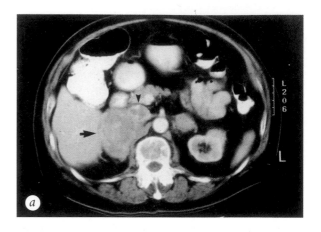

Advances in imaging also permit a better understanding of aortic invasion in patients with lung and oesophageal carcinoma. Determination of invasion of the aorta has been based on the extent of tumour contact on conventional CT. Recent applications of cine CT may better define whether tumour-aorta contact is significant through respiratory or cardiac motion studies.[58] Advances in intravascular ultrasound may better grade the importance of tumour-vessel contact also. Imaging with an intra-aortic probe was recently used in a small series of oesophageal tumours and allowed direct aortic wall characterization. This allowed the authors to identify adventitial tumour spread, preoperatively, in 3 patients who would have been graded as having no tumour invasion by standard CT guidelines.[59] The application of direct imaging of vessel walls appears to be the logical next step to cancer staging and planning. This approach is valuable for evaluating other tumours which involve the mediastinum such as superior sulcus tumours.[60]

## Differential diagnosis of cardiac tumours

A number of disorders must be considered in the differential diagnosis of cardiac tumours. Modern diagnostic imaging methods are not only able to display and characterize cardiac wall and chamber anatomy, but also they can evaluate cardiac function and flow, and these techniques may be able to distinguish between such mass lesions.[61–64] There are a number of infiltrative diseases which may mimic cardiac tumours. Cardiomyopathy is the commonest and causes difficulty when there is asymmetrical myocardial involvement.

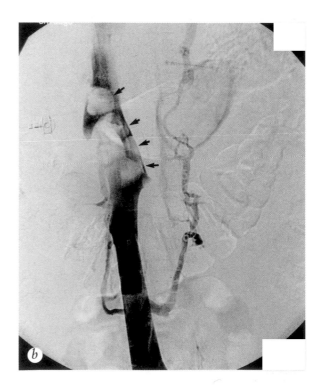

*Figure 14.6* — a) Contrast-enhanced CT in an elderly male with metastatic prostate carcinoma. A mixed attenuation mass arises in the right adrenal bed (arrow). This process extends into the inferior vena cava (arrowhead). b) Digital subtraction inferior vena cavogram. A polylobulated mass (arrows) produces near occlusion of the inferior vena cava. At the time of this exam, the patient had developed new bilateral lower extremity oedema.

Cross-sectional imaging provides the best diagnostic approach in these patients and has been discussed in the literature for MRI and for CT.[65,66] Sarcoidosis, amyloidosis and tuberculosis may also produce masses, often impinging upon the right heart, and these lesions may produce symptoms of pericardial constriction.[67–69] Both MRI and CT provide excellent diagnostic capability in these patients.[70–72] Tumours of the pericardium such as mesothelioma can produce a similar clinical picture.[73] Pseudotumours due to a variety of other uncommon lesions also occur, such as parasitic echinococcal cysts. However, a thorough history and physical examination will often suggest the diagnosis.

Involvement of the great vessels may occur either by direct invasion or by propagation of tumour along the great veins and this may extend into the right heart chambers. Pulmonary embolism can also occur and be safely identified by these non-invasive studies.[74,75]

# Future impact of digital imaging on tumour diagnosis

The revolution in microprocessors in terms of speed, size and reduced cost has led to rapid and more sophisticated medical imaging equipment with faster image acquisition with CT, MRI, ultrasound, positron emission tomography (PET) and single photon emission tomography (SPECT). However, of equal importance and perhaps even more exciting is the development of 3D displays, including the use of colour Doppler, reproducible quantitation, integration of images from different modalities, and most recently, the presentation of this data in virtual reality. This area has particular relevance to an organ as complex in structure and function as the beating heart. It also has special implications for radiation therapy planning using modern computerized linear accelerators with 'beam's eye view' treatment ports. Both CT and MRI offer 3D displays of the vascular tree as well as high spatial and contrast resolution of adjacent soft tissues.[76,77] Echocardiography has recently become a digital imaging modality with advanced 3D imaging capability. These technologies are continually being refined and improved. Furthermore, the ability to measure organ tissue perfusion appears closer to clinical application as the pharmaceutical industry has started to develop new contrast media for all of these modalities. MRI spectroscopy has the capability to study tumour chemistry and also to identify anatomic structure and function. Measurements of tumour oxygen consumption and the patterns of tumour blood flow are also being explored

by several research teams and this area appears to be promising.[78]

Technological advances have not been solely confined to high profile imaging modalities such as CT, ultrasound, MRI, PET and SPECT. Digital radiography using photostimulable phosphor technology is being employed increasingly and will have a significant impact by converting all conventional radiography to digital media, which accounts for approximately 80% of the total radiology workload in a general hospital. Computer-aided diagnosis in conjunction with digital radiography has the potential for improved diagnosis and treatment of cancer patients. Computer programs have been developed that can identify abnormalities such as nodules, interstitial infiltrates and cardiomegaly by automated analysis of a digital radiograph. Though the accuracy of these programs still falls short of that of an experienced radiologist, these techniques have been shown to improve the ability of most observers to detect subtle abnormalities in simulated clinical situations. Temporal subtraction is a digital technique that registers and subtracts a previous from a current chest radiograph to enhance detection of interval change. Energy subtraction, on the other hand, exploits the differential absorption of specific components of the X-ray beam to produce separate 'bone' and 'soft tissue' images from a single exposure (Fig. 14.7a and b). As image interpretation migrates from the viewbox to the computer workstation in the future, the increasingly more powerful computer programs are likely to play an important role.

# Conclusion

Although cardiac tumours are rare, they nevertheless represent an important subgroup, the diagnosis of which is challenging for the primary care physician. Symptoms are not characteristic and serious complications including stroke, myocardial infarction and even sudden death from arrhythmia may be the first signs of the tumour.

The most common primary cardiac neoplasm is the benign myxoma and the most frequent primary malignant lesion is sarcoma. Cardiac metastases from distant primary carcinomas are now frequently encountered. Echocardiography until the past decade was the only consistently reliable and available non-invasive diagnostic tool. New non-invasive CT and MRI exams now exist and have greatly limited the use of echocardiography and angiocardiography with or without coronary arteriography in the evaluation of cardiac neo-

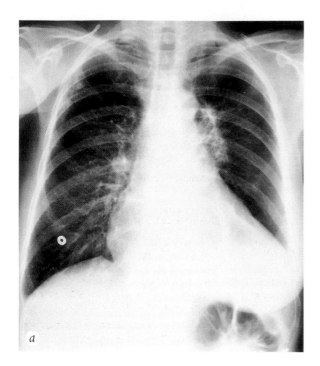

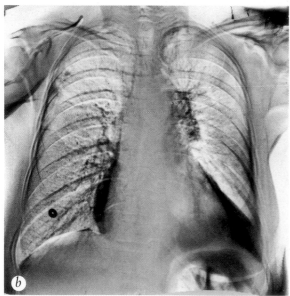

*Figure 14.7* — a) Routine chest radiograph: Increased cardiac size has developed in this woman with known breast carcinoma since the previous chest radiograph. (*Courtesy of Heber MacMahon, MD*) b) Temporal subtraction image, obtained by automated digital registration and subtraction of the previous from the current radiograph shows a change in the cardiac silhouette due to pericardial effusion, indicated by a black halo surrounding the heart. Areas of new opacity appear dark while unchanged areas are light grey in the subtraction image.

plasms.[79–84] These techniques provide additional diagnostic information and are regarded as essential for adequate treatment planning, particularly when surgical resection is being considered.

# References

1. McAllister HA Jr, Fenoglio JJ Jr. *Tumors of the Cardiovascular System. Fascicle 15, Second Series, Atlas of Tumor Pathology.* Washington, DC, Armed Forces Institute of Pathology, 1978.

2. McAllister HA Jr. Tumors of the heart and pericardium. In: Silver MD (ed) *Cardiovascular Pathology,* vol I. New York: Churchill Livingstone, 1983, ch. 35.

3. Markel ML, Waller BF, Armstrong WF. Cardiac myxoma. *Medicine* 1987; **66**: 114–125.

4. Peters MN, Hall RJ, Cooley DA, Leachman RD, Garcia E. The clinical syndrome of atrial myxoma. *JAMA* 1974; **230**: 695–701.

5. St. John Sutton MG, Mercier LA, Giuliani ER, Lie JT. Atrial myxomas: A review of clinical experience in 40 patients. *Mayo Clin Proc* 1980; **55**: 371–376.

6. Vidaillet HJ Jr, Seward JB, Fyke FE III, Su WPD, Tajik AJ: 'Syndrome myxoma': A subset of patients with cardiac myxoma associated with pigmented skin lesions and peripheral and endocrine neoplasms. *Br Heart J* 1987; **57**: 247–255.

7. Danoff A, Jormark S, Lorber D, Fleischer N. Adrenocortical micronodular dysplasia, cardiac myxomas, lentigines, and spindle cell tumors. Report of a kindred. *Arch Intern Med* 1987; **147**: 443–448.

8. Burke AP, Virmani R. Cardiac myxoma, a clinicopathologic study. *Am J Clin Pathol* 1993; **100**: 671–678.

9. Boussen K, Moalla M, Blondeau P, Ayed HB, Lie JT. Embolization of cardiac myxomas masquerading as polyarteritis nodosa. *J Rhematol* 1991; **18**: 283–285.

10. Pindyck F, Pierce EC II, Baron MG, Lukban SB. Embolization of left atrial myxoma after transseptal cardiac catheterization. *Am J Cardiol* 1972; 30: 569–571.

11. Tomora H, Hoshia Furu H, Kuribayashi S *et al.* Evaluation of intracardiac thrombus with computed tomography. *Am J Cardiol* 1983; **51**: 843–852.

12. Tuna IC, Julsrud PR, Click RL, Tazelaar HD, Bresnahan DR, Danielson GK. Tissue characterization of an unusual right atrial mass by magnetic resonance imaging. *Mayo Clin Proc* 1991; **66**: 498–501.

13. Barberger-Gateau P, Paquet M, Desaulniers D, Chenard J. Fibrolipoma of the mitral valve in a child: Clinical and echocardiographic features. *Circulation* 1978; **58**: 955–958.

14. Spooner EW, Farina MA, Shaher RM, Foster ED. Left ventricular rhabdomyoma causing subaortic stenosis. The two-dimensional echocardiographic appearance. *Pediatr Cardiol* 1982; **2**: 67–71.

15. Guereta LG, Burgueros M, Elorza MD, Alix AG, Benitor F, Gamallo C. Cardiac rhabdomyoma presenting as fetal hydrops. *Pediatr Cardiol* 1986; **7**: 171–174.

16. Kuehl KS, Perry LW, Chandra R, Scott LP III. Left ventricular rhabdomyoma. A rare cause of subaortic stenosis in the newborn infant. *Pediatrics* 1970; **46**: 464–468.

17. Violette EJ, Hardin NJ, McQuillen EN. Sudden unexpected death

due to asymptomatic cardiac rhabdomyoma. *J Forensic Sci* 1981; **26**: 599–604.

18. Pillai R, Kharma N, Brom AG, Becker AE. Mitral valve origins of pedunculated rhabdomyomas causing subaortic stenosis. *Am J Cardiol* 1991; **67**: 663–664.

19. Fisher MR, Higgins CB, Andereck W. Magnetic resonance imaging of an intrapericardial pheochromocytoma. *J Comput Tomogr* 1985; **9**: 1103–1105.

20. Hamilton BH, Francis IR, Gross BH et al. Intrapericardial paragangliomas (pheochromocytomas): Imaging features. *AJR* 1997; **168**: 109–113.

21. Putman JB Jr, Sweeney MS, Colon R, Lanza LA, Frazier OH, Cooley DA. Primary cardiac sarcomas. *Ann Thorac Surg* 1991; **51**: 906–910.

22. Schmaltz AA, Apitz J. Primary rhabdomyosarcoma of the heart. *Pediatr Cardiol* 1982; **2**: 73–75.

23. MacDonald S, Fay JE, Lynn RM. Intrapericardial teratoma: A continuing challenge. *Can J Surg* 1983; **26**: 81–82.

24. Maeta H, Hiyama T, Okamura K et al. Successful excision of intracardiac teratoma. *J Thorac Cardiovasc Surg* 1982; **83**: 909–913.

25. Yilling FP, Schlant RC, Hertzler GL, Krzyaniak R. Pericardial mesothelioma. *Chest* 1982; **81**: 520–523.

26. Prichard RW. Tumors of the heart: Review of the subject and report of one hundred and fifty cases. *Arch Pathol* 1951; **51**: 98–128.

27. DeLoach JF, Haynes JW. Secondary tumors of heart and pericardium: Review of the subject and report of one hundred thirty-seven cases. *Arch Intern Med* 1953; **91**: 224–249.

28. Kutalek SP, Panidis IP, Kotler MN, Mintz GS, Carver J, Ross JJ. Metastatic tumors of the heart detected by two-dimensional echocardiography. *Am Heart J* 1985; **109**: 343–349.

29. el Allaf D, Burette R, Pierard L, Limet R. Cardiac tamponade as the first manifestation of cardiothoracic malignancy: A study of 10 cases. *Eur Heart J* 1986; **7**: 247–253.

30. Kadir S, Coulam CM. Intracaval extension of renal cell carcinoma. *Cardiovasc Intervent Radiol* 1980; **3**: 180–183.

31. Penn I. Malignancies associated with immunosuppressive or cytotoxic therapy. *Surgery* 1978; **83**: 492–502.

32. Penn I. Tumor incidence in human allograft recipients. *Transplant Proc* 1979; **11**: 1047–1051.

33. Lipton MJ. Rejection in the cardiac transplant ' The role of X-ray examination. In: *Cardiac Imaging: X-ray, MR and Ultrasound*. Amsterdam: Excerpta Medica,1991, pp.159–170.

34. Schiller V₁, Fishbein MC, Siegel RJ. Unusual cardiac involvement in carcinoid syndrome. *Am Heart J* 1986; **112**: 1322–1323.

35. Strickman NE, Hall RJ. Carcinoid heart disease. In: Kapoor AS, Reynolds RD (eds) *Cancer and the Heart*. New York: Springer-Verlag, 1986, pp.135–136.

36. Artaza A, Beiner JA, Gonzalez M, Aranda I, de Teresa EG, Pulpon LA. Carcinoid heart disease: Report of a case secondary to a pure carcinoid tumor of the ovary. *Eur Heart J* 1985; **6**: 800–805.

37. Sane DC, Feldman JM. A blush from the heart. *Chest* 1987; **92**: 360–361.

38. Mattingly TW. The functioning carcinoid tumor: A serendipity in diagnosis. *Trans Am Clin Climatol Assoc* 1965; **77**: 190–204.

39. Topol EJ, Fortuin NJ. Coronary artery spasm and cardiac arrest in carcinoid heart disease. *Am J Med* 1984; **77**: 950–952.

40. Millward MJ, Blake MP, Byrne MJ, Hung J, Gibson P. Left heart involvement with cardiac shunt complicating carcinoid heart disease. *Aust NZ J Med* 1989; **19**: 716–717.

41. Kvols LK, Moertel CG, O'Connell MJ, Schutt AJ, Rubin J, Hahn RG. Treatment of the malignant carcinoid syndrome. Evaluation of a long-acting somartostatin analogue. *N Engl J Med* 1986; **315**: 702–704.

42. Oates JA. The carcinoid syndrome. *N Engl J Med* 1986; **315**: 702–704.

43. Mullins PA, Hall JA, Shapiro LM. Balloon dilatation of tricuspid stenosis caused by carcinoid heart disease. *Br Heart J* 1990; **63**: 249–250.

44. Abner A. Approach to the patient who presents with superior vena cava obstruction. *Chest* 1993; **103**: 394S-97S.

45. Armstrong BA, Perez CA, Simpson JR et al. Role of irradiation in the management of superior vena cava syndrome. *Int J Radiat Oncol Biol Phys* 1987; **13**: 531–39.

46. Gooding GAW, Hightower DR, Moore EH, Dillon WP, Lipton MJ. Obstruction of the superior vena cava or subclavian veins: sonographic diagnosis. *Radiology* 1986; **159**: 663–665.

47. Bechtold RE, Wolfman NT, Karstaedt N, Choplin RH. Superior vena caval obstruction: detection using CT. *Radiology* 1985; **157**: 485–487.

48. Kim H-J, Kim HS, Chung SH: CT diagnosis of superior vena cava syndrome: importance of collateral vessels. *AJR* 1993; **161**: 539–542.

49. Bigsby R, Greengrass R, Unruh H. Diagnostic algorithm for acute superior vena caval obstruction (SVCO). *J Cardiovasc Surg* 1993; **34**: 347–350.

50. Crowe MTI, Davies CH, Gaines PA. Percutaneous management of superior vena cava occlusions. *Cardiovasc Intervent Radiol* 1995; **18**: 367–372.

51. Oudkerk M, Kuijpers TJA, Schmitz PIM, Loosveld O, deWit R. Self-expanding metal stents for palliative treatment of superior vena caval syndrome. *Cardiovasc Intervent Radiol* 1996; **19**: 146–151.

52. Shah R, Sabanathan S, Lowe RA, Mearns AJ. Stenting in malignant obstruction of superior vena cava. *J Thorac Cardiovasc Surg* 1996; **112**: 335–340.

53. Tassi A, Cirocchi R, Volpi G, Pacifici A, Goracci G. Preoperative evaluation of inferior vena cava involvement secondary to malignant abdominal neoplasms. *J Cardiovasc Surg* 1993; **34**: 241–247.

54. Savarese DMF, Rohrer MJ, Pezzella T, Davidoff A, Fraire AE, Menon M. Successful management of intracardiac extension of tumor thrombus in a patient with advanced nonseminomatous germ cell testicular cancer. *Urology* 1995; **46**: 883–887.

55. Uemoto S, Fleming W, Keogh BE, Habib NA. Case report. Combined pulmonary tumour embolectomy and extended right hepatectomy with inferior vena cava resection for advanced hepatocellular carcinoma. *Br J Surg* 1995; **82**: 127–128.

56. Ljungberg B, Stenling R, Osterdahl B, Farrelly E, Aberg T, Roos G. Vein invasion in renal cell carcinoma: impact on metastatic behavior and survival. *Urology* 1995; **154**: 1681–1684.

57. Langenburg SE, Blackbourne LH, Sperling JW et al. Management of renal tumours involving the inferior vena cava. *J Vasc Surg* 1994; **20**: 385–388.

58. Ohtsuka T, Minami M, Nakajima J, Kohno T, Yagyu K, Furuse A. Cine computed tomography for evaluation of tumors invasive to the thoracic aorta: seven clinical experiences. *J Thorac Cardiovasc Surg* 1996; **112**: 190–192.

59. Akiyama S, Kodera Y, Sekiguchi H *et al*. Preoperative intra-aortic ultrasonography to determine resectability in advanced oesophageal cancer. *Br J Surg* 1995; **82**: 1671–1674.

60. Laissy JP, Soyer P, Sekkal SR *et al*. Assessment of vascular involvement with magnetic resonance angiography (MRA) in Pancoast syndrome. *Mag Reson Imag* 1995; **13**: 523–530.

61. Mavroudis C, Way LW, Lipton MJ, Gertz EW, Ellis RJ. Diagnosis and operative treatment of intracavitary liposarcoma of the right ventricle. J Thorac Cardiovasc Surg 1981; **81**: 137–140

62. Kircher B, Abbott JA, Pau S *et al*. Left atrial volume determination by biplane two-dimensional echocardiography: validation by cine computed tomography. *Am Heart J* 1991; **121**: 864–871.

63. van der Velde ET, van Dijk AD, Steendijk P *et al*. Left ventricular segmental volume by conductance catheter and cine-CT. *Eur Heart J* 1992; **13 (Suppl)**: 15–21.

64. Wood AM, Hoffmann K, Lipton MJ: Cardiac function ' Quantification with MR and CT. In: Link K (ed) *The Radiological Clinics of North America*. Philadelphia: WB Saunders, 1994, vol 32(3), pp. 553–579.

65. Higgins CB, Byrd B, Stark D *et al*. Magnetic resonance imaging of hypertrophic cardiomyopathy. *Am J Cardiol* 1985; **55**: 1121–1126.

66. Diethelm L, Simonson JS, Dery R, Gould RG, Schiller NB, Lipton MJ. Determination of LV mass with ultrafast CT and 2-D echocardiography. *Radiology* 1989; **171**: 213–217.

67. Sechtem U, Higgins CB, Sommerhoff BA, Lipton MJ, Huycke EC. Magnetic resonance imaging of restrictive cardiomyopathy. *Am J Cardiol* 1987; **59**: 480–482.

68. Schwartz AB, Mitchell RS, Higgins CB, Lipton MJ, Klausner SC: . Invasive calcific constrictive pericarditis simulating a left ventricular mass. *Am Heart J* 1986; **112**: 861–863.

69. Stark D, Higgins CB, Lanzer P *et al*. MRI of the pericardium: Normal and pathological findings. *Radiology* 1984; **150**: 469–474.

70. Smiseth OA, Frais MA, Junemann M *et al*. Left and right ventricular diastolic function during acute pericardial tamponade. *Clin Physiol* 1991; **11**: 61–71.

71. Moncada R, Bates M, Salinas M *et al*. Diagnostic role of computed tomography in pericardia disease: congenital defects, thickening, neoplasms and effusions. *Am Heart J* 1982; **103**: 263–282.

72. RienmŸller R, GŸrgan M, Erdmann E, Kemkes B, Kreutzer E, Weinhold C. CT and MR evaluation of pericardial constriction: A new diagnostic and therapeutic concept. *J Thoracic Imag* 1993; **8**: 108–121.

73. Thomason R, Schlegel W, Lucca M, Cummings S, Lee S. Primary malignant mesothelioma of the pericardium: Case report and literature review. *Texas Heart Inst J* 1994; **21**: 170–174.

74. DiCarlo LA, Schiller NB, Herfkens RJ, Brundage BH, Lipton MJ. Noninvasive detection of proximal pulmonary artery thrombosis by two-dimensional echocardiography and computerized tomography. *Am Heart J* 1982; 104: 879–881.

75. Leef JA, Lipton MJ. Pulmonary artery imaging. In: Schlant RC, Alexander RW, Lipton MJ (eds) *Diagnostic Atlas of the Heart*. New York: McGraw-Hill. 1996 pp. 333–350.

76. Giger ML, Pelizzari C. Advances in tumor imaging. *Sci Am* 1996; **275**: 76–78.

77. Hoffmann KR, Chen SY, Carroll JD, Lipton MJ. Digital imaging of the heart. In: Schlant RC, Alexander RW, Lipton MJ (eds) *Diagnostic Atlas of the Heart*. New York, McGraw-Hill. 1996 New York, pp. 351–374.

78. Karczmar GK, Lipton MJ, Kuperman V, River JN, Lewis MZ. MR measurement of response to hyperoxia differentiates tumors from normal tissue and may be sensitive to oxygen consumption. *Invest Radiol* 1994; **29 (Suppl)**: S161-S163.

79. Cassidy MM, Schiller NB, Lipton MJ, Higgins CB: Interaction of echocardiography with recent noninvasive cardiovascular imaging modalities. *Cardiology*, Sept/Oct: 29–47, 1987.

80. Higgins CB, Lipton MJ. Computed tomography and magnetic resonance imaging of cardiac and paracardiac tumours. In: Taveras JM, Ferucci JT Jr (eds) *Radiology: Diagnosis/Imaging/Intervention*. Philadelphia: JB Lippincott Company. 1984 Vol 2, Section 59, pp 1–4.

81. Lipton MJ. The thorax: heart and mediastinum. In: Burgener F, Kormano M (eds) *Differential Diagnosis in CT*. Stuttgart: Georg Thieme, 1996, pp. 222–245.

82. Baron M. MRI of pericardium, cardiomyopathy and cardiac masses. In: Casarella WJ (ed) *Syllabus for the Categorical Course on Cardiovascular Imaging*. American Roentgen Ray Society, 1990.

83. Carrol CL, Higgins CB, Caputo GR. Magnetic resonance imaging of acquired cardiac disease. *Texas Heart Inst J* 1996; **23**: 144–154.

# INDEX

## A

Abscesses, brain, 9, 14

Acinar cell carcinoma, pancreas, 122

Acinar cell cystadenocarcinoma, pancreas, 122

Acoustic Schwannoma, 17, 19

Acromegaly, 20–21, 141, 142

ACTH
  assay, 141
  ectopic secretion, 142

Adenocarcinomas
  bladder, 135
  bronchus, 49
  ethmoid sinus, 41 (Fig.)
  gallbladder, 120, 120 (Table)
  metastases to brain, 14
  nasosinusal, 40
  oesophagus, 81
  small intestine, 90
  transpyloric spread, 88
  see also Renal cell carcinoma

Adenoid cystic carcinoma, 44

Adenomas
  colon, 101–102 (see also Familial adenomatous polyposis)
  gallbladder, 119–120
  liver, 114, 116–117

Adenopathy
  bronchial carcinomas, 49
  hilar, 121

neck, 39–40

pelvis, MRI, 155

Adjuvant chemotherapy
  colorectal cancer, 104
  primary bone tumours, 183

Adrenal glands, 145–148

Adrenal vein sampling, 148

Adrenocortical adenomas, 147–148

Adrenocortical carcinoma, vs adenoma, 147

Aerodigestive tract, upper, head and neck tumours, 35–40

AIDS
  lymphoma, 169
    CNS, 14
    thorax, 56
  tissue characterization of lesions, 30
  see also Kaposi's sarcoma

Air contrast see Double contrast

Airway mucosa, head and neck tumours, 35

AJC (American Joint Committee), testicular cancer staging, 137

Aldosterone, Conn's syndrome, 147

Algorithms, 3–4

A-fetoprotein
  hepatocarcinoma, 117
  liver adenomas, 116

American Joint Committee, testicular cancer staging, 137

Amiodarone, thyroid scintigraphy, 145

Ampulla of Vater, carcinoma, 87

Amputation, osteosarcoma, 180

Amyloidosis, vs cardiac tumours, 199

Anaplastic astrocytoma, 9, 11 (Fig.)

Anaplastic carcinoma of thyroid, 145

Androgenic steroids, liver adenoma, 116

Aneurysmal bone cysts, 177

Angiocardiography, 199–200

Angiography
  cardiac myxoma, 193–194
  hepatocarcinoma, 118
  primary bone tumours, 182
  small intestine, 90
  see also CT arteriography; Flush aortography

Angiography (magnetic resonance), 17, 30

Angiomyolipoma, kidneys, 134

Angioplasty, superior vena cava syndrome, 197

Angiosarcoma, heart, 191 (Table)

Anterior cranial fossa, 40

Anterior craniofacial resection, 42

Aorta, tumour invasion, 197–198
  oesophageal carcinoma, 82

Aortography, and phaeochromocytoma, 146

Apical tumours, 53–54

APUD cell tumours, 143
  SST analogue scintigraphy, 149

Arsenal diagnostique, 3

Arterial waveform patterns, duplex Doppler ultrasound, 155

Arteriography see Angiography; CT arteriography; Flush aortography

Asbestos workers, mesothelioma, 59–60, 195

Ascites, 93

    liver metastases, 118

    ovarian carcinoma, 158

Astrocytomas, 9–11

    *vs* central neurocytoma, 12

    spinal cord, 25

Atrial myxoma, 192–194

Audit, 4

### B

Balkan nephropathy, 134

Balloon valvuloplasty, carcinoid syndrome, 197

Barium enemas

    acromegaly, 142

    cervical carcinoma, 163

    double contrast, 101–102, 103

Barium meals, 85

Barium studies, small intestine, 89–90

Barium swallows, 81

Basioccipital region, 23

BCRA1, BCRA2 genes, 65

Benign prostatic hypertrophy, 135

Bile duct tumours, 119–121

Biliary cystadeno(carcino)mas, 119

Biliary cysts, 113

Biopsy

    bone tumours, 180, 182

    breast, 67, 68

    ductal adenocarcinoma of pancreas, 122

    haemangioma, 114

    hepatocarcinoma, 118

    liver adenoma, 117

    liver metastases, 119

    lymph nodes, ovarian carcinoma staging, 156

    neck masses, 44

    pleura, 60

    soft-tissue sarcomas, 187

Biphasic helical computed tomography, carcinoid tumours, 108

Bladder tumours, 135

Bleomycin toxicity, 58 (Fig.)

Blood flow impedance, endometrial cancer, 160

Blood vessels, tumour spread along, 37

Body coil *vs* endorectal coil MRI, prostate cancer, 137

Bone, 150

    invasion, head and neck tumours, 37–38

    metastases, 183–185

        colorectal cancer, 105

        treatment, 185

    pain, 183

    primary tumours, 177–183

        benign, 178

        biopsy, 182

            closed, 182

            needle, 182

            open, 182

        distant staging, 182

        local staging, 180–182

    scintigraphy, 178, 180, 182

    metastases, 184

        breast cancer, 75, 76

Brainstem gliomas, 15

Brain tumours

    bronchial carcinoma metastases, 49

    extra-axial, 15–19

    intra-axial, 9–15

Branchial cleft cysts, 43

Breast

    symptomatic, 65–66, 67

    tumours, 65–77

        heart involvement, 191, 196

        male breast, 73–74

        from mammography, 67–68

        small intestine, 94

        stomach, 87

Bronchi, oesophageal carcinoma spread, 82

Bronchial adenoma, ectopic ACTH secretion, 142

Bronchial carcinomas, 49–51

    ectopic ACTH secretion, 142

    heart

        invasion, 195–196

        metastases, 191

    pleura, 60

    small intestine, 95

    solitary pulmonary nodules, 52

    superior sulcus tumours, 53–54

    superior vena cava syndrome, 197

Bronchiectasis, 51

Bronchiolo-alveolar carcinoma, 49

Bronchogenic cysts, heart, 191 (Table)

Bull's eye appearance, gastric melanoma, 87

### C

CA125 testing, ovarian carcinoma screening, 155, 156

Caecal carcinoma, 93

Calcification

    islet cell tumours of pancreas, 123

    liver metastases, 106

    meningioma, 17

    oligodendroglioma, 11

    Paget's disease of breast, 73

    solitary pulmonary nodules, 53

    thyroid masses, 143

Calcium injection, intra-arterial, portal venous sampling, 148

Calculi, squamous cell carcinoma of kidneys, 135

*Candida albicans* pneumonia, 57

Carcinoid syndrome, 148

    heart, 196–197

Carcinoid tumours

    colorectal, 108

    peptide receptors, 149

    small intestine, 91–92

    stomach, 86–87

Carcinoma *in situ*, 162 (Fig.)

Carcinomas
   choroid plexus, 20
   skull base, 23
   *see also Specific types and sites*

Carcinosarcoma
   kidneys, 127
   oesophagus, 83

Cardiac tumours, 191–197, 198–200

Cardiomyopathy, 198–199

Cartilage invasion, head and neck tumours, 37–38

Cavernoma, brain, 9

C-cells, thyroid, 143

Central nervous system, 9–32
   *see also* Brain tumours

Central neurocytoma, 12

Central scar, focal nodular hyperplasia, 114

Cerebellar haemangioma, von Hippel Lindau syndrome, 141

Cerebellopontine angle tumours, 17, 19

Cerebrospinal fluid seeding, 15
   ependymoma, 13
   pineal teratoma, 23

Cervical adenopathy, metastases, 39–40

Cervix uteri
   carcinoma, 161–164
      *vs* endometrial cancer, 160
   stenosis, 159

Chemicals, transitional cell carcinoma, 134

Chemotherapy
   bone scintigraphy, 75
   breast cancer response, MRI, 69
   lung toxicity, 57
   primary bone tumours, 182–183
   soft-tissue sarcomas, 187
   *see also* Adjuvant chemotherapy

Chest radiography, gastric carcinoma staging, 85

Children
   neck masses, 43
   primary bone tumours, 177

Cholangiocarcinoma, 120–121

Cholangiography, 121

Cholesteatoma, kidney, 135

Chondroblastoma, 178

Chondrosarcoma
   incidence, 177
   prognosis, 178
   skull, 23

Chordoma, 178
   skull, 23, 24 (Fig.)

Choriocarcinoma
   metastases to brain, 14
   testes, 137

Choristoma, 20
   *see also* Granular cell tumours

Choroid plexus papilloma, 20
   *vs* meningioma, 17

Chromaffin cells *see* Phaeochromocytoma

Chromophobe cell carcinoma, kidney, 127

Cirrhosis
   CA125 elevation, 156
   hepatocarcinoma, 117

Classifications
   Dukes, colorectal cancer, 101, 104
   Eggel's, hepatocarcinoma, 117
   Jewitt & Whitmore, prostate cancer, 136
   primary bone tumours, 177
   Rye, Hodgkin's disease, 169 (Table)
   *see also* Staging; TNM classification

Collecting tubule carcinoma, kidney, 127

Colloid scintigraphy, focal nodular hyperplasia of liver, 114

Colography, computed tomography, 103

Colon, 108
   hydrosonography, 104

Colonoscopy, 101, 103
   acromegaly, 142

Colorectal cancer, 101–109
   acromegaly, 142
   caecum, 93
   duodenal spread, 88
   metastases, surgery and lymphadenectomy, 119

Colour Doppler ultrasound
   breast, 68
   gynaecology, 155, 156
      transvaginal, 157

Computed tomography
   bone lesion excision guidance, 180
   bone tumour needle biopsy, 182
   bronchial carcinomas, 51
      staging, 50
   colorectal cancer, 102–103
   densitometry, solitary pulmonary nodules, 53
   gastric carcinoma, 85
   gynaecology, 155
   myelography, 25
   *see also* CT arteriography; Spiral computed tomography

Computer-aided diagnosis, 199

Congenital cysts, pancreas, 122

Conn's syndrome, 147–148

Contraceptives, oral, liver adenoma, 114, 116

Contrast media
   bowel opacification, 155
   injection for CT
      bronchial carcinoma staging, 50
      colorectal cancer, 103
      focal nodular hyperplasia of liver, 114
      hepatocarcinoma, 127
      liver metastases, 119
      solitary pulmonary nodules, 53
   *see also* Ultrasound contrast media

Cord compression *see* Spinal cord compression

Core biopsy, breast, 67

Coronary arteriography, 199–200
   cardiac myxoma, 193–194
   cardiac sarcomas, 195

Corpora lutea, 155

Corticotrophinoma, 141

Corticotrophin releasing factor, for inferior petrosal sinus sampling, 142

Cost *vs* benefit, 3–4

Craniofacial resection, anterior, 42

Craniopharyngioma, 20, 22

Cribriform plate, 42

CT arteriography, liver metastases, 106–107

Cushing's disease, 141–142

Cushing's syndrome, 20–21, 21

Cyclosporin, tumours, 196

Cystadeno(carcino)mas, biliary, 119

Cystadenoma, bile ducts, 120 (Table)

Cystic tumours of pancreas, 122–123

Cysts
biliary, 113
in brain tumours, 9
bronchogenic, heart, 191 (Table)
intramedullary, 25
kidneys, 127, 132–133 (Fig.)
liver, 113, 114
ovaries, 156–157
papillary carcinoma of breast, 73
pericardial, 191 (Table), 194, 195
pineal, 23
thyroid, 143

Cytomegalovirus pneumonia, 57

**D**

Dacron grafts, and fibrous histiocytoma, 195

DCIS *see* Ductal carcinoma, *in situ*

Decision analysis, 3

Deep cervical fascia, 43

Demyelination, 9

Densitometry, CT, solitary pulmonary nodules, 53

De Quervain's thyroiditis, 143

Dermoid tumours, 17, 19, 20

Diabetes insipidus, 22

Dietary factors, ovarian carcinoma, 155

Diffusion imaging, functional MRI, 30

Digital mammography, 68

Digital radiography, 199

Digital subtraction inferior vena cavogram, 198 (Fig.)

Doppler ultrasound
focal nodular hyperplasia of liver, 114
gynaecology, 155
primary bone tumours, 182
*see also* Colour Doppler ultrasound; Pulsed Doppler ultrasound

Double contrast
barium enema, 101–102, 103
barium swallow, 81

Double duct sign, 122

Double reading examinations, radiology, 102

Ductal adenocarcinoma, pancreas, 121–122

Ductal carcinoma
infiltrating, 73
*in situ*, 65, 72
microcalcifications, 68, 69, 72
invasive, 70–72

Duct cell adenocarcinoma, pancreas, 122

Ductography, breast, 70

Dukes classification, colorectal cancer, 101, 104

Duodenum, 87–88
carcinoma, 87–88, 120
gastric carcinoma spread, 85, 88
gastric lymphoma spread, 86, 88
intubation, 90

Duplex Doppler ultrasound, gynaecology, 155

Dural tail, meningioma, 17

Dura mater, ethmoid roof, 42

Dye injections, breast cancer surgery, 75

Dysembryoplastic neuroepithelial tumours, 12–13
*vs* oligodendroglioma, 11

Dysphagia, 81

Dysplasia, colon adenomas, 101

Dyspnoea, 49

**E**

Early gastric cancer, 85

Echinococcal infection, 113
heart, 199
liver, 113

Echocardiography, 192, 194

Ectopic ACTH secretion, 142

Eggel's classification, hepatocarcinoma, 117

Emboli, cardiac myxoma, 192

Embolization, hepatic, carcinoid syndrome, 148, 197

Embryonal carcinoma, testes, 137

Embryonal rhabdomyosarcoma, bile ducts, 120 (Table)

Embryonic cell carcinoma, mediastinum, 58–59

Empty sella syndrome, 141

Enchondroma, 177, 178, 179 (Fig.), 180

Endocrine tumours, 141–151
and cardiac myxoma, 192
pituitary, 20–22

Endometrial cancer, 159–161

Endometriosis
bladder, 135
CA125 elevation, 156

Endoprostheses, primary bone tumour management, 182, 183
magnetic resonance imaging, 181

Endorectal coils, MRI, 137
cervical carcinoma, 162

Endoscopic retrograde cholangiography, 121

Endoscopic retrograde pancreatography, 122

Endoscopic sonography
colorectal cancer, 104
oesophagus, 82–83 (*see also* Transoesophageal echocardiography)

Endoscopy, 35
gastric carcinoma, 85
nasosinusal tumours, 40

Endovaginal coils, MRI, cervical
carcinoma, 162

Endovaginal ultrasound, 155, 156
colour flow, 157

Energy subtraction, 199

Enteroclysis, 89–90

Ependymoma, 13, 16 (Fig.)
*vs* central neurocytoma, 12
cerebellopontine angle, 19
infratentorial, 15
spinal cord, 25

Epidermoid tumours, 17, 19, 20

Epiglottis, 37

Epithelial neoplasms, pancreas, 122

Epstein-Barr virus, cyclosporin-induced
tumours, 196

Esthesioneuroblastoma, 23

Ethmoid sinus, adenocarcinoma, 41 (Fig.)

Ewing's sarcoma, 178
5-year survival rates, 178
follow-up, 183
incidence, 177
metastases, 182
treatment, 182–183

Extranodal spread, 40

Extraosseous bone tumours, magnetic
resonance imaging, 181

Extrathoracic metastases, bronchial
carcinomas, 49

**F**

Fab'2 antibody fragments, ovarian
carcinoma imaging, 158

Familial adenomatous polyposis, 107–108

Familial ovarian carcinoma, 155

Family history, colorectal cancer, 107–108

Fetus, cardiac rhabdomyoma, 194

Fibre-optic bronchoscopy, 49–50, 51

Fibrillary astrocytoma, 9

Fibroadenoma, breast, 65, 68

Fibroma
bladder, 135

cardiac, 191 (Table)

Fibromatosis, 185, 186

Fibrosarcoma
bladder, 135
heart, 191 (Table), 195

Fibrous dysplasia, 177, 180

Fibrous histiocytoma *see* Malignant
fibrous histiocytoma

FIGO staging
cervical carcinoma, 162 (Fig.)
endometrial carcinoma, 159
ovarian carcinoma, 157 (Table)

Fine needle aspiration cytology
breast masses, 66
bronchial carcinomas, 50, 53 (Fig.)
neck masses, 43, 44
recurrent endometrial cancer, 161

5-year survival rates, primary bone
tumours, 178

Flat adenoma, 107–108

Flexible sigmoidoscopy, 102

Fluorodeoxyglucose-PET, 30
breast cancer, 69, 76
ovarian carcinoma, 158

Fluoroscopy, bone tumour needle biopsy,
182

Flush aortography, and
phaeochromocytoma, 146

Focal nodular hyperplasia, liver, 114
*vs* adenoma, 116–117

Foetus, cardiac rhabdomyoma, 194

Follicular adenoma, *vs* thyroid carcinomas,
143

Follow-up
breast cancer, 75–76
colorectal cancer, 107–108

Foramen of Monro, compression, 9

Fractures
pathological, 184
stress fractures, 180

Frameless MR stereotaxy, 30

Frostberg, reverse '3' sign, 88

Functional magnetic resonance imaging, 30
radiation effects *vs* recurrent tumours,
29

**G**

Gadolinium enhancement, MRI, 13, 14, 17
breast, 69

Gallbladder
adenocarcinoma, 120
adenoma, 119–120

Gallium scintigraphy, hepatocarcinoma, 117

Gangliocytoma, 11–12

Ganglioglioma, 11–12

Gastrinoma, 148
pancreas, 122, 123
SST analogue scintigraphy, 149

Gastrointestinal tract, gut hormone
tumours, 148–149

Germ cell tumours
mediastinum, 58–59
testes, 149–150

Germinoma
pineal, 23
metastases, 29 (Fig.)
pituitary, 20

Giant-cell astrocytoma, subependymal, 11

Giant-cell tumours of bone, 177, 178, 180

Giant haemangioma, 114

Glioblastoma, *vs* oligodendroglioma, 11

Glioblastoma multiforme, 9

Gliomas
brainstem, 15
cerebellopontine angle, 19
*vs* dysembryoplastic neuroepithelial
tumours, 13
optic pathway, 20
orbit, 20
pituitary gland, 20
from radiotherapy, 30
spinal cord, 25

Gliomatosis cerebri, 9, 14

Glomus jugulare tumours, 23

Glomus tympanicum tumours, 23

Glosso-tonsillar squamous cell carcinoma, 36 (Fig.)

Glottis, squamous cell carcinoma, 37 (Fig.)

Glucagonoma, 148
    pancreas, 122, 123
    SST analogue scintigraphy, 149

Glycogenosis, liver adenoma, 116

Gradient echo imaging, MRI, bronchial carcinoma staging, 50

Grading, radiographic, primary bone tumours, 179

Grafts, vascular, and fibrous histiocytoma, 195

Granular cell tumours
    bile ducts, 120 (Table)
    gallbladder, 120 (Table)
    heart, 191 (Table)
    *see also* Choristoma

Granulomas, lung, 52, 53

Graves' disease, 143

Gut hormone tumours, 148–149

Gynaecology, 155–166

Gynaecomastia, 73

## H

Haemangioblastoma
    brain, 13
    spinal cord, 25
    von Hippel Lindau syndrome, 141

Haemangioma, 185, 186
    bladder, 135
    cardiac, 191 (Table)
    liver, 113–114
    vertebral, 27
    von Hippel Lindau syndrome, 141

Haemangiopericytoma
    heart, 195
    *vs* meningioma, 17

Haematuria, 127

Haemolytic anaemia, cardiac myxoma, 192–194

Haemoperitoneum, hepatocarcinoma, 117

Haemoptysis, 49, 50–51

Haemorrhage
    brain tumours, 9, 15
    endometrial cancer, 159
    leptomeningeal, 15
    ovarian cysts, 157
    pituitary gland, 22

Hamartoma
    cardiac rhabdomyoma, 194
    lung, 52, 53

Hands, acromegaly, 142

Head and neck, 35–45

Heart *see* Cardiac tumours

Helical computed tomography
    biphasic, carcinoid tumours, 108
    colorectal cancer, 102
    *see also* Spiral computed tomography

Hemilaryngectomies, planning, 36–37

Hepatic artery blood flow, *vs* portal vein blood flow, 106

Hepatic embolization, carcinoid syndrome, 148, 197

Hepatic lymph nodes, colorectal cancer metastases, 105

Hepatic metastases *see under* Liver

Hepatic reserve, metastases, 118

Hepatocarcinoma, 117

Hepatoma, venous extension, 191

Herbicides, ovarian carcinoma, 155

Hereditary non-polyposis colorectal cancer, 107–108

Heterotopic gastric mucosa, bile ducts, 120 (Table)

High-resolution ultrasound
    breast cancer staging, 74
    thyroid carcinoma, 143

Hilar adenopathy, 121

Histiocytoma *see* Malignant fibrous histiocytoma

Hodgkin's disease, 169–173

kidneys, 135
    thorax, 55, 56

Hormone replacement therapy, and endometrial cancer, 159, 160

Hormones
    gastrointestinal tract, 148
    sampling, 141

Horner's syndrome, 54

Hydrocephalus, brain tumours, 9

Hydronephrosis, cervical carcinoma, 163

Hydrosonography, colonic, 104

Hypernephroma *see* Renal cell carcinoma

Hyperostosis, meningioma, 17

Hyperparathyroidism, primary, 145

Hypoalbuminaemia, pericardial effusion, 191

Hypophysectomy, investigations, 141

Hypopituitarism, 22

Hypoxia, cardiac rhabdomyoma, 194

Hysterectomy, cervical carcinoma histology, 163

## I

Imaging strategies, 3–4

Immunoimaging, 39

Immunoscintigraphy
    colorectal cancer, 105
    ovarian carcinoma, 158
    *see also* Monoclonal antibodies

Immunosuppression, cyclosporin-induced tumours, 196

Incidentaloma, pancreas, 148

Infections
    endoprostheses, 183
    thoracic lymphoma therapy, 57–58

Inferior petrosal sinus sampling, 141–142

Inferior vena cava, tumour invasion, 197–198

Infiltrating ductal carcinoma, 73

Inflammatory disease, *vs* tumours, 30
    facial structures, 42

Infrared light, breast imaging, 70

Insulinoma, pancreas, 122, 123, 148

Interval cancers, breast, 65

Intestinal obstruction, 93

Intra-arterial calcium injection, portal venous sampling, 148

Intracavitary coils, MRI, cervical carcinoma, 161–162

Intradural tumours, spine, 25–27

Intramedullary tumours, 25

Intramuscular lipoma, 185

Intraoperative ultrasound, liver metastases, 106, 119

Intraosseous bone tumours, magnetic resonance imaging, 181

Intrauterine echocardiography, cardiac rhabdomyoma, 194

Intravenous urography, cervical carcinoma, 163

Invasive ductal carcinoma of breast, 70–72

Invasive lobular carcinoma of breast, 72

Invasive pulmonary aspergillosis, 57

*In vitro* sonography, lymph nodes, colorectal cancer, 104–105

Iodine, isotopes, 142–143, 145

Iodocholesterol scintigraphy, Conn's syndrome, 147–148

Islet cell tumours, pancreas, 123

## J

Jaundice, 113

    bile duct tumours, 119

    hepatocarcinoma, 117

    liver metastases, 118

    ultrasound, 120–121

Jejunum, carcinomas, 87

Jewitt & Whitmore classification, prostate cancer, 136

Juvenile angiofibroma, 23

Juvenile pilocytic astrocytoma, 15

## K

Kaposi's sarcoma

    colon, 108

    small intestine, 92

Kidneys, tumours, 127–135

    vascular invasion, 198

Klatskin's tumour, 120

Krukenberg tumour, 85

## L

Laminated calcification, solitary pulmonary nodules, 53

Laparoscopy, ovarian tumours, 150

Laparotomy, ovarian carcinoma staging, 156

Large cell carcinoma, bronchus, 49

Laryngeal cartilages

    proton density SE magnetic resonance imaging, 38

    tumour spread, 37

Laryngectomies, planning, 36–37

Larynx, tumour spread, 35, 36–37

Laser spectroscopy, breast masses, 70

Laser therapy, colorectal cancer, 104

Left atrial enlargement, myxoma, 192

Leiomyomata

    bladder, 135

    *vs* endometrial cancer, 160

Leiomyosarcoma

    bladder, 135

    colorectal, 108

    duodenum, 88

    heart, 191 (Table)

    oesophagus, 83

    small intestine, 92

Leptomeningeal haemorrhage, 15

Leukaemias

    heart involvement, 191

    kidneys, 135

Limb salvage surgery

    magnetic resonance imaging, 181

    osteosarcoma, 180

Lingual septum, tongue neoplasms, 36

Linitis plastica, 85, 87

Lipiodol, hepatocarcinoma, 117

Lipoma, 186

    cardiac, 191 (Table), 194

    intramuscular, 185

    neck, 44

Liposarcoma, 185, 186

    heart, 191 (Table), 195

Liver

    cirrhosis, CA125 elevation, 156

    embolization, carcinoid syndrome, 148, 197

    metastases, 118–119

        breast cancer, 75, 76

        colorectal cancer, 105, 106–107

            resection for, 105

        ovarian carcinoma, 158

    transplantation, hepatocarcinoma, 118

    tumours, 113–119

Lobular carcinomas

    *in situ*, 65, 72–73

    invasive, 72

Lodwick grading, primary bone tumours, 179

Logic in medicine, 4

Loosening, endoprostheses, 183

Lungs

    metastases, 54–55

        colorectal cancer, 105

        primary bone tumours, 178, 183

    tumours, 49–55

Lymphadenectomy, and surgery for colorectal cancer metastases, 119

Lymphadenitis, neck, 43

Lymphangiography

    cervical carcinoma, 163

        staging, 161

    lymphomas, 170

    testicular tumours, 137

Lymphangioma

    cardiac, 191 (Table)

    neck, 43

Lymphangitis carcinomatosa, 55

pleura, 60

Lymphatic spread
    gastric cancer, 85
    oesophageal carcinoma, 81
    to small intestine, 93
    testicular tumours, 137

Lymphatic system, 169–173
    colon, 101

Lymph nodes
    breast cancer staging, 74–75
    cervical carcinoma, 163
    colorectal cancer staging, 104–105
    gastric cancer, 85
    hepatic, colorectal cancer metastases, 105
    metastases, 173
    neck, 43
    oesophageal carcinoma, 81, 82
    oesophageal compression, 84
    ovarian carcinoma, 158
        staging biopsy, 156
    see also Adenopathy

Lymphoedema
    breast, 69
    breast cancer treatment, 75

Lymphomas, 169–173
    bone, age incidence, 178
    brain, 9, 13–14, 20
    colon, 108
    duodenum, 88
    head and neck, 43
    heart, 191, 195
    kidneys, 135
    mediastinum, 59
    vs meningioma, 17
    orbit, 20
    peptide receptors, 149
    pleura, 60
    posterior fossa, 17
    small intestine, 90–91
    spine, 27

stomach, 86, 88
    superior vena cava syndrome, 197
    thorax, 55–58
    tissue characterization, 30
Lymphopenia, chest infections, 57
Lymphoscintigraphy of breast, 69, 75
Lynch Type I variant, hereditary non-polyposis colorectal cancer, 107–108

**M**

Macroadenomas, pituitary, 21–22, 142
Macrocystic adenoma, pancreas, 122–123
Magnetic resonance angiography, 17, 30
Magnetic resonance cholangiography, 121
Magnetic resonance imaging
    acoustic Schwannoma, 17
    breast, 69–70
    bronchial carcinoma staging, 50
    disadvantages, 181
    gynaecology, 155
    primary bone tumour follow-up, 182
    vs scintigraphy, vertebral metastases, 27
    soft-tissue sarcoma recurrence, 187
Magnetic resonance spectroscopy, 30, 199
    radiation effects vs recurrent tumours, 29
Malignant fibrous histiocytoma, 185
    age incidence, 178
    heart, 195
Mammography, 66–68
    screening, 65
Masses see Soft tissue masses
Mastectomy, lobular carcinoma in situ, 73
Matrix mineralization, bone tumours, 179, 180 (Fig.)
Maxillary sinus, squamous cell carcinoma, 43 (Fig.)
Maxillonasal tumours, vs nasoethmoidal tumours, 40–41
MDP scanning see Bone, scintigraphy
Mechanical loosening, endoprostheses, 183
Mediastinum

lymphomas, 55
    oesophageal carcinoma spread, 82
    tumours, 49, 58–59
        heart involvement, 195–196
Medullary carcinoma of breast, 71 (Fig.), 73
Medullary thyroid carcinoma, 143, 145
    SST analogue scintigraphy, 149
Medulloblastoma, 15
Melanoma
    duodenum, 88
    metastases
        brain, 14
        heart, 191, 195
        stomach, 87
    peptide receptors, 149
    small intestine, 94
Meningeal haemorrhage, 15
Meningioma, 17, 18 (Fig.)
    vs acoustic Schwannoma, 19
    orbit, 20
    pituitary region, 20
    from radiotherapy, 30
    skull base, 23
    spine, 25
Menopause
    endometrial cancer, 159
    and ovarian carcinoma, 155
MEN syndromes see Multiple endocrine neoplasia syndromes
Mesenchymal sarcoma, gallbladder, 120 (Table)
Mesenchymal tumours
    bile ducts, 120 (Table)
    gallbladder, 120 (Table)
Mesenteric fibrosis, carcinoid tumours, 92
Mesenteric lymph nodes, computed tomography, 91
Mesorectal excision, total, 105
Mesothelioma, 59–60
    AV node, 191 (Table)
    heart, 191 (Table), 195, 199
Metaiodobenzylguanidine scanning

medullary carcinoma of thyroid, 145

phaeochromocytoma, 145–147, 194

thyroid scintigraphy, 143

Metaplasia, oesophageal carcinoma, 83

Metastases

from bone, 181

to bone, 150

to brain, 9, 14–15

bronchial carcinomas, 49–50

cerebellopontine angle, 19

cervical adenopathy, 39–40

cervical carcinoma, 163

colorectal cancer, 105–107

cranial, extra-axial, 20

to duodenum, 88

gallbladder, 120 (Table)

to heart, 191, 195–196

hepatocarcinoma, 117

intramedullary, 25

to kidneys, 135

liver, 118–119

lungs, 54–55

vs meningioma, 17

oesophageal carcinoma, 81

to oesophagus, 84

ovarian carcinoma, 158

pleura, 60

posterior fossa, 17

skip, 181

skull

base, 23

extra-axial cranial, 20

to small intestine, 94–95

spine, 23–25, 26 (Fig.), 27, 29 (Fig.)

to stomach, 87

see also Lymph nodes, metastases

Methoxy-iso-butyl-isonitrile scanning, breast, 69

MIBG see Metaiodobenzylguanidine scanning

Microadenomas, pituitary, 20–21, 141, 142

Microcalcifications, breast, 68, 69

ductal carcinoma in situ, 72

invasive ductal carcinoma, 70

Microcystic adenoma, pancreas, 122–123

Micrometastases

breast cancer, 74

colorectal cancer, 105

Mitral valve, cardiac myxoma, 192

Mixed neural/glial cell tumours, 11–12

Mixed pattern teratocarcinoma, testes, 137

Monoclonal antibodies, radiolabelled

breast scanning, 69

ovarian carcinoma, 157–158

at surgery, 108

see also Immunoscintigraphy

Mortality rates, primary bone tumours, 178

Mucinous adenocarcinoma, kidneys, 135

Mucinous carcinoma of breast, 71 (Fig.), 73

Mucinous cystadenoma, pancreas, 122–123

Mucinous cystic adenoma, pancreas, 122

Mucoceles, paranasal sinuses, 41

Multiple endocrine neoplasia syndromes, 141, 143

phaeochromocytoma, 146

Multiple myeloma, 150, 183–185

Myelography (computed tomography), 25

Myeloma

extradural spinal, 27

multiple, 150, 183–185

Myocardium, cardiac myxoma, 192–193

Myometrium, endometrial cancer invasion, 159–160

Myositis ossificans, 180

Myxoid sarcoma, 186

Myxoma, 186

cardiac, 191 (Table), 192–194

### N

Nasoethmoidal tumours, vs maxillonasal tumours, 40–41

Nasopharyngeal tumours

detection of spread, 37, 38 (Fig.)

skull base, 23

Nasosinusal neoplasms, 40–43

Neck, soft tissue masses, 43–44

Needle aspiration

salivary tumours, 44

thyroid masses, 43

see also Fine needle aspiration cytology

Needle biopsy

bone metastases, 184

primary bone tumours, 182

Neoadjuvant chemotherapy, primary bone tumours, 182

Nerves, tumour spread along, 37

Nerve sheath tumours, 17–18, 185, 186

skull base, 23

see also Schwannomas

Neural/glial cell tumours, mixed, 11–12

Neuroblastoma, 20

Neuroendocrine tumours, peptide receptors, 149

Neuroepithelial tumours, dysembryoplastic, vs oligodendroglioma, 11

Neurofibroma, 28 (Fig.)

cardiac, 191 (Table)

neck, 44

spine, 25

Neurofibromatosis, 17, 25

phaeochromocytoma, 146

Neurogenic sarcoma, heart, 191 (Table)

Neurogenic tumours, mediastinum, 59

Neurotransmitters, from gastrointestinal tract, 148

Neurovascular bundle

magnetic resonance imaging, 181

osteosarcoma involvement, 180

Neutropenia, chest infections, 57

Nipples

discharge, retraction, 73

Paget's disease of breast, 73

Nodal necrosis, 39

Non-Hodgkin's lymphoma, 14, 21 (Fig.), 169–173
  kidneys, 135
  thorax, 55, 56
Non-ossifying fibroma, 180
Non-seminomatous tumours, testes, 137
Non-small cell carcinoma, bronchus, 49
Nulliparity, ovarian carcinoma, 155

## O

Octreotide
  gut hormone tumour scintigraphy, 148–149
  medullary carcinoma of thyroid, 145
Oesophagus, 81–84
  carcinoma, 81–83
  gastric carcinoma spread, 85
  secondary neoplasms, 83–84
Oestrogens, and endometrial cancer, 159
Olfactory neuroblastoma, skull base, 23
Oligodendroglioma, 9, 11
  vs central neurocytoma, 12
Omentum, ovarian carcinoma, 156
Oncocytoma, kidneys, 134
Opportunistic infections, thoracic lymphoma therapy, 57
Optic chiasm, tumours compressing, 20, 142
Oral contraceptives
  liver adenoma, 114
  ovarian carcinoma protection, 155
Oral tumours, detection of spread, 37
Orbits, 20
  exenteration, 42
  nasosinusal tumours, 40
  tumour assessment, 41–42
Osteoblastoma, 178, 180, 182
Osteochondroma, 177, 180
Osteoid osteoma, 177, 178, 180, 182
Osteonecrosis, 183
Osteoporosis, multiple myeloma, 150
Osteosarcoma, 178

extraskeletal, heart, 191 (Table)
follow-up, 183
incidence, 177
metastases, 182
  to brain, 14
Paget's disease, 150
surgery, 180
treatment, 182–183
Ovarian tumours, 150, 155–158
  carcinoma, 155–158
  Krukenberg tumour, 85

## P

Paget's disease of bone, 150
Paget's disease of breast, 73
Pancoast's tumours, 53–54
Pancreas
  gastrinoma, SST analogue scintigraphy, 149
  tumours, 120, 121–123
    duodenum, 88
    MEN 1 syndrome, 141
Papilla of Vater, carcinoma, 87
Papillary adenoma, bile ducts, 120 (Table)
Papillary carcinoma of breast, 73
Papillary epithelial neoplasms, pancreas, 122
Papillary fibroelastoma, cardiac, 191 (Table)
Papilloma see Choroid plexus papilloma
Paraganglioma, 23
  cardiac, 194
Paraglottic spaces, 35
Paralaryngeal spaces, 37
Parametrium, cervical carcinoma invasion, 162–163
Paranasal sinuses
  head and neck tumours, 35
  hyperostosis, 17
  magnetic resonance imaging, 41
  tumours, skull base, 23
  see also Nasosinusal neoplasms
Parapharyngeal spaces, salivary tumours, 44

Parasitic cysts
  cardiac, 194, 199
  see also Echinococcal infection
Parathyroid tumours, 145
  MEN syndromes, 141, 143 (Table)
Paravertebral masses, 27
Parinaud's syndrome, 23
Pathological fractures, 184
Pelvis
  adenopathy, MRI, 155
  bone tumour assessment, 182
  computed tomography, testicular tumours, 149–150
  lymphangiography, cervical carcinoma, 163
Periampullary tumours, 120, 121
Pericardial cysts, 191 (Table), 194, 195
Pericardium
  cardiac tumours, 191, 195
  metastases to, 196
Periorbita, 41
Periosteum
  nasosinusal tumours, 41
  reaction to bone tumours, 179
Perirectal fascia see Total mesorectal excision
Perirectal lymph nodes, colorectal cancer, 105
Peritoneum
  colorectal cancer metastases, 105
  gastric carcinoma, 85
  ovarian carcinoma, 158 (see also Omentum)
  small intestine involvement, 93
Peritumoural reaction, colorectal cancer, 104
Petrous vein sampling, 21
Phaeochromocytoma, 145–147
  bladder, 135
  heart, 194
  MIBG uptake, 143, 194
  von Hippel Lindau syndrome, 141

Phased array multicoil, gynaecology, 155

Phenacetin, transitional cell carcinoma, 134

Phleboliths, 186

Pigmentation, and cardiac myxoma, 192

Pineal cysts, 23

Pinealoblastoma, 23

Pinealocytoma, 23

Pineal tumours, 22–23

Piriform sinus, squamous cell carcinoma, 40 (Fig.)

Pituitary adenomas, 20–22, 141

 *vs* meningioma, 17

Pituitary apoplexy, 22, 141

Pituitary gland, 141–142

Pituitary region, tumours, 20–22

Plasmacytoma, 184

Pleomorphic xanthoastrocytoma, 11

Pleura

 effusions, 51, 60

 tumours, 49, 59–60

*Pneumocystis carinii* pneumonia, 57

Pneumonias, 49

 thoracic lymphoma therapy, 57

Pneumonitis, radiotherapy, 56–57

Pneumosinus dilatans, 17

Pneumothorax, osteosarcoma metastases, 182

Polycystic kidney disease, 113

Polypoid tumours, endometrial cancer, 160

Polyposis Registry, 107

Polyps

 colon, 101–102 (*see also* Familial adenomatous polyposis)

 lymphomas, 108

 gastric carcinoid, 86–87

'Popcorn' calcification, solitary pulmonary nodules, 53

Porcelain gallbladder, 120

Portal circulation, colorectal cancer metastases, 105

Portal vein blood flow, *vs* hepatic artery blood flow, 106

Portal venous phase, CT arteriography, 106–107

Portal venous sampling, intra-arterial calcium injection, 148

Positron emission tomography, 39–40, 199

 lymphomas, 170

 *see also* Fluorodeoxyglucose-PET

Posterior fossa neoplasms, 15

 CT *vs* MRI, 17

Postnecrotic cirrhosis, hepatocarcinoma, 117

Postoperative changes, intracranial tumours, 27

Power Doppler ultrasound, 127

Pre-epiglottic space, 37

Pregnancy, CA125 elevation, 156

Primary treatment, breast cancer, ultrasound, 75

Primitive neuroectodermal tumours, 15, 23

Prolactin, assay, 142

Prolactinoma, 20, 141, 142

Prostate, 135–137

 benign hypertrophy, 135

 carcinoma, 136–137

 bone metastases, 150

Prostatectomy, radical, 136

Prostatic specific antigens, 136

Prostheses, magnetic resonance imaging, 181

Proton density SE magnetic resonance imaging, laryngeal cartilages, 38

Proton emission tomography, radiation effects *vs* recurrent tumours, 29

Pseudosarcoma, oesophagus, 83

Pseudotumours, heart, 199

Pterygo-palatine fissure, nasosinusal tumours, 40

Pulmonary aspergillosis, invasive, 57

Pulmonary fibrosis, radiotherapy, 56–57

Pulmonary hypertension, cardiac myxoma, 192

Pulmonary valve, carcinoid syndrome, 196–197

Pulsatility index

endometrial cancer, 160

 *vs* resistance index, ovarian tumour vascularity, 156

Pulsed Doppler ultrasound, hepatocarcinoma, 117

Punctate calcification, liver metastases, 106

Pylorus, gastric tumour spread, 85, 88

**R**

Radiation doses, mammography, 67

Radical hysterectomy, cervical carcinoma histology, 163

Radical prostatectomy, 136

Radiographic grading, primary bone tumours, 179

Radiography, digital, 68, 199

Radionuclide scanning *see* Scintigraphy

Radiosurgery, stereotactic, 15

Radiotherapy

 enteritis, 93

 intracranial effects, 27, 29

 pneumonitis, 56–57

 soft-tissue sarcoma recurrence, 187

Rathke's cleft cysts, 22

Receiver-operator characteristic curves, pulsatility *vs* resistance index, ovarian tumour vascularity, 156

Rectal carcinoma, 104, 105

Rectal ultrasound, 103–104

Rectovaginal pelvic examination, ovarian carcinoma screening, 155

Recurrence, superior vena cava syndrome, 197

Recurrent tumours

 breast cancer, 75–76

 cervical carcinoma, 163–164

 endometrial cancer, 160

 primary bone tumours, 183

 *vs* radiation effects, 29

Regional cerebral blood flow, functional MRI, 30

Renal adenoma, 134

Renal cell carcinoma, 127, 128–131 (Fig.), 134 (Fig.)

metastases

bone, 184

duodenum, 88

heart, 191

small intestine, 95

von Hippel Lindau syndrome, 141

Resistance index, *vs* pulsatility index, ovarian tumour vascularity, 156

Retained secretions, *vs* tumours, facial structures, 42–43

Retromolar trigone, squamous cell carcinomas, 38 (Fig.)

Retropharyngeal lymph nodes, 39

Reverse '3' sign of Frostberg, 88

Rhabdomyoma, cardiac, 191 (Table), 194

Rhabdomyosarcoma

chemotherapy, 187

head and neck, 43

heart, 191 (Table), 195

skull base, 23

Risk factors, breast cancer, 65

Rye classification, Hodgkin's disease, 169 (Table)

## S

Salivary glands, head and neck tumours, 35, 44

Salpingo-oophorectomy, ovarian carcinoma staging, 156

Sarcoidosis

*vs* cardiac tumours, 199

*vs* lymph node metastases, 56

Sarcomas

heart

metastatic, 191

primary, 195

soft-tissue, 185–187

Schwannomas

acoustic, 17, 19

neck, 44

spine, 25, 28 (Fig.)

Sciatica, bone tumours, 178

Scintigraphy

breast, 69

cancer metastases, 75, 76

cardiac paraganglioma, 194

gut hormone tumours, 148–149

iodocholesterol, Conn's syndrome, 147–148

liver

focal nodular hyperplasia, 114

haemangioma, 114

and liver metastases, 119

*vs* magnetic resonance imaging, vertebral metastases, 27

parathyroid disease, 145

phaeochromocytoma, 145–147

small intestine, 90

thyroid masses, 43, 143–145

*see also* Monoclonal antibodies, radiolabelled

Scirrhous gastric carcinoma, 85

Sclerosis, bone, head and neck tumours, 37

Scoliosis, bone tumours, 178

Screening

breast cancer, 65, 69

cervical cytology, 161

endometrial cancer, 159

lung cancer, 49

ovarian carcinoma, 155

stomach cancer, 85

Secretions *see* Retained secretions

Seeding, ovarian carcinoma, 156

Seminal vesicles, 136

Seminoma

mediastinum, 58–59

testes, 137

Sentinel node, breast cancer, 75

Septum pellucidum, central neurocytoma, 12

Seroma, 187

Serotonin, 148

Serous cystadenoma, pancreas, 122–123

Sestamibi scanning, parathyroid disease, 145

Short T1 inversion recovery sequences, MRI, pelvic adenopathy, 155

Sigmoidoscopy, flexible, 102

Silicone breast implants, magnetic resonance imaging, 69

Simple bone cysts, 177

Single photon emission tomography, 39–40, 199

liver metastases, 119

phaeochromocytoma, 147

*see also* Thallium-SPECT

Sipple syndrome, 141

Skeleton *see* Bone

Skin pigmentation, and cardiac myxoma, 192

Skip metastases, 181

Skull base, 23

approach to nasosinusal tumours, 40

Small cell carcinoma, bronchus, 49

Small intestine

barium studies, 89–90

carcinoma, 90

neoplasms, 87, 88–90

secondary neoplasms, 93–95

Small parts tissue imaging, breast ultrasound, 68

Smoking, transitional cell carcinoma, 134

Soft-tissue masses

breast, 65–66

neck, 43–44

Soft-tissue tumours, primary, 185–187

Solid epithelial neoplasms, pancreas, 122

Solitary bone metastasis, 183–184

Solitary pulmonary nodule, 51–53

Somatostatinoma, pancreas, 122, 123

Somatostatin receptor ligand, gut hormone tumour scintigraphy, 149

Spectroscopy, breast masses, 70

Sphenoid region, 23

Spiculated mass, invasive ductal carcinoma of breast, 70

Spinal cord compression, 27

Spine, 23–27

 haemangioma, von Hippel Lindau syndrome, 141

 magnetic resonance imaging, 181–182

 primary bone tumours, 178

Spiral computed tomography

 bronchial carcinoma staging, 50

 lung metastases, 54

 phaeochromocytoma, 147

 thyroid masses, 143

 see also Helical computed tomography

Squamous cell carcinomas, 38 (Fig.)

 bone invasion, 37

 bronchus, 49

 head and neck, 35, 36 (Fig.)

 kidneys, 135

 maxillary sinus, 43 (Fig.)

 nasosinusal, 40

 oesophagus, 81

 piriform sinus, 40 (Fig.)

 skull base, 23

Staging

 bone tumours, 180–182

 breast tumours, 74–75

 bronchial carcinomas, 49–50

 cervical carcinoma, 161, 162 (Fig.)

 colorectal cancer, 103–105

 Dukes classification, 101, 104

 endometrial cancer, 159

 gastric carcinoma, 85–86

 lymphomas, 170–173

  thorax, 55–56

 nodal, 39 (Table)

 oesophageal carcinoma, 81–83

 ovarian carcinoma, 156

 primary bone tumours, 182

 prostate cancer, 136

 soft-tissue sarcomas, 187

 thoracic tumours, 49

Stents, superior vena cava syndrome, 197

Stereotactic cross-sectional imaging, 30

Stereotactic mammography, 67

Stereotactic radiosurgery, 15

Steroid therapy, chest infections, 57

STIR (short T1 inversion recovery sequences), MRI, pelvic adenopathy, 155

Stomach

 lymphoma, spread to duodenum, 86, 88

 oesophageal carcinoma spread, 81

 primary carcinoma, 84–86

  spread to duodenum, 85, 88

 secondary neoplasms, 87

Stress fractures, 180

Subependymal giant-cell astrocytoma, 11

Subtraction, digital radiography, 199

Subtraction scanning, parathyroid disease, 145

Sulphur colloid scintigraphy, hepatocarcinoma, 117

Superior orbital fissure, nasosinusal tumours, 40

Superior sulcus tumours, 53–54

Superior vena cava syndrome, 197

Superscan, bone scintigraphy, 184

Surgery

 bone metastases, 184–185

 soft-tissue sarcomas, 187

 see also Amputation

Surgical staging, primary bone tumours, 182

Synchronous lesions, colorectal cancer, 103

Synovial sarcoma, 185

 chemotherapy, 187

 heart, 191 (Table)

## T

Talc, ovarian carcinoma, 155

Tamponade, metastases to pericardium, 196

Target lesions, liver ultrasound, 75

Task activation studies, functional MRI, 30

TC5 monoclonal antibody, ovarian carcinoma imaging, 158

Technetium-99m see Scintigraphy

Temporal subtraction, 199

Teratocarcinoma, mixed pattern, testes, 137

Teratodermoids, pituitary region, 20

Teratoma

 cardiac, 191 (Table), 195

 mediastinum, 58–59

 pineal, 23

 testes, 137

Testicular tumours, 137, 149–150

Thallium scintigraphy

 breast cancer, 69

 parathyroid disease, 145

 thyroid masses, 145

Thallium-SPECT, 30, 39

Thermography, breast, 70

Thorax, tumours, 49–61 3D displays, 199 3D volume imaging, cervical carcinoma, 162

Thrombi

 hepatocarcinoma, 117

 intracardiac, 194

 from tumours, 191

Thrombocytopenia, lung haemorrhage, 57

Thrombosis, stents, 197

Thymoma, 58

 heart, 191 (Table)

 vs lymph node metastases, 56

 pleura, 60

Thyroglobulin assays, 143

Thyroglossal duct cysts, 43

Thyroid carcinomas, 143–145

Thyroiditis, De Quervain's, 143

Thyroid masses, 43–44, 142–145

 mediastinum, 59

Thyrotoxicosis, 143

Thyrotropin assay, 141–142

Thyroxine therapy, and thyroid scintigraphy, 145

Time factors, imaging strategies, 3–4

Tissue characterization, 30

TNM classification

bladder cancer, 135

bronchial carcinomas, 49, 50 (Table)

colorectal cancer, 103–105

prostate cancer, 136

renal cell carcinoma, 127

testicular cancer, 137

transitional cell carcinoma, 134–135

Tongue

squamous cell carcinoma, 36 (Fig.)

tumour spread from, 35–36, 37

Total mesorectal excision, 105

Toxoplasmosis, *vs* CNS lymphoma, 14

Trachea, oesophageal carcinoma spread,
82

Transabdominal ultrasound

cervical carcinoma staging, 161

gynaecology, 155

Transhepatic cholangiography, 121

Transitional cell carcinoma

bladder, 135

kidneys, 134–135

Transoesophageal echocardiography, 194

Transplantation

heart, 196

liver, hepatocarcinoma, 118

and lymphomas, 169

Transrectal ultrasound, 136

cervical carcinoma, 161

recurrent endometrial cancer, 160–161

Transthoracic echocardiography, 194

Transvaginal sonography *see* Endovaginal
ultrasound

Tricuspid valve

carcinoid syndrome, 196–197

cardiac myxoma, 192

Trigeminal nerve, 37

Trigeminal Schwannoma, 19, 23

Tri-iodothyronine therapy, thyroid
scintigraphy, 145

Triple assessment, breast masses, 66

Tuberculosis, *vs* cardiac tumours, 199

Tuberous sclerosis

angiomyolipoma of kidneys, 134

cardiac rhabdomyoma, 194

tumours, 11

Tubular carcinoma of breast, 73

Tubulo-papillary carcinoma, kidney, 127

Tumour rests, rectal cancer, 105

## U

UICC (*Union Internationale Contre le
Cancer*), testicular cancer staging, 137

Ulcers

gastric carcinoma, 85

gastric lymphomas, 86

Ultrasound

bone tumour needle biopsy, 182

breast cancer, 74–76

breast masses, 68–69 (*see also Named
tumours*)

disappearing haemangioma, 113

gastric carcinoma, 86

gynaecology, 155

intraoperative, liver metastases, 106

jaundice, 120–121

kidneys, 127

liver metastases, 119

neck masses, 43

thyroid tumours, 44

pleural effusion aspiration, 51

rectal, 103–104

soft-tissue sarcoma biopsy, 187

*see also* Doppler ultrasound;
Echocardiography; Endoscopic
sonography; High-resolution
ultrasound; Transrectal ultrasound

Ultrasound contrast media, 76, 119

*Union Internationale Contre le Cancer*,
testicular cancer staging, 137

Upper aerodigestive tract, head and neck
tumours, 35–40

Ureteric obstruction, cervical carcinoma,
163

Urinogenital system, 127–138

Uterus, 158–164

## V

Vagina

atresia, 159

*see also* Endovaginal coils; Endovaginal
ultrasound

Valve disease

carcinoid syndrome, 196–197

*vs* cardiac myxoma, 193

Variant carcinomas, pancreas, 122

Vascular invasion, 197–198

Vasoactive intestinal peptide receptor
scintigraphy, 149

Vasogenic oedema, brain tumours, 9, 14

Vasovagal attacks, breast diagnosis, 67, 69

Venography, superior vena cava
syndrome, 197

Venous extension, tumours, 191, 197–198

Verner–Morrison syndrome, 148

Vertebrae, 27

*see also* Spine

Villous adenoma, colorectal, 104

VIPoma, 148

pancreas, 122, 123

VIP receptor scintigraphy, 149

Viral hepatitis, hepatocarcinoma, 117

Virchow-Robin spaces, lymphoma spread,
14

Virtual reality, 199

Visceral metastases, ovarian carcinoma, 158

Vocal cords, 35, 36–37

Volume rendering, colorectal cancer,
102–103

Volumetry, cervical carcinoma, 162

Von Hippel Lindau syndrome, 13, 25, 141

phaeochromocytoma, 146

renal cell carcinoma, 127

## W

Wrecking ball phenomenon, cardiac myxoma, 192

## X

Xanthoastrocytoma, 11

## Y

Yolk sac carcinoma, testes, 137

## Z

Zollinger-Ellison syndrome, 148

# IMAGING IN ONCOLOGY